Ethics, Social Responsibility and Quality of Life in Times of Crisis

Ethics, Social Responsibility and Quality of Life in Times of Crisis

Guest Editors

Audrey J. Murrell
Ray Jones
Xiaoping Zhao

MDPI

Basel • Beijing • Wuhan • Barcelona • Belgrade • Novi Sad • Cluj • Manchester

Guest Editors
Audrey J. Murrell
School of Business
University of Pittsburgh
Pittsburgh
USA

Ray Jones
Katz Graduate School of Business
University of Pittsburgh
Pittsburgh
USA

Xiaoping Zhao
Antai College of Economics and Management
Shanghai Jiao Tong University
Shanghai
China

Editorial Office
MDPI AG
Grosspeteranlage 5
4052 Basel, Switzerland

This is a reprint of the Special Issue, published open access by the journal *International Journal of Environmental Research and Public Health* (ISSN 1660-4601), freely accessible at: https://www.mdpi.com/journal/ijerph/special_issues/Times_of_Crisis.

For citation purposes, cite each article independently as indicated on the article page online and as indicated below:

Lastname, A.A.; Lastname, B.B. Article Title. *Journal Name* **Year**, *Volume Number*, Page Range.

ISBN 978-3-7258-5925-2 (Hbk)
ISBN 978-3-7258-5926-9 (PDF)
https://doi.org/10.3390/books978-3-7258-5926-9

Contents

About the Editors

Audrey J. Murrell

Audrey J. Murrell is currently Professor of Business Administration, Psychology, Public and International Affairs, and Clinical and Translational Science at the University of Pittsburgh, School of Business. She attended Howard University (B.A. in psychology) and the University of Delaware (M.S. and Ph.D. in social psychology). Dr. Murrell conducts research on mentoring, diversity, equity, and inclusion, along with ethical and social issues in management. She also serves as a consultant in the areas of mentoring, organizational effectiveness, diversity, and leadership development.

Ray Jones

Ray Jones is a Professor of Business Administration and Ethics at the University of Pittsburgh School of Business within the Organizations and Entrepreneurship group. His expertise is in business ethics and organizational behavior, as well as social responsibility and corporate governance. He earned his Bachelor's degree from Purdue University, and his MPA and PhD from the University of Pittsburgh. Previously, he served as coordinator of the Certificate Program in Leadership and Ethics (CPLE) at the University of Pittsburgh.

Xiaoping Zhao

Xiaoping Zhao is a Professor at Southwestern University of Finance and Economics in Chengdu, Sichuan, China. He received his Ph.D. from Virginia Tech University and was a post-doctoral fellow at the University of Pittsburgh, School of Business, within the David Berg Center for Ethics and Leadership. His research explores stakeholder relationships and their impact on firm performance and corporate social performance. His teaching covers important topics for organizational effectiveness, such as corporate governance, ethics, and strategic management.

Preface

This special collection of research and theory papers focuses on how organizations and their stakeholders respond, adjust, and manage crisis situations that are either internal or external to the organization. This collection of research and conceptual papers examines and advances important topics such as ethics, corporate social responsibility, crisis communication and stakeholder engagement. These topics are significant as part of the daily operations of any effective organization. However, issues of leadership, stakeholder engagement, ethics, and social responsibility play an important and strategic role during times of organizational and societal crisis. While some organizations focus on preventing or minimizing crisis situations, others leverage crises as opportunities for leaders and organizational development, along with stakeholder learning and engagement. This collection of research and theory papers is both timely and timeless. It addresses the lessons learned from the past while also posing innovative approaches to crisis situations as a type of "learning laboratory" for leaders, employees, and other key stakeholders. From self-sacrificial leadership to global crises such as the COVID-19 pandemic to ongoing hunger and food insecurity to stakeholder trust, the diverse array of papers examines both the challenges and opportunities that crises provide to organizations, its leadership and stakeholders. The collection of research, theory and practice in this volume seeks to enhance leadership impact and organizational effectiveness on both a local and global scale. We hope that researchers, policy makers, and organizational leaders are informed, engaged, and challenged by the collection of papers in this important and timeless volume.

Audrey J. Murrell, Ray Jones, and Xiaoping Zhao
Guest Editors

International Journal of
Environmental Research and Public Health

MDPI

Article

Food Security as Ethics and Social Responsibility: An Application of the Food Abundance Index in an Urban Setting

Audrey J. Murrell [1,*], Ray Jones [1], Sam Rose [2], Alex Firestine [3] and Joe Bute [2]

[1] David Berg Center for Ethics and Leadership, School of Business, University of Pittsburgh, Pittsburgh, PA 15260, USA
[2] Food21 of Pennsylvania, Pittsburgh, PA 15139, USA
[3] College of Business Administration, University of Pittsburgh, Pittsburgh, PA 15260, USA
* Correspondence: amurrell@pitt.edu; Tel.: +1-412-648-7835

Abstract: High levels of food insecurity signal the presence of disparities and inequities in local food access that have been shown to negatively impact the health and well-being of individuals and communities. Some argue that the lack of healthy, affordable and culturally relevant food within a community represents a troubling social and ethical concern for any society. The current research conducts an assessment of a specific community utilizing the framework outlined by the Food Abundance Index (FAI) scorecard. Combined with contemporary regional data on the demographics of the area, data revealed extremely low scores for both access and density dimensions. Our findings can help business, community and policymakers better understand and target evidence-based solutions to address the issue of food insecurity within this region.

Keywords: food insecurity; ethics; food systems; social responsibility; social inequalities

1. Introduction

Food insecurity has been identified as a significant health and nutrition issue within the United States and globally [1]. High food insecurity has been associated with key health outcomes such as risk factors for children's health and educational outcomes [2], long-term adverse consequence for overall health of children, maternal depression [3] and health status, mental health conditions [4], subsequent weight gain [5], poor sleep outcomes [6], chronic disease [7] and suicide ideation [8]. These data have led to research calling for immediate action to address food insecurity from a health, economic and social equality perspective. Some argue that the lack of healthy, affordable and culturally relevant food within a community represents an important social and ethical issue [9]. Food is considered a basic human right—as echoed by the United Nations, Declaration of Human Right, "people have a right to freedom from hunger, and everyone has a right to have access to adequate food" [10]. A right to food is a claim that is accepted and acknowledged by individuals and all of society [11]. This is because food, which is essential to all our lives, fulfills a basic biological need (along with water and oxygen) without which an individual would not survive or maintain their well-being [12,13].

Using this perspective, the current research agrees that satisfying this need for food is crucial for an individual and a community to maintain health, dignity and well-being. We see high food insecurity as a violation of one's rights to a healthy and secure life and a denial of the opportunity to realize one's full potential in society [14]. Consistent with the rights and common good approaches to ethics, access to food is part of society's ethical and social responsibility as well as a necessary component of social sustainability [15]. In addition to an individual's right to basic health and well-being, food insecurity may point to issues of disparity, discrimination or inequality [16]. For example, in the United States, food insecurity tends to be higher among households with incomes near or below the federal poverty line and black and Hispanic minority groups. Due to a variety of historical, political and social reasons, households with incomes near or below the poverty line are most likely to be minority households, single parent households, inner city or rural residents, elderly and people with disabilities [17]. The incidence of food insecurity among an economically and socially disadvantaged group raises concerns about ethics, social responsibility and economic equality [18].

1.1. Food Insecurity: An Ethics Analysis

A right to food access is a claim that is accepted and acknowledged by individuals and all of society. This is because food, which is essential to all our lives, fulfills a basic biological need without which an individual would not survive or maintain their well-being. Some theorized that ethics, public health and human rights are inextricably linked, and that people could not have rights and dignity if they could not maintain a healthy lifestyle [13]. This is similar to views that environmental, economic and social sustainability are linked as their collectively impact business and society. Clearly food insecurity with its negative consequences and its prevalence across community wide areas termed as "food deserts" are seen as a violation of ethics and social responsibility from a human rights perspective [19].

In addition to an individual's right to basic health and well-being, food insecurity may point to issues of disparity, discrimination, or inequality [20]. For example, in the United States, food insecurity tends to be higher among households with incomes near or below the federal poverty line and black and Hispanic minority groups [21]. Due to a variety of historical, political and social reasons, households with incomes near or below the poverty line are most likely to be minority households, single parent households, inner city or rural residents, elderly and people with disabilities [22]. The incidence of food insecurity among an economically and socially disadvantaged group raises concerns about social justice, economic equality and discrimination within the current food system [23]. The inequitable distribution of benefits and burdens and the impact of these benefits and burdens that span all dimensions of social life including income, economic wealth, food, power, education, shelter, and health care brings to the forefront a number of basic ethical issues and concerns pertaining to food security [24].

1.2. Food Insecurity: A Social Responsibility Issue

Some would argue that high rates of food insecurity within the U.S. are the result of a fundamental conflict between a competitive market-driven food system and the overall needs of local communities and global societies [25]. A common good is often defined as certain or general conditions that are distributed equally to everyone's advantage. The common good approach to ethics argues that social systems and environments on which we all depend must work in a manner that benefits all people [26]. But, current business practices are contrary to what one would argue are socially responsible business practices from a common goods perspective and has resulted in globally disparities, which have marginalized those at the bottom of the income distribution. For example, the current global food system consists of large-scale corporations whose strategy results in the marginalization of the small-scale producer thus reducing diversity in the number of firms involved across the food supply chain [27]. Other food retail practices like marketing unhealthy foods to kids and minority groups, higher pricing for organic and healthy foods, and a deliberate targeting of effluent and suburban consumers over those in low-income neighborhoods are all practices that are fail to recognize the interdependence between the health and welfare of communities and the competitiveness of businesses [28].

Clearly, food is one such common good that has been deemed important for the welfare of society. This is crucial for an individual to maintain his/her health and dignity and realize one's full potential in society. Not only is food security a complex ethical issue but is also what is referred to as a "wicked problem". A wicked problem is one that is tough to describe, has innumerable causes and require non-traditional approaches and processes in order to understand and solve complex wicked problems [29]. Food security also represents a wicked problem because it has a number of causes, has multiple perspectives that can be used to describe it, and doesn't have a right answer for solving the consequences of this complex problem. Thus, any solution to the ethical and wicked problem of food insecurity, must involve multidimensional models and solutions in order to be effective [30]. Also, while the public sector has traditionally shouldered the responsibility for addressing issues related to hunger and food insecurity, increasingly studies have shown that private sector involvement and investment is critical to achieve comprehensive food security and build sustainable communities that co-create value for a wide array of stakeholders and that provides opportunities for economic and social security to all [31].

Therefore, the main objective of this paper is to describe a community-based study that utilized a data-driven tool that can help businesses, communities' as well as policy-makers identify areas of needs to target efforts to eliminate/reduce food insecurity. An understanding of the complex problem of food security, investigating the prevalence of food insecurity and identifying food insecure areas is an essential first step in executing transformational and socially responsible solutions to the complex issue of food insecurity. While awareness of the increase in the number of communities that are impacted by low food security has increased, existing tools to measure or track level of food security are complicated, limited in scope, expensive and not made available to local communities who need reliable information in order to address these negative conditions. Thus, a need for more reliable and accessible evaluation tools prevails [32].

Previous research has developed such as tool that is aimed at shedding additional light on the issue of food security called the "Food Abundance Index (FAI)" that integrates food deserts as one way of examining food security in geographic regions. The FAI, which uses a scorecard for assessing levels of food security across five key dimensions has been designed for broad use by individuals, communities, policy makers and businesses and reflects our unique approach to food security as a matter of both social responsibility and sustainability. The development and use of the FAI tool is based on studies on food deserts including geographic measures of food access in food deserts and prior efforts that examine retail food environments. Prior research on measures of food insecurity focus on key dimensions such as availability, affordability and quality of healthy nutritious foods and its effect on consumption behaviors [33]. These efforts are critical in order to provide an evidence-based assessment of food insecurity that can better direct solutions that take into account dimensions of food insecurity along with neighborhood demographics, impact on health and well-being and the impact of existing government interventions within targeted communities [34].

Clearly. solutions to address problems of food security need to be based on robust data about the extent of the problem and its consequences. While academics and scholarly researchers have been studying these issues for nearly two decades now, the peer reviewed academic research in which these studies and data is published is often not accessed by practitioners and policymakers [35]. On the other hand, reports on research by practitioners are often published in proprietary reports that come with costs not often within the reach of traditional academic researchers [36]. Our current research makes an initial attempt to bridge this gap by applying the Food Abundance Index to a local community as a test of its utility as a potential tool for understanding and driving business and social interventions to address food insecurity as an issue of ethics and social responsibility.

2. Research Setting

The Mid-Mon Valley region was selected for this particular research due to its unique history of rapid growth and targeted attention by public, private and community organizations concerned with the need for economic and environmental recovery. The decline of key industries such as steel had a substantial negative socio-economic impact on the region producing a systemic shock to the infrastructure of the region. In addition, the presence of revitalization projects specifically addressing food insecurity, most of which experienced significant volume increases during the COVID-19 pandemic, provided an indication that this region would provide an important test and application of the FAI framework.

The Mid-Mon Valley region was one of the largest and most complete steel making regions in the world for a period of nearly one hundred years [37]. Uniquely situated for access to coal, limestone and iron ore, it became one of the largest vertically integrated production centers in industrial history. At any one time every facet of steelmaking was going on continuously along the Monongahela River. Prominent manufacturing corporations had previously employed thousands of workers in the region throughout the 20th century. By the early 1970s only one significant corporation remained providing employment for up to 30,000 workers across all Mid-Mon Valley factories. As a result, the local economies and every other aspect of the community was directly tied to these facilities in the area which were operated by a single large manufacturer. Within the next decade, this corporation experienced over $561 million in losses which led to significant job and tax revenue loss. Layoffs and facility closures followed which results in severe loss in tax revenue, income, and population. During this time, unemployment rose to 20% and a significant number of residents lost their jobs due to the decline. Several regional initiatives and public policy efforts were created to address the economic, social and employment issues with the region [38].

The Financial Recovery Act of 1987 and the Mon Valley Initiative (MVI) sought to uplift economic activity in the region and have a significant impact on working towards a recovery in the region [39]. From a food security perspective, the Greater Pittsburgh Area Food Bank whose headquarters was located within the region was an important resource for food within these effected communities. These series of revitalization projects spark the potential for a resurgence of economic growth in the area for the future [40]. This provided an appropriate context for testing the FAI index together with regional data to examine this issue and identify targets areas for comprehensive solutions and additional regional investments.

For the size of the population, several of the ZIP codes within the Mid-Mon Valley have a significantly lower average income per household than the Allegheny County average. This region also has a higher minority population compared to the county as a whole. The region contained only one significant food production industry sector that was also one of the top ten employers in the region. According to the U.S. Bureau of Labor Statistics, the average food at home/away from home budget is approximately $8000 per year per household. However, the US census published that 12% of households are enrolled in Supplemental Nutrition Assistance Program (SNAP) benefits [41]. These SNAP benefits in the Mid-Mon Valley pay for approximately half of a family's total food budget per year on average. This leaves these families with an additional expense of approximately $4000 per year, which can translate to close to 25% of their income. Lastly, the food industry sector as well as overall employment in the region, has been significantly negatively impacted by COVID-19 [42].

3. Methods

The Food Abundance Index (FAI)

The original Food Abundance Index (FAI) was developed to measure the level of 'food security' and uses the presence of 'food deserts' as the key metric for assessing potential levels of food insecurity in a specific community [43]. The measure has been designed for broad use by individuals, communities, policymakers, businesses and corporations and reflects a unique approach to measuring food insecurity as a matter of both business responsibility and social responsibility. The FAI focuses on five dimensions that prior research show are key drivers of food insecurity.

Access. The access dimension is defined as the availability and ease of contact to healthy, nutritious and balanced food sources. When evaluating for access, the presence of food outlets selling at a minimum fresh produce, meat and dairy products are taken into consideration. These include mainstream grocery stores (large and small) and alternative food sources such as farmer markets, organic food outlets and local food source outlets like community supported agriculture, food cooperatives, farm stands, pick your own operation, etc. But the mere presence of such food sources is not enough, if people do not have direct access to the grocery store or food outlet. Since minority or economically disadvantaged communities often lack access to supermarkets within a short walking distance people have to rely on public transit to gain access to grocery stores. It was decided that to be classified as accessible, grocery stores must have a serviced bus stop within a five-minute or short walking distance within the designated study area.

Diversity. The diversity dimension first analyses the availability of multiple food sources selling healthy nutritious foods within the study area. Diversity of sources is important to look at because areas with high food insecurity usually lack healthful food sources like grocery stores, organic outlets, farmer markets, etc. which typically are outlets that have sell nutritious food items like fresh produce, meat, and dairy. This is also an issue of great concern because residents of food insecure areas would have to travel further to get essential food items or may have to depend on the one food outlet (in the absence of diversity) within the neighborhood offering unhealthy food products. Diversity also refers to the presence and availability of a variety of healthy and nutritious food items based on most relevant government sanctioned dietary and nutrition guidelines.

Quality. The duality dimension refers to the presence and availability of appropriately prepared, transported and preserved food that meets dietary needs of relevant community. At a minimum everyone should have access to adequately prepared and edible foods. A neighborhood without quality food forces residents to rely on fast food sources or convenience stores or travel outside of their neighborhood to achieve quality food for their family. This FAI dimension determines whether a food outlet sells fresh edible foods and no out-of-date or expired products from each food group of the relevant federal guidelines within the study area. A produce quality rating system is utilized to determine the freshness and appearance of products sold. One can also use existing consumer data on food quality from agencies like the health department to determine the quality of food available within the study area. Food stores can also play a significant role in promoting healthy buying, eating and consuming habits in their consumers. For example, the presence of healthy dietary intake promotion displays within the store like signage promoting low calorie foods, fruits and vegetables, organic or locally grown foods; labels near the food displays giving nutritional content of the food item; information on the food guide pyramid or tips for proper food storage and preservation creates a high-quality in-store food environment. Hence, healthy food promotion is also used as a part of the quality dimension.

Density. Density refers to the proportion of unhealthy food sources to healthy food sources present within the study area relative to health food sources. Food insecure communities typically have an imbalance between unhealthful and healthful food destinations and residents must rely on venues that sell highly processed foods and foods that are high in salt, fat and sugar. As a result, food insecure residents are more vulnerable to economic, social and physical consequences of living in areas with a dearth of outlets that sell nutritious foods. An ideal food environment should have a greater number of food outlets like grocery stores, produce vendors, organic and local food outlets like farmer markets, community supported agriculture, farm stands, etc. that provide a constant and reliable source for fresh produce, meat/poultry and dairy items as compared to convenience and fast-food stores.

Affordability. The final element of 'affordability' refers to the concentration and availability of healthy and nutritious food sources given the income and purchasing power of residents within the relevant geographic location. Firstly, affordability can be examined by the availability of healthy and nutritious foods at costs less than or equal to the national average cost of purchasing a 'standard market basket' of food items. The assessment uses the food list from the relevant federal guidelines, which provides a list of foods items plus condiments needed to prepare a week's worth of food for an individual or a family. Store surveys can also be conducted to collect information on the lowest price at which food included in the market basket is sold for in the study area. Affordability can then be determined by comparing the cost of purchasing the complete market basket within the study area to the national average cost of purchasing based on the federal or government guidelines for the relevant assessment area.

The FAI is designed to provide a multi-dimensional tool for measuring the level of food security and especially whether a 'food desert' may exist within a specific community or neighborhood area. It attempts to combine the strengths of existing measures of food access and availability and examines food security across the multiple dimensions of access, diversity, quality, density and affordability. The FAI uses a scorecard approach similar to the LEED certification (Leadership in Energy and Environmental Design) for communities that awards points for actions across the five dimensions that enhance a community's level of food security [44]. The scorecard approach allows individuals, communities and organizations to measure for levels of food security present in a geographic region, identify where problems or gaps may exist and track changes or progress across multiple dimensions [45].

For the current research. an updated version of the original Food Abundance Index (FAI) was used as the framework to identify and aggregate data directly from multiple public, research and community-based data sources. Our purpose was to apply the revised FAI tool as a framework for pooling relevant data and to combine, share and use these data resources to make decisions pertaining to local and regional food related policies and program efforts. This approach provides a better reflection of the key factors within each community related to the dimensions of the FAI that can provide a more detailed assessment of the level of food insecurity. There is a clear need for this type of aggregate data is in order to address potential gaps related to measuring food insecurity that exist with single item or single source data. With the current research, we used the framework of the FAI to select, collect and then aggregate existing data within current and publicly available data sets. To assess the Mon Valley region, the revised FAI tool was applied via a digital platform that included an interactive GIS map database that displays the region's food outlets, which is updated monthly by the Western Pennsylvania Regional Data Center (http://www.wprdc.org/) (last accessed on 5 August 2022).

The enhanced FAI design provides numerous additional benefits. The sheer cost and contributed effort to conduct and maintain this program have been significantly reduced from the original assessment tool both by innovations in the aggregation of existing sources of data that can be updated more rapidly as conditions change and new information becomes available. By centralizing data from multiple sets in one application, and incorporating existing public and proprietary data sources many of the gaps in previous approaches can be addressed. Thus, the FAI tool combines pooling, sharing and using existing sources of data in order to use the current scorecard to collect, analyze, and employ these data to provide a more comprehensive examining of food insecurity pertaining to local and regional communities.

4. Results

Our results using the aggregated data as defined by the FAI framework focuses on two of the key dimensions: access and density. As with the prior research, each dimension is measured by three levels: Required, Suggested, and Innovative. If the study area meets the required criteria, it is awarded one point, and if not, it is deducted one point. Meeting the suggested or innovative requirements awards two or three points respectively, and do not subtract points if not present. For each dimension, the highest obtainable score is a 7, and the lowest is a -1. Scores for aggregated data are summarized based on these two key dimensions (density and access) as defined by the FAI scorecard are provided below.

4.1. Density Evaluation Findings

The Density dimension of the Food Abundance Index focuses on the proportion of nutritious, healthy food outlets to non-nutritious alternatives within the study area. For this analysis, we calculated a series of ratios that corresponded with the three levels of analysis in the Food Abundance Index. The factors, point assignments, and raw ratios are described in Table 1.

Table 1. FAI Density Dimension Results.

Density Factor Criteria	FAI Points for Region	Mid-Mon Valley Ratio
Higher number of grocery stores to convenience stores	−1	1 grocery store to 7 convenience stores
Higher number of grocery stores and produce vendors to convenience stores	0	2 grocery stores/organic food outlets to 7 convenience stores
Higher number of local organic food source outlets to fast food and convenience stores	0	1 organic food outlet to 94 fast food/convenience stores

From the analysis, this region was awarded the lowest possible score for the Density dimension, earning a −1, as the ratio calculated between grocery stores and convenience stores was below the required threshold. In addition, there is a low quantity of organic food outlets and grocery stores in the communities in the Mid-Mon Valley region compared to fast food and convenience stores. The majority of food outlets in the Mid-Mon Valley are restaurants, as full service and fast-food restaurants account for 84.57% of food outlets. Excluding restaurants, there is a high concentration of convenience stores, corner stores, and food bank distribution centers in the area. This district also has a geographic challenge of food outlets being distributed on both sides of the Monongahela River, with limited bridge and transportation access between the district communities. This exacerbates the problem of a smaller amount of accessible healthier food outlets (e.g., limited assortment stores, supermarkets, grocery stores). While physical distance from these sparse stores may be minimal, the travel times can be extended due to heavy bridge traffic, congestion and lack of public transportation options.

4.2. Access Evaluation Findings

The Access dimension of the Food Abundance Index focuses on the ability to contact healthy, nutritious food with ease. The required level for this dimension is the presence of a mainstream grocery store within walking distance of a public transportation stop. The suggested level awards two points for the presence of a farmer's market or organic store, and the innovative level requires members of the community to have access to community-based nutrition education and support. An analysis of the Mid-Mon Valley region reveals it has all these qualities, and thus earns six of six possible points. However, additional findings from the application reveal there may be underlying issues despite the positive scoring.

The latest Food Abundance Index application data (see Table 2) shows nine locations in this region lacking public transportation stops within 0.25 miles out of a total of 61 known food outlets (14.75%). In addition, seven of the census tracts in the district have an estimated less than 30% of households owning at least one car. For households with vehicles, auto congestion may inhibit access, as it is relatively high throughout this district. This high rate of congestion may also increase travel times for residents that have to take a bus to their primary food outlet. Food outlets reside on both sides of the river that splits this district, which poses a challenge to people traveling across bridges to access them. The sparsity of bridges, high congestion, and presence of food outlets without nearby transportation stops act as barriers for residents to acquire healthy food thus, reducing overall access. The findings from our data aggregation for the access dimension of the FAI are summarized in Table 2.

Table 2. FAI Access Dimension Results.

Access Factor Requirement	FAI Points for Region
Presence of a mainstream grocery store within walking distance of a public transportation stop in the region	1
Presence of a farmer's market or organic store in the region	2
Presence of community-based nutrition education support in the region	3

4.3. Key Findings from the FAI Analysis

Aggregated data for both access and density reveal that the Mid-Mon Valley is susceptible to experiencing significantly low levels these two dimensions of food security. Within our aggregated data we noted that there were several factors that contributed to the low scores for access and density. These contributing factors include lack of walkable public transportation to area food outlets, lack of vehicle ownership, and traffic congestion in the area. In addition, lack of availability of a diverse variety of local food outlets were also identified as critical factors contributing to low scores for both access and density dimensions. The aggregation across multiple existing data sources in our evaluation of the access and density dimensions also yielded specific targeted areas of focus that are highlighted as part of our findings (see Figure 1).

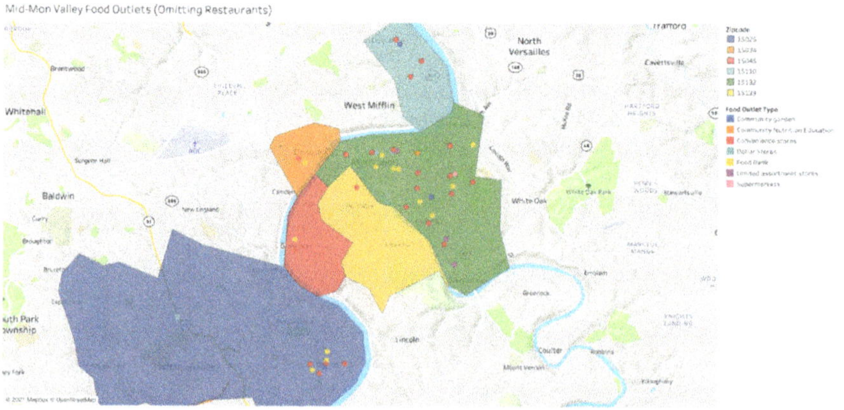

Figure 1. FAI Access to and Density Dimensions by Public Transportation Resources.

The presence of community-based food education programs and limited organic stores reveal potential and the need for further community-based development. While some outlets did not have adequate access to public transportation, this accounted for some of the outlets in the area. External data revealed other access challenges, such as congestion and lack of access may be defined by factors outside of the specific FAI scoring methodology and calculation. This further suggests the necessity for future qualitative community surveying as a complement to the FAI scorecard in order to address issues such as how individuals and families cope with lack of access, density and transportation resources that may not be apparent in the existing data sources used in the current calculations and scoring of the FAI dimensions (access and density).

5. Discussion

Our application of the enhanced FAI tool provides valuable insight into key dimensions of access and density that should be addressed for the community studied within the current research. Based on the findings from research, the Food Abundance Index provides a robust measurement tool to assess the extent of food insecurity within a community or neighborhood. A major contribution of this work is to present a new multi-dimensional measure of food insecurity that strengthens the link between the level of food security as both an ethical and social responsibility issue. We suggest that the adoption and utilization of data produced by the FAI offers a number of policy and management implications to help bring about sustainable social change in the food supply chain and address this as a wicked social problem [46].

The FAI can help communities understand that strategies like opening a mainstream grocery store in a food desert are just a starting point. Food security is a complex multi-dimensional issue and a host of strategies that address all aspects of food security will be needed to eliminate this social problem. These include working with stores to add healthy, nutritious foods to their inventory, working with businesses to market healthy foods, providing educational support for healthy consumption, incentivizing people to buy healthy foods and making alternate sources of healthy foods like farmers markets accessible to all, especially low-income populations by acceptance of food stamps at farmer markets [47]. It also suggests that business and workforce development efforts are needed to build capacity across all aspects of sustainability (economic, social and environmental) [48]. Resident's food needs can also be used as an economic driver to undertake sustainable policies and market-based enterprises that allow equitable food access. Our unique scorecard approach used by the FAI to measure food security can also be useful to communities to track improvement in levels of food insecurity over time based on intervention strategies implemented over time.

An ethics and social responsibility perspective asserts that 'life' in community is a public good, which should benefit all and be available to all in society [49]. Food security is one such good that has been deemed important for the welfare of society. However, the present food system models of production, distribution and supply chain management can negatively impact power and minoritized communities. While the public sector has traditionally shouldered the responsibility for addressing issues related to hunger and food insecurity, the private sector if it does not provide for the marginalized and food insecure, is losing out on a whole market of value-demanding consumers [50].

Identifying food insecure areas is the first steps in helping communities reach the ultimate goal of building an ethical and equitable food system. The information, awareness and understanding of the current state of access to and availability of healthy, affordable foods gathered through tools such as the Food Abundance Index could provide the basis for change, action and future direction to academics and practitioners. Thus, our work in developing and distributing the FAI tool reflects our attempt to bridge the gap and expand the boundaries between academia and practitioners using robust methodology and innovative assessment tool.

Our tool has been designed to be accessible and easy to use by practitioners, especially those with limited financial and research resources to study the problems of food security, identify shortcoming in the local food system and also develop evidence-based solutions/policies. In addition, the FAI tool considers food security across multiple dimensions and provides a complete picture of food security in a community as related to key dimensions (access and diversity) examined in the current research and the additional dimensions of quality, density and affordability not measured in this research but provide opportunity for future research. As a measurement tool, the FAI can not only assess whether a food desert exists within a particular community, but as our current findings indicate, it can also be used to identify where gaps or problems may exist that may cause a breakdown in food security in the future. Lastly, the FAI uses a scorecard approach to measure for different levels of food security, track improvement in levels of food security over time and provide a benchmark that practitioners can use for addressing the issue of food security in other geographic areas.

We argue that the adoption and utilization of data produced by the FAI offers a number of potential contribution and benefits. Analysis of geographic areas using the FAI will help lay the foundation for reducing communities' food insecurities and improving economic status, health, and overall well-being. We expect that use of the FAI to also stimulate additional academic research by providing researchers with a comprehensive tool to measure levels of food security as well as outcomes and the impact of change efforts. Lastly, we anticipate use of the FAI tool to facilitate collaboration, knowledge sharing and dialog between academic and community-based research based on the common language, methodology and focus provided by this new approach to understand the dimensions and impact of food insecurity as a key social issue.

6. Conclusions

Our analysis identified several issues and assets that can be utilized by business, community and public sector organizations to address the issue of access and density to develop both ethical and socially responsible solutions within this region. These issues and assets are summarized below as key implications of our work using the expanded FAI tool within this area examined in the current research.

6.1. Key Gaps and Issues Identified in the Mid-Mon Valley

a. Collapse of industrial era economic infrastructure.
b. Legacy of limited attention to environmental sustainability in industrial practices.
c. Gap in availability of and reasonable access to healthy affordable food.
d. Diminished regional food infrastructure related to transformation.
e. Lack of investment on the regional level in food systems infrastructure.
f. Disproportionate representation of lower income, lower levels of business ownership and employment by the age and race/ethnicity demographic groups.
g. Community negatively impacted by the COVID-19 global pandemic.
h. Higher number of health disparities associated with poor nutrition and lack of healthy, affordable food options.

6.2. Key Assets and Opportunities Identified in the Mid-Mon Valley

a. A greater metro region marketplace of over 1.2 million people, with a total of 537,000 households, spending approximately $3 billion plus per year combined on food and beverage needs.
b. A "foodshed" region with the soils, water, people and production capable of supplying an estimated potential of at least 25% ($750 million in sales) or more of the annual total food and beverage market demands of the greater metro area this district resides within.
c. Greater Foodshed region contains over 7 million acres in production is already in the top ten agriculture producing regions in the US.
d. A capable workforce with embedded historical experience in industrial production, that can be evolved and adapted to in region food production.
e. An extensive business network of entrepreneurs tied to former and existing industrial and retail enterprises that could be resources to rebuild the local food economy.

7. Future Directions

While the use of aggregated data to examine the dimensions of the Food Abundance Index as a tool are important indicators, it should be viewed not only as a one-time snapshot but as a way of measuring continued progress and ongoing improvement. The use of the FAI tool as the framework for collecting and aggregating existing data can help to curate data in real time as an integral part of developing comprehensive policies, programs, and projects to address challenges and deficiencies. Our current work points to the future potential of the FAI tool to shape ongoing efforts to leverage new and existing data in a meaningful way that can provide direction and feedback to policymakers, community members and business leaders.

The use of existing data that is shaped and informed by the FAI framework can become an invaluable tool for developing a resilient and sustainable food economy both regionally and globally. Bringing together data from a multitude of sources is an important contribution of the current work for both research and practice. This tool can be beneficial in the future to move away from previous attempts to address food desert with single efforts solutions such as a single grocery or food outlet. The FAI framework together with comprehensive data sources can fill a critical need for evidence-based approaches that not only shape decision making but also measure its ongoing impact and effectiveness The further refinement of the FAI tool reflects our ongoing efforts to shape the conversation and efforts toward building a more resilient and sustainable food ecosystem that reduces disparities and moves us forward to a more equitable and just food ecosystem.

Author Contributions: Conceptualization, A.J.M., R.J., S.R., A.F. and J.B.; methodology, A.J.M., S.R. and A.F.; software, S.R. and A.F.; validation, S.R. and A.F.; formal analysis, S.R. and A.F.; investigation, A.J.M., R.J., S.R. and A.F.; resources, A.J.M., R.J. and J.B.; data curation, S.R. and A.F.; writing—A.J.M., R.J., S.R. and A.F.; writing—review and editing, A.J.M., R.J., S.R., A.F. and J.B.; visualization, S.R. and A.F.; supervision, A.J.M., R.J. and J.B.; project administration, A.J.M. and J.B.; funding acquisition, A.J.M. and J.B. All authors have read and agreed to the published version of the manuscript.

Funding: This research received no external funding.

Institutional Review Board Statement: The project does not include any interaction or intervention with human subjects or include any access to identifiable private information, thus the project does not require IRB review.

Informed Consent Statement: Not applicable.

Data Availability Statement: The data presented in this study are available on request from the corresponding author.

Conflicts of Interest: The authors declare no conflict of interest.

References

1. Kirkpatrick, S.I.; McIntyre, L.; Potestino, M.L. Child hunger and long-term adverse consequences for health. *Arch. Pediatrics Adolesc. Med.* **2010**, *164*, 7554–7562. [CrossRef] [PubMed]
2. Howard, L.L. Does food insecurity at home affect non-cognitive performance at school? A longitudinal analysis of elementary student classroom behavior. *Econ. Educ. Rev.* **2011**, *30*, 157–176.
3. Garg, A.; Toy, S.; Tripodis, Y.; Cook, J.; Cordella, N. Influence of maternal depression on household food insecurity for low-income families. *Acad. Pediatrics* **2015**, *15*, 305–310. [CrossRef] [PubMed]
4. Heflin, C.M.; Ziliak, J.P. Food insufficiency, food stamp participation and mental health. *Soc. Sci. Q.* **2008**, *89*, 706–727. [CrossRef]
5. Jones, S.L.; Frongillo, E.A. Food insecurity and subsequent weight gain in women. *Public Health Nutr.* **2007**, *10*, 145–151. [CrossRef]
6. Ding, M.; Keiley, M.K.; Garza, K.B.; Duffy, P.A.; Ziza, C.A. Food insecurity is associated with poor sleep outcomes among US adults. *J. Nutr.* **2015**, *145*, 615–621. [CrossRef]
7. Seligman, H.K.; Laraia, B.A.; Kushel, M.B. Food insecurity is associated with chronic disease among low-income NHANES participants. *J. Nutr.* **2010**, *140*, 304–310. [CrossRef] [PubMed]
8. McIntyre, L.; Williams, L.V.; Lavorato, D.H.; Patten, S. Depression and suicide ideation in late adolescence and early adulthood are an outcome of child hunger. *J. Affect. Disord.* **2013**, *150*, 123–129. [CrossRef]
9. Pollard, C.M.; Booth, S. Food insecurity and hunger in rich countries- It is time for action again inequality. *Int. J. Environ. Res. Public Health* **2019**, *16*, 1804. [CrossRef] [PubMed]
10. United Nations. Declaration of Human Right. 1948. Available online: http://www.ohchr.org/en/udhr/pages/introduction.aspx (accessed on 5 August 2022).
11. Dowler, E.A.; O'Connor, D. Rights-based approaches to addressing food poverty and food insecurity in Ireland and U.K. *Soc. Sci. Med.* **2012**, *74*, 44–51. [CrossRef]
12. Anderson, C.A.M.; Thorndike, A.N.; Lichtenstein, A.H.; Van Horn, L.; Kris-Etherton, P.M.; Foraker, R.; Spees, C. Innovation to create a health and sustainable food system. *Circulation* **2019**, *139*, e1025–e1032. [CrossRef] [PubMed]
13. Birkenmaier, J.; Huang, J.; Kim, Y. Food insecurity and financial access during economic recession: Evidence from the 2008 SIPP. *J. Poverty* **2016**, *20*, 194–213. [CrossRef]
14. Odunitan-Wayas, F.A.; Alaba, O.A.; Lambert, E.V. Food insecurity and social injustice: The plight of urban poor African immigrants in South Africa during the COVID-19 crisis. *Glob. Public Health* **2021**, *16*, 149–152. [CrossRef]
15. Granillo-Macías, R. Logistics optimization through a social approach for food distribution. *Socio-Econ. Plan. Sci.* **2021**, *76*, 100972. [CrossRef]

16. Walker, R.J.; Garacci, E.; Dawson, A.Z.; Williams, J.S.; Ozieh, M.; Egede, L.E. Trends in food insecurity in the United States from 2011–2017: Disparities by age, sex, race/ethnicity, and income. *Popul. Health Manag.* **2021**, *24*, 496–501. [CrossRef]
17. Nord, M.; Andrews, M.; Carlson, S. Measuring Food Security in the United States: Household Food Security in the United States, 2008. ERR-83 2009, U.S. Department of Agriculture, Economic Research Service. Available online: www.ers.usda.gov/publications/err83/err83.pdf (accessed on 5 August 2022).
18. Bowen, S.; Elliott, S.; Hardison-Moody, A. The structural roots of food insecurity: How racism is a fundamental cause of food insecurity. *Sociol. Compass* **2021**, *15*, e12846. [CrossRef]
19. Sharma, A.; Jolly, P.M.; Chiles, R.M.; DiPietro, R.B.; Jaykumar, A.; Kesa, H.; Monteiro, H.; Roberts, K.; Saulais, L. Principles of foodservice ethics: A general review. *Int. J. Contemp. Hosp. Manag.* **2022**, *34*, 135–158. [CrossRef]
20. Zenk, S.; Schutz, A.; Israel, B.; James, S.; Bao, S.; Wilson, M. Neighborhood composition, neighborhood poverty, and the spatial accessibility of supermarkets in Detroit. *Am. J. Public Health* **2005**, *95*, 660–667. [CrossRef] [PubMed]
21. Morland, K.; Wing, S.; Roux, A.D.; Poole, C. Neighborhood characteristics associated with the location of food stores and food service places. *Am. J. Prev. Med.* **2002**, *22*, 23–29. [CrossRef]
22. Zenk, S.; Schulz, A.; Israel, B.; James, S.; Bao, S.; Wilson, M. Fruit and vegetable access differs by community racial composition and socioeconomic position in Detroit, Michigan. *Ethn. Dis.* **2006**, *16*, 275–280.
23. Gallagher, M. *Examining the Impact of Food Deserts on Public Health in Chicago*; Gallagher Research Consulting Group: Chicago, IL, USA, 2006.
24. Banerjee, S.; Radak, T.; Khubchandani, J.; Dunn, P. Food insecurity and mortality in American adults: Results from the NHANES-linked mortality study. *Health Promot. Pract.* **2021**, *22*, 204–214. [CrossRef] [PubMed]
25. O'Hara, S.; Toussaint, E.C. Food access in crisis: Food security and COVID-19. *Ecol. Econ.* **2021**, *180*, 106859. [CrossRef]
26. Naranova-Nassauer, A. Stakeholder relations of sustainable banks: Community benefit above the common good. *Bus. Ethics Environ. Responsib.* **2021**, 1–15. [CrossRef]
27. Yadav, V.S.; Singh, A.R.; Gunasekaran, A.; Raut, R.D.; Narkhede, B.E. A systematic literature review of the agro-food supply chain: Challenges, network design, and performance measurement perspectives. *Sustain. Prod. Consum.* **2022**, *29*, 685–704. [CrossRef]
28. Backholer, K.; Gupta, A.; Zorbas, C.; Bennett, R.; Huse, O.; Chung, A.; Isaacs, A.; Golds, G.; Kelly, B.; Peeters, A. Differential exposure to, and potential impact of, unhealthy advertising to children by socio-economic and ethnic groups: A systematic review of the evidence. *Obes. Rev.* **2021**, *22*, e13144. [CrossRef]
29. Camillus, J.C. Strategy as a wicked problem. *Harv. Bus. Rev.* **2008**, *86*, 98–101.
30. Lönngren, J.; Van Poeck, K. Wicked problems: A mapping review of the literature. *Int. J. Sustain. Dev. World Ecol.* **2021**, *28*, 481–502. [CrossRef]
31. Mui, Y.; Headrick, G.; Raja, S.; Palmer, A.; Ehsani, J.; Porter, K.P. Acquisition, mobility and food insecurity: Integrated food systems opportunities across urbanicity levels highlighted by COVID-19. *Public Health Nutr.* **2022**, *25*, 114–118. [CrossRef]
32. Glanz, K.; Sallis, J.F.; Saelens, B.E.; Frank, L.D. Nutrition Environment Measures Survey in Stores (NEMS-S): Development and Evaluation. *Am. J. Prev. Med.* **2007**, *32*, 282–289. [CrossRef]
33. Larsen, K.; Gilliland, J. Mapping the evolution of 'food deserts' in a Canadian city: Supermarket accessibility in London, Ontario, 1961–2005. *Int. J. Health Geogr.* **2008**, *7*, 16. [CrossRef]
34. Cohen, B. Community Food Security Assessment Toolkit. U.S. Department of Agriculture 2002, Economic Research Service. Available online: http://www.ers.usda.gov/publications/efan02013/efan02013.pdf (accessed on 5 August 2022).
35. Carrillo-Álvarez, E.; Salinas-Roca, B.; Costa-Tutusaus, L.; Milà-Villarroel, R.; Shankar Krishnan, N. The measurement of food insecurity in high-income countries: A scoping review. *Int. J. Environ. Res. Public Health* **2021**, *18*, 9829. [CrossRef] [PubMed]
36. Bjorn, A.; Lee, B.; Born, B.; Monsivais, P.; Kantor, S.; Sayre, R. Mapping Food Insecurity and Access in Seattle and King County. University of Washington and Washington State University King County Extension. Prepared on Behalf of the Seattle and King County Acting Food Policy Council. 2008. Available online: http://www.b-sustainable.org/built-environment/access-to-local-food-by-neighborhood/AFPCFoodAccessIssuePaperNo.4_000.pdf (accessed on 5 August 2022).
37. Deitrick, S.; Briem, C. The Pittsburgh transition: Not quite so simple. *Econ. Dev. Q.* **2021**, *35*, 197–201. [CrossRef]
38. Hill, E. Development starts with historical endowments: Industrial policy and leadership are catalysts. *Econ. Dev. Q.* **2021**, *35*, 202–215. [CrossRef]
39. Polson, D. Building a bigger "We": Reflections on more than a decade of building community power in Pittsburgh. In *Igniting Justice and Progressive Power*; Routledge: New York, NY, USA, 2021; pp. 154–178.
40. Deitrick, S.; Briem, C. Quality of life and demographic-racial dimensions of differences in most liveable Pittsburgh. *J. Urban Regen. Renew.* **2022**, *15*, 193–209.
41. Parum, F.; Dharmasena, S. US Consumers' Intake of Food at Home (FAH) and Food Away from Home (FAFH) As a Complex Economic System. *J. Food Distrib. Res.* **2021**, *52*, 77–85.
42. Morales, D.X.; Morales, S.A.; Beltran, T.F. Racial/ethnic disparities in household food insecurity during the COVID-19 pandemic: A nationally representative study. *J. Racial Ethn. Health Disparities* **2021**, *8*, 1300–1314. [CrossRef]
43. Murrell, A.J.; Jones, R. Measuring food insecurity using the Food Abundance Index: Implications for economic, health and social well-being. *Int. J. Environ. Res. Public Health* **2020**, *17*, 2434. [CrossRef]
44. U.S. Green Building Council's LEED Certification. Available online: www.usbgc.org/LEED (accessed on 5 August 2022).

45. Treuhaft, S.; Karpyn, A. The Grocery Gap: Who Has Access to Healthy Food and Why It Matters. PolicyLink and the Food Trust. 2020. Available online: http://www.bench-marks.org/downloads/070625_platinum_research_full.pdf (accessed on 5 August 2022).
46. Dabone, C.; Mbagwu, I.; Muray, M.; Ubangha, L.; Kohoun, B.; Etowa, E.; Nare, H.; Kiros, G.; Etowa, J. Global food insecurity and African, Caribbean, and Black (ACB) populations during the COVID-19 pandemic: A rapid review. *J. Racial Ethn. Health Disparities* **2021**, *9*, 420–435. [CrossRef]
47. Ekenga, C.C.; Tian, R. Promoting Food Equity in the Context of Residential Segregation. *Environ. Justice* **2021**, 1–6. [CrossRef]
48. Toussaint, M.; Cabanelas, P.; Blanco-González, A. Social sustainability in the food value chain: An integrative approach beyond corporate social responsibility. *Corp. Soc. Responsib. Environ. Manag.* **2021**, *28*, 103–115. [CrossRef]
49. Prahalad, C.K. *Fortune at the Bottom of the Pyramid: Eradicating Poverty through Profits*; Wharton School Publishing: Philadelphia, PA, USA, 2004.
50. Utami, H.N.; Alamanos, E.; Kuznesof, S. 'A social justice logic': How digital commerce enables value co-creation at the bottom of the pyramid. *J. Mark. Manag.* **2021**, *37*, 816–855. [CrossRef]

International Journal of
Environmental Research and Public Health

MDPI

Article

The Role of Social Responsibility and Ethics in Employees' Wellbeing

Claudiu George Bocean [1,*], Michael Marian Nicolescu [2], Marian Cazacu [2] and Simona Dumitriu [2]

[1] Department of Management, Marketing and Business Administration, Faculty of Economics and Business Administration, University of Craiova, 13 AI Cuza Street, 200585 Craiova, Romania
[2] Doctoral School, University of Craiova, 13 AI Cuza Street, 200585 Craiova, Romania; nicolescumichaelmarian@gmail.com (M.M.N.); cazacumariantbm@gmail.com (M.C.); simonadumitriu1969@gmail.com (S.D.)
* Correspondence: claudiu.bocean@edu.ucv.ro; Tel.: +40-7-2629-9522

Abstract: Social responsibility (SR) is a concept or practice by which organizations take into account the interest of society by taking responsibility for the impact of their activities on all stakeholders. The SR of organizations implies ethical behavior concerning all stakeholders and a company's commitment to the sustainable economic development of society. Organizational ethics is a set of written and unwritten codes of principles and values that govern decisions and actions within an organization. Ethics has a rather internal perspective, while social responsibility has a rather external perspective. This study examines the impact of social responsibility and organizational ethics on employees' wellbeing. To perform the empirical analysis, we conducted a survey among 423 employees from Romanian organizations. Using the structural equation modeling, we analyzed the relationships between social responsibility, organizational ethics, and employees' wellbeing, emphasizing the positive impact of ethical and responsible behavior of the organization on the employees' wellbeing. The organization's employees play a dual role: firstly, they are all internal stakeholders, and secondly, they are constituents of an external stakeholder essential for the organization—the community. The results show a significant positive influence of social responsibility and organizational ethics on employees' wellbeing as a result of a responsible and ethical behavior in relation to the organizational stakeholders.

Keywords: social responsibility; organizational ethics; wellbeing; employees; community; structural equation modeling

1. Introduction

The modern organization is an entity with a substantial social impact due to its ability to mobilize productive resources and create new wealth. However, the organization's legitimacy depends not only on success in creating wealth but also on its ability to meet the expectations of the various stakeholders that contribute to its existence and success.

Social responsibility (SR) concerns implementing ethical behavior and attitude in the organization, providing a perspective on core values and organizational culture to promote responsible behavior towards staff. Organizational ethics (OE) influence practices in the field of social responsibility. It is in the interest of every organization to develop and incorporate elements of both OE and SR into its agenda, as the challenges of an increasingly globalized economy with stringent sustainability requirements will require an integrated approach of OE and SR to support the sustainable development of organizations [1,2].

To be sustainable, organizations need to identify innovative ways to balance the social and environmental needs of internal and external stakeholders (employees, unions, community) with the economic (financial) needs of internal and external stakeholders (shareholders, employees, suppliers, customers, tax administrations) [3–5]. External SR extends to the community and society, including environmental concerns, while internal

SR addresses the organization's human resources [6]. In addition, internal SR focuses on strategies and practices to improve employee health and wellbeing (WB) [7], human rights [8], training and development [9,10], ensuring equal opportunities in business [11], and work–life balance [12].

Although most studies show a significant relationship between SR and OE practices, these relationships are neither universal nor consistent [13]. Therefore, investigating the different dimensions of SR practices concerning the dimensions of OE is necessary to integrate the two concepts and evaluate the combined effects on the employees' WB and the community in which the organization operates.

Although the impact of SR and OE on economic, social, and environmental performance has long been analyzed, not many studies examine the effects of SR and OE on employees' WB. Despite the awareness that employees are a key internal stakeholder whose motivation depends on the organizational success, being at the same time a constituent part of a critical external stakeholder (the community in which the organization operates), there are a few studies in the area.

The research gap that the paper aims to cover comes from the lack of work to study the combined effect of OE and SR on employees' WB. Since organizational employees are an essential category of internal stakeholders, the organization must pay special attention to SR and OE; these significantly affect employees' WB. This study's objectives involve analyzing the direct relationships among employees' perceptions of SR, OE, and WB, and the mediation effects between the variables considered. By studying these objectives, this study aims to understand better cause-and-effect relationships on how SR and OE can influence employee WB. The paper structure has six sections. The introduction and literature review approach the research topic from a theoretical point of view. Sections 3 and 4 describe the research design and results. The last two sections provide discussions and conclusions of the research.

2. Literature Review

2.1. Social Responsibility

SR is the moral responsibility of an organization toward the community in which it operates in particular and towards society in general [4,14]. SR is a concept that has received multiple definitions, and there are various classifications of its dimensions: the economic, legal, ethical, and philanthropic dimensions [15] and the economic, social, environmental, stakeholder, and volunteer dimensions [16]. Davis and Blomstrom argue that the substance of SR stems from the ethical "obligation" of the organization to assess the effects of its decisions and actions on the entire social system [17]. At the same time, [18] identifies the gap between the concept of SR and practice. Other authors [15,19,20] looked at SR in terms of organizational efforts to meet the needs of different categories of stakeholders. For example, McWilliams and Siegel [21] saw in SR an increase in the social interests of business organizations or a commitment to increase the reputation and improve the image by diminishing the community's negative perception of the organization [22]. Matten and Moon considered SR to be a component of the organization's strategic policy that illustrates its interest in social issues, not just the primary goal of profit maximization [13]. Aguinis considers that SR represents those actions and policies that meet stakeholders' expectations to maximize results in three areas: economic, social, and environmental [6].

An issue increasingly addressed by an employer is employee involvement in SR actions [23]. Such employer behavior brings social benefits and plays an essential role in ensuring employees' WB, directly affecting the satisfaction, commitment, and loyalty of current employees and leading to greater motivation, increased productivity, and a greater propensity to innovate [24,25]. In addition, when employees identify the organization's commitment to socially responsible behavior, they tend to have more responsible attitudes that correlate with better performance due to improved relationships between employees and other stakeholders [26].

2.2. Relationships between Organizational Ethics and Social Responsibility

According to [27], philanthropic responsibilities stem from the philosophical, ethical tradition of concern for what is good for society and justify organizations to help improve the quality of life of different stakeholders and the community. Reich points out that SR is nothing more than intelligent management covered by the language of morality and ethics. Only organizations which aim to adhere to all universally accepted ethical standards can expect a positive attitude and support from society [26,28]. Moreover, solving the problems that affect the community and society leads to competitive advantages for the organization. Nord and Fuller saw corporate SR as a matter of higher-level strategy. They linked it to the conceptualization of organizational change, raising awareness of an alternative model that would complement the strategic vision and add an ethical dimension [23,24,29].

At the same time, managers have developed practices related to OE and SR within their organizations. There are many reasons why organizations implement these practices: reducing costs, mitigating risks, gaining legitimacy, gaining a competitive advantage, and creating new value [30]. In addition, researchers and managers have recommended aligning these practices within organizations [23,24,26,31–34]. Still, there is little empirical research exploring the impact of alignment or why it has not become a common practice within organizations. Based on these considerations, we formulated the following research hypothesis:

Hypothesis 1 (H1). *Employees' perception of OE directly positively affects employees' perception of SR.*

2.3. Employees' WB

The community includes individuals in constant interaction in a particular space where they live and work [35]. In addition to the spatial dimension, a community may be determined by the common interest of its members [36]. Given that interactions between individuals within the community include several dimensions (psychological, cultural, spiritual, social, economic, and natural) [37], meeting all the needs of individuals related to these dimensions confers a WB status. Consequently, WB also includes the social, economic, environmental, cultural, and political dimensions [38].

The concepts of health and WB are often used together and sometimes even interchangeably. However, health refers to an individual's physiological or psychological indicators [39], while WB is a more comprehensive concept that aim to describe the individual's general condition in a social context [40,41]. Therefore, WB consists appropriately of non-contextual measures of life (e.g., life satisfaction, happiness), general considerations (e.g., job satisfaction), and more specific dimensions (e.g., salary satisfaction, good workplace).

WB includes the individual's general satisfaction regarding privacy, social relationships, work environment, and reduced stress [42–44]. Therefore, employers' concern for ensuring a better job for their employees and a WB status was considered a component of SR, which is part of ethical behavior.

The concept of WB has therefore been approached in the paradigm of the multidimensionality of human, social, and economic capital [45]; physical, psychological, social, and economic WB [46]; and social, environmental, economic, health, political, physical, and residential dimensions [47]. The economic dimension is manifested by providing sufficient income, job stability, and existing opportunities in the labor market [47,48]. The social dimension includes income and profession that offer a certain social status [37,49] and concepts such as security, community spirit, cohesion, trust, reciprocity, involvement, and informal interaction [5,37,47].

Employers want to improve employee wellbeing because lowering WB can lead to unhappiness, decreased productivity, and increased stress and anxiety, eventually leading to a high turnover [44,50–52]. Therefore, as a dimension of relationships and social status, employees' WB can be considered an objective of SR concerning its human resources and work environment [53].

The WB concept integrates employees' status at and outside the workplace: job satisfaction or dissatisfaction, reward, working relationships, working conditions, friendly work environment, promotion opportunities, care for the environment, and interest in the general health community. WB is a complex and multifaceted construct [54], balancing between objective indicators (life standards) and subjective measures (psychological, social, and spiritual aspects) [55].

Other authors have added to the social dimension the interaction between individuals in the family, at home, and in neighborhoods [56] or education [38]. The environmental dimension includes the perception of individuals about the place where they live, with a solid psychological load for individuals. McCrea et al. [47] suggested that environmental satisfaction, green areas, transport, air quality, energy quality, and sustainability are crucial indicators of WB [37,45,47,57–59].

2.4. Relationships between Employees' WB, SR, and OE

SR is a social obligation of the organizations to decide and act responsibly following the objectives and values of society [60]. Currently, SR is perceived as a continuous commitment of organizations to behave ethically and contribute to the economic development of the community and society in which the organization operates by improving the quality of human WB, through involvement in the local community and society. SR is the basis of sustainability, competitiveness, and innovation and is a strategic advantage of any organization [61–64]

Due to the potential impact of organizations on WB employees and the community in which they operate, ethical behavior and SR programs are of great importance for overall WB [65]. In this context, Chowdhury et al. proposed an SR and OE reporting on stakeholder health and WB [66], based on the Global Reporting Initiative (GRI) sustainability reporting standards. Cheng et al. [67] suggest that if SR activities do not live up to employees' expectations, they generate mistrust of organizations, leading to reduced commitment [34,67,68] and WB and increasing turnover rates [67]. Various authors [67–71] have studied the impact of employees' perceptions regarding CSR and organizational ethics on outcome measures: employee satisfaction, turnover rates, and overall organization sustainability. Consequently, examining and monitoring employees' perceptions regarding SR and OE is beneficial for the organization's human resources management and strategic management to meet the expectations of all stakeholders, especially employees [67–69,72].

Based on the relationships between OE, SR, and WB described in the literature, we formulated the following research hypothesis:

Hypothesis 2 (H2). *Employees' perception of SR and OE directly positively affects employees' perception of WB.*

Internal stakeholder-oriented SR programs target WB employees by obtaining employee satisfaction based on meeting the expectations of their organizations [73]. Employees have an ethical expectation towards their organizations in terms of job stability, recognition and appreciation, fairness of rewards, opportunities for professional and personal development, freedom of association in trade unions, work–life balance, involvement in decisions, autonomy, participation in organizational decisions, and involvement of the organization in the community [74]. In addition, organizations will invest in ethical health and safety management practices that impact the company's performance [75].

Occupational health and safety (OHS) promote human resource management, safety, occupational safety, physical and mental health, and in general, an essential part of the WB of human resources [76–79]. WB incorporates the employee's physical, emotional, and mental wellbeing, exerting a significant positive impact on achieving objectives [74, 77,80,81]. However, several authors [82,83] have highlighted the need to see the health and wellbeing of employees beyond the work environment by taking into account other ethical factors related to other areas of human resources: the process of training and development [9,10], ensuring equal opportunities in business [11], work–life balance [12], job stability, and existing options in the labor market [47,48].

Researching employees' perceptions and attitudes towards SR, OE, and WB is important [34,84,85] because it can lead to seeking opportunities for better implementation of responsible and ethical social practices and initiatives. In addition, companies are increasingly recognizing the strategic importance of OE and SR in ensuring employees' WB and the sustainability of their business [69,84,86], as well as employee satisfaction in implementing SR programs and ethical conduct.

Based on these considerations, we formulated the following research hypothesis:

Hypothesis 3 (H3). *Employees' perception of OE has significant indirect positive effects on their perception of WB, mediating their perceptions of SR.*

Figure 1 shows the conceptual model of the research on the relations between SR, OE, and WB.

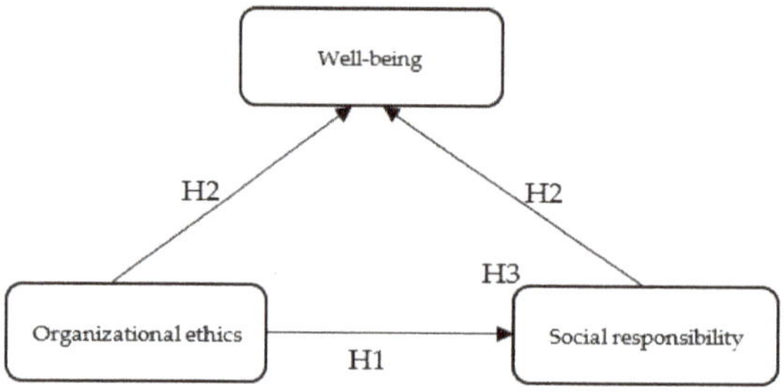

Figure 1. Conceptual model. Source: designed by authors.

3. Methodology

3.1. Research Design

To study the impact of SR and OE on employees' WB, we conducted quantitative research in a survey among employees of Romanian companies.

The data collected in a database were subjected to descriptive and inferential statistical analyses. To determine the intensity and meaning of the relationships between the research variables, we used structural equation modeling and artificial neural network analysis. Finally, the obtained results confirmed the hypotheses' validity based on the literature. Figure 2 illustrates the research process.

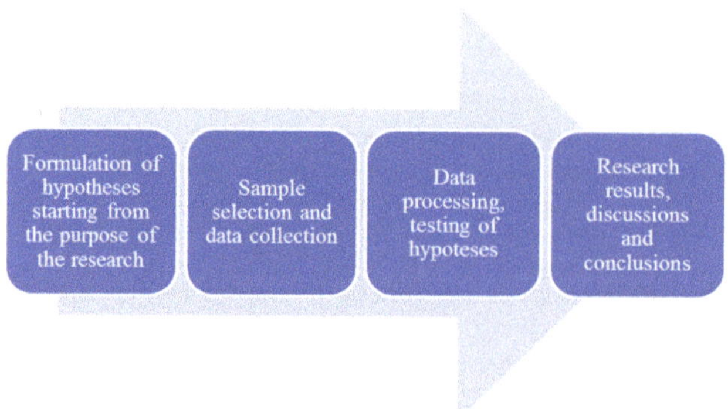

Figure 2. Research process. Source: own construction.

3.2. Selected Sample

To perform the empirical analysis, we conducted a survey based on a questionnaire filled by 423 employees from Romanian organizations, small and medium enterprises, and large corporations between March 2022 and May 2022. The sampling method chosen was random stratified sampling. The target population of the research is the employees in Romanian private companies, comprising 4,500,000 individuals. The sample of 423 individuals was selected with a level of confidence of 95%, with a margin of error of 4.762%. Table 1 describes the descriptive statistics for the selected sample.

Table 1. Descriptive statistics.

	Min	Max	Mean	Std. Deviation	Skewness	Kurtosis
Economic sector	1	4	2.81	0.981	−0.239	−1.048
Size	1	3	1.80	0.748	0.345	−1.146
Gender	1	2	1.30	0.459	0.875	−1.241
Age	1	5	2.70	1.099	0.606	−0.250
Education	1	5	3.30	1.101	−0.615	−0.237
Experience in work	1	5	2.30	1.345	0.669	−0.762
Experience in organization	1	5	2.91	1.136	0.187	−0.752
Position	1	2	1.20	0.399	1.517	0.301
Income category	1	5	2.91	1.512	−0.012	−1.443

Source: designed by authors using SPSS v.20 (SPSS Inc., Chicago, IL, USA).

Employees were selected in the sample using the economic sector criterion: 9.9% in agriculture, 29.8% in industry, and 60.3% in services (including technology and communications). The sample structure according to the size of the companies from which the employees come is as follows: 40% of the employees come from small and medium companies, 40.2% come from large companies, and 19.8% come from multinational companies. Within the sample, 68.15% are male and 31.85% are female. Regarding the age, 9.95% are under 30 years old, 69.93% are between 31 and 55 years old, and 20.12% are over 55. In addition, 19.8% of respondents have received secondary education, and 80.2% have studied a higher degree. Over 60.3% of respondents have more than ten years of work experience, and over 60.2% have more than ten years of experience in the organization. Most respondents are subordinates, with only 19.81% being managers. Depending on the income category, over 43.32% of respondents have a net income above the average net salary in the economy.

3.3. Research Tools and Methods

The design of this study involved conducting a survey based on a questionnaire applied to employees of Romanian organizations. The questionnaire contains the socio-economic-demographic variables that characterize SR, OE, and WB. We evaluated the impact of SR and OE on WB empirically by using statistical methods for modeling structural equations (SEMs) in the partial least squares (PLS) variant using a procedure described by [87,88], similarly used by [89,90]. The initial literature review established measures for each construct and the reliability and validity of variables using various statistical tests (Cronbach's Alpha, Composite Reliability, and Average Variance Extracted). We built items for SR and OE based on previous research. SR includes five dimensions describing the levels of responsibility: responsibilities to shareholders (increasing the organizational value); responsibilities to employees, unions, customers, and suppliers (societal welfare, organizational SR philosophy); responsibilities to central and local public authorities and the community (organizational citizenship); and responsibilities to society (societal contribution). The items concerning SR, which define the levels of responsibility, were defined based on [15,91–93]. OE includes five dimensions describing the ethical principles in the organization: transparency, fair competition, respect for the customer, employees' wellness, and sustainability, as stated in other research [8,15,33,89]. The WB scale was established based on the TINYpulse questionnaire [94], using the eight dimensions for WB: general WB, emotional WB, environmental wellness, intellectual WB, occupational WB, physical health, and social WB. To measure the variables SR, OE, and WB, we used a five-level Likert scale (5—total agreement, 4—partial agreement, 3—agreement, 2—partial disagreement, 1—total disagreement).

The exogenous variables (the items of the questionnaire) which characterize SR, OE, and WB are presented in Table 2.

Table 2. Exogenous variables.

Latent Variables	Exogenous Variables	
	Code	Description
WB	GWB	General WB
	EWB	Emotional WB
	EW	Environmental wellness
	IWB	Intellectual WB
	OWB	Occupational WB
	PH	Physical health
	SWB	Social WB
	SW	Spiritual wellness
OE	OE1	Transparency
	OE2	Fair competition
	OE3	Respect for the customer
	OE4	The organization treats employees well
	OE5	Sustainability
SR	RS1	Organizational citizenship
	RS2	Societal contribution
	RS3	Societal welfare
	RS4	Organizational SR philosophy
	RS5	Increasing the organizational value

Source: designed by authors based on [75–78].

The self-administered questionnaire results can be affected by common method bias (CMB) [95]. We tested all variables using Harman's single-factor test using principal component analysis. The extracted variance was below 50% (45.329%), attesting to no significant common method bias effects [95].

4. Results

We used structural equation modeling (SEM) in the partial least square variant (SmartPLS 3.0 software: SmartPLS GmbH, Oststeinbek, Germany) to validate the three hypotheses. The model has three unobservable latent variables: SR, OE, and WB. Each of the three latent variables depends on a series of observable exogenous variables defined by the items in the questionnaire. Figure 3 shows the exogenous variables for each latent variable.

Following the methodology described by [88], we eliminated from the model those items that have an outer loading below 0.7, considering the lower influence of these items on the latent determinant variables. Figure 4 presents the resulting model.

The validity and reliability of the model were tested following the procedure described in [87,88]. All three indicators, namely Cronbach's Alpha, Composite Reliability, and Average Variance Extracted), recorded good values (Table 3). In the model, SRMR recorded a value of 0.048, and NFI recorded a value of 0.934.

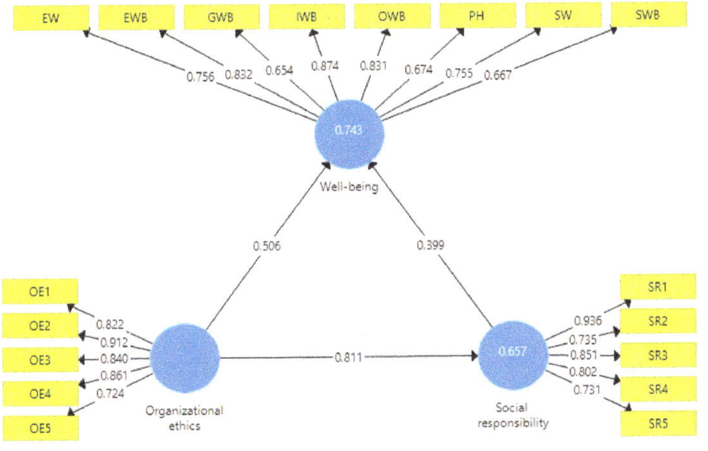

Figure 3. Preliminary model. Source: designed by authors using SmartPLS 3.0 (SmartPLS GmbH, Oststeinbek, Germany).

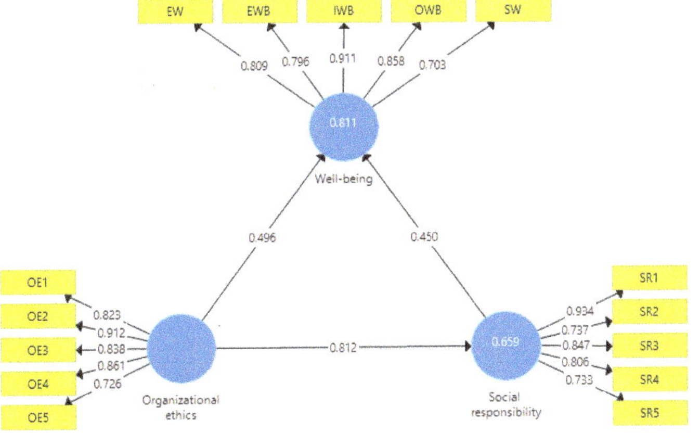

Figure 4. Model applied. Source: designed by authors using SmartPLS 3.0 (SmartPLS GmbH, Oststeinbek, Germany).

Table 3. Validity and reliability.

	Cronbach's Alpha	Composite Reliability	AVE
Organizational ethics	0.889	0.919	0.696
Social responsibility	0.875	0.907	0.664
Wellbeing	0.879	0.910	0.670

Source: designed by authors using SmartPLS 3.0 (SmartPLS GmbH, Oststeinbek, Germany).

Finally, running a bootstrapping process, we determined the path coefficients and specific indirect effects in our model for assessing the role of SR and OE in ensuring employees' WB (Table 4).

Table 4. Path coefficients and specific indirect effects.

	Original Sample	Standard Deviation	T Statistics	p Values
Organizational ethics → Social responsibility (H1)	0.812	0.011	71.746	0.000
Organizational ethics → Wellbeing (H2)	0.496	0.033	15.031	0.000
Social responsibility → Wellbeing (H2)	0.450	0.033	13.462	0.000
Organizational ethics → Social responsibility → Wellbeing (H3)	0.365	0.023	15.637	0.000

Source: designed by authors using SmartPLS 3.0 (SmartPLS GmbH, Oststeinbek, Germany).

Analyzing the path coefficients and specific indirect effects in Table 4, we affirm that all three hypotheses are valid. The organizations' ethical practices positively affect SR programs in employees' perception. The two sustainability constructs (OE and SR) positively impact employees' WB. In addition to the direct effect on WB, the organization's ethical behavior has substantial indirect effects on WB, with an SR program based on ethical principles and values as a mediating variable.

5. Discussions

The relationship between SR, OE, and WB has not frequently been subject to an evaluation process in the literature on SR and OE. However, there is a recognition that this relationship can contribute to establishing sustainable jobs to ensure WB at the individual level and welfare at the societal level. In recent years, several researchers have conducted empirical studies to determine the impact of SR programs on work results from the perspective of stakeholders (including employees) [34,96–99]. Employees are key stakeholders who, once satisfied, can positively influence the implementation of SR programs [97]. Therefore, employees' perceptions of SR shape the community's view of organizations [96]. In addition, employees with a good level of WB can improve and stimulate SR programs and ethical behavior that promotes all stakeholders' wellbeing, including employees [34].

Employers improve employee WB because low WB can produce unhappiness, lower productivity, and increased stress and anxiety, eventually leading to a high turnover rate [44,50–52,67]. Therefore, employees' WB is an objective of SR programs concerning its human resources and work environment [53], ensuring employee commitment [68]. Researching the relationships between the variables of the researched model, SR and OE can contribute to increasing economic, social, and environmental performance and the health and wellbeing of employees, as we have demonstrated by confirming the validity of the H2 hypothesis.

The conceptual model in this study, which reveals the relationship between corporate SR and OE, also aims to help integrate and facilitate the implementation of SR activities and tools to ensure ethical conduct in organizations. Various authors have pointed out the need for a unified theory regarding SR and OE because there is much confusion and redundancy between the dimensions of the two concepts [27,30,33,89]. In our research, we tested the relationship established between SR and OE by confirming the validity of the H1 hypothesis. Combining these two areas can provide sustainability to organizations and ensure employees' WB and that of the community they operate in [20].

Many studies have attempted to understand the impact of SR and ethical practices on employees' satisfaction, a constituent of employees' WB [34,84,85,100–107]. Researching employees' perceptions and attitudes towards SR, OE, and WB is important [34,84,85] because it can lead to seeking opportunities for better implementation of responsible and ethical social practices and initiatives. In addition, employees' satisfaction provides an insight into the emotional state of work experience and environment [108], directly contributing to organizational performance [73]. Although employees' satisfaction is an essential component of employee WB, it is not just about satisfaction. There are several areas of SR that address job satisfaction aspects: job stability; employee status; fair pay; social benefits; occupational safety and health; work–life balance and employment opportunities; training and personal development; cordial labor relations; and a work environment characterized by communication, transparency and social dialogue, equal treatment, and equal opportunities [34,75,84,109]. Satisfaction is directly related to work, while WB also covers general aspects of general physical and mental health, relationships in the social environment, social status, care for the environment in which they live, and the individual's connection to the community and society in general.

Programs in the SR area stimulate the improvement of health, the environment, and involvement in educational activities, acting as an essential mechanism for mediating between the organization's ethical practices and improving employees' and communities' WB [110], as demonstrated by the confirmation of the validity of Hypothesis H3. Companies are increasingly recognizing the strategic importance of OE and SR in ensuring employees' WB and the sustainability of their business [69,84,86], as well as employee satisfaction in implementing SR programs and ethical conduct. Organizations that promote health and safety management practices and ensure an adequate work environment [88] benefit from increased employee engagement, as the organization demonstrates an interest in employees' WB. Rela et al. showed that other factors, such as community capacity and motivation, government policy, and other stakeholders' contributions, influenced WB [5].

The results of our research are in line with the results of previous research showing that ethical issues can have a significant impact on physical health and spiritual wellbeing.

6. Conclusions

The research results indicate that the variables SR and OE have significant and positive influences on WB dimensions, consistent with previous studies showing a significant relationship between these constructs [4,111–117]. SR contributes to the satisfaction of employees' interests related to WB dimensions (health, education, economy) and OE by inducing ethical behavior and attitudes that contribute to increasing WB. Research results confirm that SR programs and ethical behavior contribute to the employees' wellbeing.

6.1. Practical Implications

Although OE activities and SR programs target both stakeholders, the present research focused on critical internal stakeholders (employees), given their dual nature. Employees are also constituents of an essential category of external stakeholders—the community. The research results confirmed the importance of SR and OE for improving employee wellbeing, SR being a mediating factor between OE and WB. These results support an essential mechanism by which OE activities and SR programs can increase WB, especially when the organization does not have sufficient resources to motivate employees and ensure job satisfaction. Employee satisfaction with job stability issues, guaranteeing a friendly work environment, caring for the environment in which they live, and organizational involvement in community social causes can all contribute to the overall WB of employees.

6.2. Theoretical Implications

Three issues can be highlighted as theoretical implications of this research. First, most studies have focused on external stakeholders [118–121], with few focusing on the positive effect of OE activities and SR programs on internal stakeholders. Second, while many types of research have addressed various facets of wellbeing (psychological, health, occupational wellbeing, etc.) [118,122–124], this study aimed at a holistic approach to the concept of WB. Although SR depends on the macroeconomic and organizational context, the main expectations for organizations are reducing poverty in the community and society in general, caring for the environment, improving public health, increasing employee WB, and an increasingly efficient educational process.

6.3. Limitations and Recommendations for Future Research

The analysis revealed a direct positive effect of SR and OE on employees' WB. However, organizational ethics have a significant indirect positive impact on WB through SR programs that induce ethical conduct and the attitude of employees. These results should take into account various limitations of the research. First, the research only targets a category of stakeholders (employees) with a dual nature (internal and external) by their presence in the organization's community. Secondly, the research was carried out only among the employees of some Romanian organizations, making it impossible to consider cultural differences between employees from different countries. Finally, the transversal approach to research provides more information through the results obtained, but does not offer a perspective on the evolutions of perceptions over time as a longitudinal approach.

Future research may address some of these limitations. In addition, future research may focus on studying the effects of moderating factors, such as communication, reputation, and organizational culture. Furthermore, there is a need for a deep investigation of the OE practices' integration and alignment with SR programs to support a more synergistic impact on WB.

Author Contributions: Conceptualization, C.G.B., M.M.N., M.C., and S.D.; methodology, C.G.B.; software, C.G.B.; validation, C.G.B., M.M.N., M.C., and S.D.; formal analysis, C.G.B.; investigation, C.G.B., M.M.N., M.C., and S.D.; writing—original draft preparation, C.G.B., M.M.N., M.C., and S.D.; writing—review and editing, C.G.B., M.M.N., M.C., and S.D.; project administration, C.G.B. All authors have read and agreed to the published version of the manuscript.

Funding: This research received no external funding.

Institutional Review Board Statement: Not applicable.

Informed Consent Statement: Not applicable.

Data Availability Statement: Not applicable.

Conflicts of Interest: The authors declare no conflict of interest.

References

1. Zizek, S.S.; Mulej, M.; Potocnik, A. The Sustainable Socially Responsible Society: Well-Being Society 6.0. *Sustainability* **2021**, *13*, 9186. [CrossRef]
2. Meseguer-Sánchez, V.; Gálvez-Sánchez, F.J.; López-Martínez, G.; Molina-Moreno, V. Corporate Social Responsibility and Sustainability. A Bibliometric Analysis of Their Interrelations. *Sustainability* **2021**, *13*, 1636. [CrossRef]
3. Choi, D.Y.; Gray, E.R. Socially responsible entrepreneurs: What do they do to create and build their companies? *Bus. Horiz.* **2008**, *51*, 341–352. [CrossRef]
4. Sciortino, R. Philanthropy in Southeast Asia: Between charitable values, corporate interests, and development aspirations. *ASEAS-Austrian J. South-East Asian Stud.* **2017**, *10*, 139–163. [CrossRef]
5. Rela, I.Z.; Awang, A.H.; Ramli, Z.; Ali, M.N.S.; Manaf, A.A. Corporate social responsibility practice and its effects on community well-being in Southeast Sulawesi, Indonesia. *Int. J. Adv. Appl. Sci.* **2020**, *7*, 54–61. [CrossRef]
6. Aguinis, H. Organizational responsibility: Doing good and doing well. In *APA Handbook of Industrial and Organizational Psychology*; Zedeck, S., Ed.; American Psychological Association: Washington, DC, USA, 2011; Chapter 24, pp. 855–879.
7. Macassa, G.; Francisco, J.C.; McGrath, C. Corporate social responsibility and population health. *Health Sci. J.* **2017**, *11*, 528. [CrossRef]
8. Chun, S.J.; Shin, Y.; Choi, N.J.; Kim, S.M. How does corporate ethics contribute to firm financial performance? The mediating role of collective organizational commitment and organizational citizenship behavior. *J. Manag.* **2013**, *39*, 853–877. [CrossRef]
9. Thang, N.N. Human resource training and development as facilitators of CSR. *J. Econ. Dev.* **2012**, *14*, 88–89. [CrossRef]
10. Ayub, A.; Iftekhar, H.; Aslam, M.S.; Razzaq, A. A conceptual framework on examining the influence of behavioral training & development on CSR: An employees' perspective approach. *Eur. J. Bus. Soc. Sci.* **2013**, *2*, 33–42.
11. Wambui, T.W.; Wangombe, J.G.; Muthura, M.W.; Kamau, A.W.; Jackson, S.M. Managing workplace diversity: A Kenyan perspective. *Int. J. Bus. Soc. Sci.* **2013**, *4*, 199–218.
12. Ozbilgin, M.F.; Beauregard, T.A.; Tatli, A.; Bell, M.P. Work-life, diversity, and intersectionality: A critical review and research agenda. *Int. J. Manag. Rev.* **2013**, *13*, 177–198. [CrossRef]
13. Matten, D.; Moon, J. "Implicit" and "explicit" CSR: A conceptual framework for a comparative understanding of corporate social responsibility. *Acad. Manag. Rev.* **2008**, *33*, 404–424. [CrossRef]

14. Sciortino, R. Philanthropy, giving, and development in Southeast Asia. *ASEAS-Austrian J. South-East Asian Stud.* **2017**, *10*, 129–138. [CrossRef]
15. Carroll, A.B. The pyramid of corporate social responsibility: Toward the moral management of organizational stakeholders. *Bus. Horiz.* **1991**, *34*, 39–48. [CrossRef]
16. Dahlsrud, A. How corporate social responsibility is defined: An analysis of 37 definitions. *Corp. Soc. Responsib. Environ. Manag.* **2008**, *15*, 1–13. [CrossRef]
17. Davis, K.; Blomstrom, R. *Business and Society: Environment and Responsibility*; Mc Graw-Hill: New York, NY, USA, 1975.
18. Robin, D.P.; Reindenbach, R.E. Social Responsibility, Ethics, and Marketing Strategy: Closing the gap between concept and application. *J. Mark.* **1987**, *51*, 44–58. [CrossRef]
19. Freeman, R.E. *Strategic Management: A Stakeholder Approach*; Pitman: Boston, MA, USA, 1984.
20. Clarkson, M.B.E. A stakeholder framework for analyzing and evaluating corporate social performance. *Acad. Manag. Rev.* **1995**, *20*, 92–117. [CrossRef]
21. McWilliams, A.; Siegel, D. Corporate social responsibility: A theory of the firm perspective. *Acad. Manag. Rev.* **2001**, *26*, 117–127. [CrossRef]
22. Truong, V.D.; Hall, C.M. Exploring the poverty reduction potential of social marketing in tourism development. *Austrian J. South-East Asian Stud.* **2015**, *8*, 125–142. [CrossRef]
23. Agudelo, M.A.L.; Jóhannsdóttir, L.; Davídsdóttir, B. A literature review of the history and evolution of corporate social responsibility. *Int. J. Corp. Soc. Responsib.* **2019**, *4*, 1–23. [CrossRef]
24. Abad-Segura, E.; Cortés-García, F.J.; Belmonte-Ureña, L.J. The Sustainable Approach to Corporate Social Responsibility: A Global Analysis and Future Trends. *Sustainability* **2019**, *11*, 5382. [CrossRef]
25. Pan, X.; Sinha, P.; Chen, X. Corporate social responsibility and eco-innovation: The triple bottom line perspective. *J. Corp. Soc. Responsib. Environ. Manag.* **2020**, *28*, 214–228. [CrossRef]
26. Crane, A.; Matten, D. COVID-19 and the Future of CSR Research. *J. Manag. Stud.* **2020**, *58*, 280–284. [CrossRef]
27. Balmer, J.T.; Fukukawa, K.; Gray, E.R. The Nature and Management of Ethical Corporate Identity: A Commentary on Corporate Identity, Corporate Social Responsibility, and Ethics. *J. Bus. Ethics* **2007**, *76*, 7–15. [CrossRef]
28. Reich, R.B. *Pink Slips Profits, and Paychecks: Corporate Citizenship in an Era of Smaller Government*; School of Business and Public Management, George Washington University: Washington, DC, USA, 1996.
29. Nord, W.; Fuller, S. Increasing Corporate Social Responsibility Through an Employee-centered Approach. *Empl. Responsib. Rights J.* **2009**, *21*, 279–290. [CrossRef]
30. Weller, A.E. Practices at the Boundaries of Business Ethics Corporate Social Responsibility. Ph.D. Thesis, Copenhagen Business School, Frederiksberg, Denmark, 2016.
31. Painter-Morland, M. Triple bottom line reporting as social grammar. *Bus. Ethics A Eur. Rev.* **2006**, *15*, 352–364. [CrossRef]
32. Rowe, M. Reputation, relationships, and risk: A CSR primer for ethics officers. *Bus. Soc. Rev.* **2006**, *111*, 441–455. [CrossRef]
33. Petry, E. Is it time for a unified approach to business ethics? *SCCE Compliance Ethics Mag.* **2008**, *5*, 45–46.
34. Hassanie, S.; Karadas, G.; Lawrence Emeagwali, O. Do CSR Perceptions InfluenceWork Outcomes in the Health Care Sector? The Mediating Role of Organizational Identification and Employee Attachment. *Sustainability* **2021**, *13*, 9840. [CrossRef]
35. Flint, C.G.; Luloff, A.E.; Finley, J.C. Where is "community" in community-based forestry? *Soc. Nat. Res.* **2008**, *21*, 526–537. [CrossRef]
36. Murphy, B.L. Locating social capital in resilient community-level emergency management. *Nat. Hazards* **2007**, *41*, 297–315. [CrossRef]
37. Christakopoulou, S.; Dawson, J.; Gari, A. The community well-being questionnaire: Theoretical context and initial assessment of its reliability and validity. *Soc. Indic. Res.* **2001**, *56*, 319–349. [CrossRef]
38. Murphy, B.L. *Community Well-Being: An Overview of the Concept*; Nuclear Waste Management Organization (NWMO): Toronto, ON, Canada, 2010.
39. Danna, K.; Griffin, R.W. Health and well-being in the workplace: A review and synthesis of the literature. *J. Manag.* **1999**, *25*, 357–384. [CrossRef]
40. Warr, P. *Work, Unemployment, and Mental Health*; Clarendon Press: Oxford, UK, 1987.
41. Warr, P. The measurement of well-being and other aspects of mental health. *J. Occup. Psychol.* **1990**, *63*, 193–210. [CrossRef]
42. Diener, E. Subjective well-being. *Psychol. Bull.* **1984**, *95*, 542–575. [CrossRef] [PubMed]
43. Diener, E. Subjective Well-being: The Science of Happiness and a Proposal for a National Index. *Am. Psychol.* **2000**, *55*, 34–43. [CrossRef] [PubMed]
44. Kuykendall, L.; Tay, L. Employee subjective well-being and physiological functioning: An integrative model. *Health Psychol. Open* **2015**, *2*, 1–11. [CrossRef] [PubMed]
45. Cuthill, M. Coolangatta: A portrait of community well-being. *Urban Policy Res.* **2002**, *20*, 187–203. [CrossRef]
46. Ramsey, D.; Smit, B. Rural community well-being: Models and application to changes in the tobacco-belt in Ontario, Canada. *Geoforum* **2002**, *33*, 367–384. [CrossRef]
47. McCrea, R.; Walton, A.; Leonard, R. A conceptual framework for investigating community well-being and resilience. *Rural Soc.* **2014**, *23*, 270–282. [CrossRef]

48. Morton, A.; Edwards, L. Community well-being indicators, survey template for local government. In *Australian Centre of Excellence for Local Government*; University of Technology: Sydney, Australia, 2012. [CrossRef]
49. Reeder, R.J.; Brown, D.M. Recreation, tourism, and rural well-being. In *Tourism and Hospitality*; Economic Research Report No. 1477-2016-121194; United States Department of Agriculture (USDA): Washington, DC, USA, 2015.
50. Boyd, A. Employee traps—corruption in the workplace. *Manag. Rev.* **1997**, *86*, 9–10.
51. Rutledge, R.B.; Skandali, N.; Dayan, P.; Dolan, R.J. Dopaminergic modulation of decision making and subjective well-being. *J. Neurosci.* **2015**, *35*, 9811–9822. [CrossRef] [PubMed]
52. Carpino, R.A.; Avramchuk, A.S. The Conceptual Relationship between Workplace Well-Being, Corporate Social Responsibility, and Healthcare Costs. *Int. Manag. Rev.* **2017**, *13*, 24–31.
53. Steiner, J.; Steiner, G. *Business, Government, and Society: A Managerial Perspective*, 13th ed.; McGraw-Hill: New York, NY, USA, 2012.
54. Tov, W. Well-being concepts and components. In *Handbook of Well-Being*; Diener, E., Oishi, S., Tay, L., Eds.; DEF Publishers: Salt Lake City, UT, USA, 2018.
55. Trudel-Fitzgerald, C.; Millstein, R.A.; von Hippel, C.; Howe, C.J.; Powers Tomasso, L.; Wagner, G.R.; Vander Weele, T.J. Psychological well-being as part of the public health debate? Insight into dimensions, interventions, and policy. *BMC Public Health* **2019**, *19*, 1712. [CrossRef] [PubMed]
56. Sirgy, M.J.; Widgery, R.N.; Lee, D.J.; Grace, B.Y. Developing a measure of community well-being based on perceptions of impact in various life domains. *Soc. Indic. Res.* **2010**, *96*, 295–311. [CrossRef]
57. Wiseman, J.; Brasher, K. Community well-being in an unwell world: Trends, challenges, and possibilities. *J. Public Health Policy* **2008**, *29*, 353–366. [CrossRef]
58. Forjaz, M.J.; Prieto-Flores, M.E.; Ayala, A.; Rodriguez-Blazquez, C.; Fernandez-Mayoralas, G.; Rojo-Perez, F.; Martinez-Martin, P. Measurement properties of the community well-being index in older adults. *Qual. Life Res.* **2011**, *20*, 733–743. [CrossRef]
59. Kim, Y.; Kee, Y.; Lee, S.J. An analysis of the relative importance of components in measuring community well-being: Perspectives of citizens, public officials, and experts. *Soc. Indic. Res.* **2015**, *121*, 345–369. [CrossRef]
60. Bowen, H.R. *Social Responsibilities of the Businessman*; University of Iowa Press: Des Moines, IA, USA, 1953.
61. World Business Council for Sustainable Development (WBCSD). *Corporate Social Responsibility: Meeting Changing Expectations*; WBCSD: New York, NY, USA, 1999.
62. Guo, H.; Lu, W. The inverse U-shaped relationship between corporate social responsibility and competitiveness: Evidence from Chinese international construction companies. *J. Clean. Prod.* **2021**, *295*, 126374. [CrossRef]
63. Kent, M.P.; Pauze, E.; Guo, K.; Kent, A.; Jean-Louis, R. The physical activity and nutrition-related corporate social responsibility initiatives of food and beverage companies in Canada and implications for public health. *BMC Public Health* **2020**, *20*, 890. [CrossRef]
64. Lee, K.; Lee, H. How does CSR activity affect sustainable growth and value of corporations? Evidence from Korea. *Sustainability* **2019**, *11*, 508. [CrossRef]
65. Nwobu, O.A. Corporate Social Responsibility, and the Public Health Imperative: Accounting and Reporting on Public Health. In *Corporate Social Responsibility*; Orlando, B., Ed.; IntechOpen: London, UK, 2021; Available online: https://www.intechopen.com/chapters/74802 (accessed on 8 March 2022). [CrossRef]
66. Chowdhury, E.H.; Backlund Rambaree, B.; Macassa, G. CSR reporting of stakeholders' health: Proposal for a new perspective. *Sustainability* **2021**, *13*, 1133. [CrossRef]
67. Cheng, Y.; Wang, Y.; Pan, F. The Impact of CSR Perceptions on Employees' Turnover Intention during the COVID-19 Crisis in China. *Int. J. Environ. Res. Public Health* **2022**, *19*, 8297. [CrossRef]
68. Loor-Zambrano, H.Y.; Santos-Roldán, L.; Palacios-Florencio, B. Relationship CSR and employee commitment: Mediating effects of internal motivation and trust. *Eur. Res. Manag. Bus. Econ.* **2022**, *28*, 100185. [CrossRef]
69. Hadj, T.B. Effects of corporate social responsibility towards stakeholders and environmental management on responsible innovation and competitiveness. *J. Clean. Prod.* **2020**, *250*, 1–10. [CrossRef]
70. Arguinis, H.; Villamor, I.; Gabriel, P.K. Understanding employee responses to COVID-19: A behavioral corporate social responsibility perspective. *Manag. Res.* **2020**, *18*, 421–438. [CrossRef]
71. Galvão, A.; Mendes, L.; Marques, C.; Mascarenhas, C. Factors Influencing Students' Corporate Social Responsibility Orientation in Higher Education. *J. Clean. Prod.* **2019**, *215*, 290–304. [CrossRef]
72. Ahmed, M.; Zehou, S.; Raza, S.A.; Qureshi, M.A.; Yousufi, S.Q. Impact of CSR and environmental triggers on employee green behavior: The mediating effect of employee well-being. *Corp. Soc. Responsib. Environ. Manag.* **2020**, *27*, 2225–2239. [CrossRef]
73. Yousaf, H.Q.; Ali, I.; Sajjad, A.; Ilyas, M. Impact of internal corporate social responsibility on employee engagement: A study of a moderated mediation model. *Int. J. Sci. Basic Appl. Res.* **2016**, *30*, 226–243.
74. Zanko, M.; Dawson, P. Occupational health and safety management in organizations. A review. *Int. J. Manag. Rev.* **2012**, *14*, 328–344. [CrossRef]
75. Macassa, G.; McGrath, C.; Tomaselli, G.; Buttigieg, S.C. Corporate social responsibility and internal stakeholders' health and well-being in Europe: A systematic descriptive review. *Health Promot. Int.* **2021**, *36*, 866–883. [CrossRef] [PubMed]
76. Amponsah-Tawiah, K.; Dartey-Baah, K. Occupational health and safety: Key issues and concerns in Ghana. *Int. J. Bus. Soc. Sci.* **2011**, *2*, 119–126.
77. Bhagawati, B. Basics of occupational safety and health. *IOSR J. Environ. Sci. Toxic Food Technol.* **2015**, *9*, 91–94.

78. Vărzaru, M.; Vărzaru, A.A. Leadership style and organizational structure in Mintzberg's vision. In Proceedings of the 7th International Management Conference: New Management for the New Economy, Bucharest, Romania, 26 August–7–8 November 2013; pp. 467–476.
79. Vărzaru, M.; Vărzaru, A.A. Knowledge Management and Organisational Structure: Mutual Influences. In Proceedings of the 13th European Conference on Knowledge Management, Unit Politecnica, Cartagena, Cartagena, Spain, 6–7 September 2012; pp. 1255–1261.
80. Vărzaru, A.A.; Vărzaru, D. Organizational performance and its control through budgets. In Proceedings of the 6th International Conference on Business Excellence, Brasov, Romania, 14–15 October 2011; Volume 2, pp. 269–272.
81. Vărzaru, A.A. Problems in the design and implementation of a costing system. In Proceedings of the 2nd International Multidisciplinary Scientific Conference on Social Sciences and Arts (SGEM 2015), Albena, Bulgaria, 26 August–1 September 2015; Volume 3, pp. 669–674.
82. WHO. *Healthy Workplaces: A Model for Action for Employees, Workers, Policy Makers, and Practitioners*; WHO: Geneva, Switzerland, 2010; pp. 1–32.
83. LaMontagne, A.D.; Martin, A.; Page, K.M.; Reavley, N.J.; Noblet, A.J.; Milner, A.J. Workplace mental health: Developing an integrated intervention approach. *BMC Psychiatry* **2014**, *14*, 131. [CrossRef] [PubMed]
84. Melovic, B.; Milovic, N.; Backovic-Vulic, T.; Dudic, B.; Bajzik, P. Attitudes, and Perceptions of Employees toward Corporate Social Responsibility in Western Balkan Countries: Importance and Relevance for Sustainable Development. *Sustainability* **2019**, *11*, 6763. [CrossRef]
85. Latif, B.; Ong, T.S.; Meero, A.; Rahman, A.A.A.; Ali, M. Employee-perceived corporate social responsibility (CSR) and employee pro-environmental behavior (PEB): The moderating role of CSR skepticism and CSR authenticity. *Sustainability* **2022**, *14*, 1380. [CrossRef]
86. Jakunskiene, E. Assessment of the Impact of Social Responsibility on Poverty. *Sustainability* **2021**, *13*, 9395. [CrossRef]
87. Hulland, J. Use of partial least squares (PLS) in strategic management research: A review of four recent studies. *Strateg. Manag. J.* **1999**, *20*, 195–204. [CrossRef]
88. Hair, J.F.; Sarstedt, M.; Ringle, C.M.; Gudergan, S.P. Advanced issues in partial least squares structural equation modeling. In *Handbook of Market Research*; Sage Publications: Thousand Oaks, CA, USA, 2017. [CrossRef]
89. Vărzaru, A.A. Assessing the Impact of AI Solutions' Ethical Issues on Performance in Managerial Accounting. *Electronics* **2022**, *11*, 2221. [CrossRef]
90. Vărzaru, A.A. Design and implementation of a management control system. *Financ. Chall. Future* **2015**, *17*, 195–200.
91. De los Salmones, M.G.; Crespo, A.H.; del Bosque, I.R. Influence of corporate social responsibility on loyalty and valuation of services. *J. Bus. Ethics* **2005**, *61*, 369–385. [CrossRef]
92. Stanaland, A.J.; Lwin, M.O.; Murphy, P.E. Consumer perceptions of the antecedents and consequences of corporate social responsibility. *J. Bus. Ethics* **2011**, *102*, 47–55. [CrossRef]
93. Alvarado-Herrera, A.; Bigne, E.; Aldas-Manzano, J.; Curras-Perez, R. A scale for measuring consumer perceptions of corporate social responsibility following the sustainable development paradigm. *J. Bus. Ethics* **2017**, *140*, 243–262. [CrossRef]
94. TINYpulse The Only Workplace Wellness Survey Template You Need to Get Real Insights. Available online: https://www.tinypulse.com/blog/employee-survey-questions-about-wellness-and-health (accessed on 7 October 2021).
95. Podsakoff, P.M.; MacKenzie, S.B.; Lee, J.Y.; Podsakoff, N.P. Common method biases in behavioral research: A critical review of the literature and recommended remedies. *J. Appl. Psychol.* **2003**, *88*, 879–903. [CrossRef] [PubMed]
96. Gond, J.P.; El Akremi, A.; Swaen, V.; Babu, N. The psychological microfoundations of corporate social responsibility: A personcentric systematic review. *J. Organ. Behav.* **2017**, *38*, 225–246. [CrossRef]
97. Asante Boadi, E.; He, Z.; Bosompem, J.; Opata, C.N.; Boadi, E.K. Employees' perception of corporate social responsibility (CSR) and its effects on internal outcomes. *Serv. Ind. J.* **2020**, *40*, 611–632. [CrossRef]
98. Luke, M.A.; Carnelley, K.B.; Sedikides, C. Attachments in the workplace: How attachment security in the workplace benefits the organisation. *Eur. J. Soc. Psychol.* **2020**, *50*, 1046–1064. [CrossRef]
99. Benitez, J.; Ruiz, L.; Castillo, A.; Llorens, J. How corporate social responsibility activities influence employer reputation: The role of social media capability. *Decis. Support Syst.* **2020**, *129*, 113223. [CrossRef]
100. Brammer, S.; Millington, A.; Rayton, B. The contribution of corporate social responsibility to organizational commitment. *The Int. J. Human Res. Manag.* **2007**, *18*, 1701–1719. [CrossRef]
101. Ruiz-Palomino, P.; Ruiz-Amaya, C.; Knorr, H. Employee organizational citizenship behavior: Ethical leadership's direct and indirect impact. *Can. J. Adm. Sci.* **2011**, *28*, 244–258. [CrossRef]
102. Vlachos, P.A.; Panagopoulos, N.G.; Rapp, A.A. Feeling good by doing good: Employee CSR-induced attributions, job satisfaction, and the role of charismatic leadership. *J. Bus. Ethics* **2013**, *118*, 577–588. [CrossRef]
103. Kowal, J.; Roztocki, N. Do organizational ethics improve IT job satisfaction in the Visegrad Group countries? Insights from Poland. *J. Glob. Inf. Technol. Manag.* **2015**, *18*, 127–145. [CrossRef]
104. Gaudencio, P.; Coelho, A.; Ribeiro, N. The role of trust in corporate social responsibility and worker relationships. *J. Manag. Dev.* **2017**, *36*, 478–492. [CrossRef]
105. Tsourvakas, G.; Yfantidou, I. Corporate social responsibility influences employee engagement. *Soc. Responsib. J.* **2018**, *14*, 123–137. [CrossRef]

106. Wisse, B.; van Eijbergen, R.; Rietzschel, E.F.; Scheibe, S. Catering to the needs of an aging workforce: The role of employee age in the relationship between corporate social responsibility and employee satisfaction. *J. Bus. Ethics* **2018**, *147*, 875–888. [CrossRef]
107. Sarfraz, M.; Qun, W.; Abdullah, M.I.; Alvi, A.T. Employees' perception of corporate social responsibility impact on employee outcomes: Mediating role of organizational justice for small and medium enterprises (SMEs). *Sustainability* **2018**, *10*, 2429. [CrossRef]
108. Barrena-Martinez, J.B.; Fernaíndez, M.L.; Fernaíndez, P.M.R. Corporate social responsibility: Evolution through institutional and stakeholder perspectives. *Eur. J. Manag. Bus. Econ.* **2016**, *25*, 8–14. [CrossRef]
109. Degie, B.; Kebede, W. Corporate social responsibility and its prospect for community development in Ethiopia. *Int. Soc. Work* **2019**, *62*, 376–389. [CrossRef]
110. Brew, Y.; Junwu, C.; Addae-Boateng, S. Corporate social responsibility activities of mining companies: The views of the local communities in Ghana. *Am. J. Ind. Bus. Manag.* **2015**, *5*, 457–465. [CrossRef]
111. Sarmila, S.M.; Zaimah, R.; Lyndon, N.; Hussain, M.Y.; Awang, A.H. Local community economic well-being through CSR project. *Mediterr. J. Soc. Sci.* **2015**, *6*, 79–87. [CrossRef]
112. Shmotkin, D. Subjective well-being as a function of age and gender: A multivariate look for differentiated trends. *Soc. Indic. Res.* **1990**, *23*, 201–230. [CrossRef]
113. Diener, E. Assessing subjective well-being: Progress and opportunities. *Soc. Indic. Res.* **1994**, *32*, 103–157. [CrossRef]
114. Suh, E.; Diener, E.; Fujita, F. Events and subjective well-being: Only recent events matter. *J. Pers. Soc. Psychol.* **1996**, *70*, 1091–1102. [CrossRef] [PubMed]
115. Munz, D.C.; Kohler, J.M.; Greenberg, C.I. Effectiveness of a Comprehensive Worksite Stress Management Program: Combining Organizational and Individual Interventions. *Int. J. Stress Manag.* **2001**, *8*, 49–62. [CrossRef]
116. Donald, I.; Taylor, P.; Johnson, S.; Cooper, C.; Cartwright, S.; Robertson, S. Work environments, stress, and productivity: An examination using ASSET. *Int. J. Stress Manag.* **2005**, *22*, 409–423. [CrossRef]
117. Jeong, J.-G.; Choi, S.B.; Kang, S.-W. Leader's Perception of Corporate Social Responsibility and Team Members' Psychological Well-Being: Mediating Effects of Value Congruence Climate and Pro-Social Behavior. *Int. J. Environ. Res. Public Health* **2022**, *19*, 3607. [CrossRef]
118. Drumwright, M.E. Socially responsible organizational buying: Environmental concern as a noneconomic buying criterion. *J. Mark.* **1994**, *58*, 1–19. [CrossRef]
119. Barone, M.J.; Miyazaki, A.D.; Taylor, K.A. The Influence of Cause-Related Marketing on Consumer Choice: Does One Good Turn Deserve Another? *J. Acad. Mark. Sci.* **2000**, *28*, 248–262. [CrossRef]
120. Bhattacharya, C.B.; Elsbach, K.D. Us versus Them: The Roles of Organizational Identification and Disidentification in Social Marketing Initiatives. *J. Public Policy Mark.* **2002**, *22*, 26–36. [CrossRef]
121. Pantani, D.; Peltzer, R.; Cremonte, M.; Robaina, K.; Babor, T.; Pinsky, I. The marketing potential of corporate social responsibility activities: The case of the alcohol industry in Latin America and the Caribbean. *Addiction* **2017**, *222*, 74–80. [CrossRef]
122. Chuang, S.; Wu, J.Y.W.; Wang, C.S.; Pan, L.H. Health-promoting Lifestyles and Psychological Distress Associated with Well-being in Community Adults. *Am. J. Health Behav.* **2017**, *42*, 446–453. [CrossRef] [PubMed]
123. Gül, Ö.; Qaglayan, H.S.; Akandere, M. The Effect of Sports on the Psychological Well-being Levels of High School Students. *J. Educ. Train. Stud.* **2017**, *5*, 72–80. [CrossRef]
124. Jeong, J.-G.; Kang, S.-W.; Choi, S.B. Employees' Weekend Activities and Psychological Well-Being via Job Stress: A Moderated Mediation Role of Recovery Experience. *Int. J. Environ. Res. Public Health* **2020**, *27*, 1642. [CrossRef] [PubMed]

International Journal of
Environmental Research and Public Health

MDPI

Article

The Impact of CSR Perceptions on Employees' Turnover Intention during the COVID-19 Crisis in China

Yang Cheng [1,*], Yuan Wang [2,*] and Feihong Pan [2]

[1] Department of Communication, North Carolina State University, Raleigh, NC 27695, USA
[2] Department of Media and Communication, City University of Hong Kong, Hong Kong, China; fhpan2-c@my.cityu.edu.hk
* Correspondence: ycheng20@ncsu.edu (Y.C.); yuan.wang@cityu.edu.hk (Y.W.)

Abstract: The COVID-19 pandemic has created tremendous challenges for organizations' corporate social responsibility (CSR), communication, and relationship management with internal stakeholders such as employees. This study conducted an online survey of 466 employees working for large Chinese corporations during the pandemic. A structural equation model based on insights from expectancy violation theory was used to examine how negative violation valence increases employees' turnover intention as mediated by uncertainty, CSR cynicism, and distrust. The survey results showed that employees' negative violation valence positively influenced their uncertainty about their organizations' CSR activities, which fostered their cynicism about CSR and distrust of their organization. Employees' CSR cynicism increased their distrust toward their organizations, which increased their turnover intention. The theoretical and practical implications of the study are discussed as well.

Keywords: CSR cynicism; China; COVID-19; turnover intention; distrust; expectancy violation

1. Introduction

Recent research has shown that organizations and their management decisions can significantly affect stakeholders' quality of life and physical and psychological well-being [1]. Stakeholders such as consumers, employees, and the community expect corporations to engage in corporate social responsibility (CSR) activities about environmental, social, and governance issues during crises [2]. For instance, the CVS drugstore gave up USD 2 billion in revenue when it stopped selling tobacco products to support public health [3]. Similarly, since the eruption of COVID-19 in China in December 2019, many corporations started active CSR activities. For instance, Microsoft in China donated over CNY 100 million to the Red Cross in Hunan Province, China on 26 January 2020 [4]. According to a survey conducted in China by McKinsey in March 2020, most of the participants and their corporations had participated in CSR activities, and around 39% of senior executives had deeply engaged in CSR activities during the pandemic [5]. By the end of January 2020, companies in China had donated a total of CNY 12.43 billion to support society during the pandemic [6]. Considering the critical role of large Chinese corporations' CSR activities in fighting against the COVID-19 pandemic, it is meaningful to examine how their employees perceive their CSR efforts and its impacts.

Although many studies [7,8] have demonstrated the positive effects of CSR on firm performance and values, such effects could become contingent on stakeholders' expectations. CSR activities during the COVID-19 pandemic, for example, might not satisfy individuals' high expectations of large corporations (i.e., those with over 250 employees) [9] during crises if these corporations do not sacrifice short-term profits as part of their CSR efforts or these efforts do not directly benefit individuals [3]. Corporations' CSR programs could face tremendous challenges if they fail to meet stakeholders' expectations [2]. Scholars have established connections between stakeholders' negative violation valence (i.e., the degree to which violations are considered to be negative expectations [10]), feelings of uncertainty, and attitudes toward corporate reputation [11]. Cheng et al. [12] found a negative relationship between consumers' CSR skepticism and their brand loyalty and preferences. However, from an internal perspective, the relationships between employees' negative violation valence, cynicism about corporate CSR, distrust, and turnover intention remain unclear. As the literature has shown, employees' attitudes and behaviors significantly influence organizations' crisis management, and more attention should be paid to internal employees during crises [13].

Scholars have found significant differences in corporations' CSR activities in Western and Eastern contexts due to their different technological, cultural, and economic systems. For instance, Tang et al. [14] found that ethics were the most cited reason for CSR engagement on American corporations' websites; employees and community were considered the most critical stakeholders in CSR communication. In Eastern contexts such as China, in contrast, CSR is regarded as ad hoc philanthropy, strategic philanthropy, or ethical business conduct, and employees are less emphasized [15]. Moreover, the Chinese public may have higher expectations of corporate CSR behaviors than American consumers [16]. Scholars [17–19] have found that in Asia, especially China, community and philanthropy are the main focus of corporate CSR activities. Shared values between the business and community are critically important in China for public perception. In contrast, in the U.S. CSR is a predictor of public trust in a business, and corporate social values might not affect stakeholders' trust and supportive behavior. Consequently, CSR activities and stakeholders' perceptions in an Eastern context such as China are distinct from those in the West, and corporate CSR communication and relationship management with internal stakeholders in the Chinese context deserve further exploration.

To fill the above research gap and enrich the crisis management literature, this paper draws on expectancy violation theory [20] and focuses on the global health crisis context. Due to the COVID-19 pandemic, employees' work environment has been disrupted and turnover intention has become unpredictable [21]. The effectiveness of CSR communication within a crisis context in China has received limited attention thus far. This study aims to fill this gap by exploring the influence of CSR perceptions on employee relationship building and turnover intention in the context of the COVID-19 pandemic. The results have practical implications for CSR communicators and human resource managers during crises.

2. Literature Review

2.1. Theoretical Framework

2.1.1. Expectancy Violation Theory

Expectancy violation theory (EVT) is a communication theory that explains how individuals deal with unexpected violations of social norms and expectations [22]. It was proposed by Burgoon and Jones [20], who used it to explain how individuals perceive and explain the invasion of their personal space. According to EVT, communication is an exchange of actions in which one person's actions can violate the expectations of the other [20]. Participants in the exchange view this violation either positively or negatively, depending on their personal relationships or perceptions of the transgression [20]. This theory predicts that expectations will affect the outcome of communication interactions in a positive or negative manner, and the positive violations will strengthen the attractiveness of violators and vice versa [22].

According to Burgoon [23], expectations are consistent patterns of predictable behavior specific to individuals, contexts, and relationships. According to EVT, individuals use expectations to describe and frame their interactions with others, and these expectations dictate how they perceive such interactions and process information and influence their subsequent behavior [23]. When one behaves in a way that deviates from typical behavior, expectations are violated [24]. When an expectancy violation happens, an individual will pay more attention to the interaction process and deal with the violation through explanations and assessments [24].

EVT has previously been applied to the field of crisis communication. Scholars have used EVT to analyze business interactions between companies or between companies and consumers. Sohn and Lariscy [25] used EVT to examine how a CSR crisis affects a corporation's reputation valence and found that higher expectations of the corporation due to its previous good reputation resulted in a more detailed investigation of expectancy violation behavior. Helm and Tolsdorf [26] documented that the public held higher expectations of companies with a better reputation and greater customer loyalty, and such companies tended to suffer more losses during crises than companies with a poorer reputation. Thus, when a company with a high reputation and customer loyalty violates customers' expectations, customers may lose their trust in it.

According to Guerrero and Burgoon [27], if someone believes that violation valence and communicators' reward valence are negative, he/she will reciprocate with negative behavior. Therefore, in the workplace, if an unpopular coworker is grouchy and unpleasant or if a disliked colleague is unhappy, people are more likely to be unhappy in return. In the business context, Kim [11] found that after an oil spill crisis at British Petroleum (BP), if BP's stakeholders had a high prescriptive expectancy of environmental CSR activities, they had more negative reactions toward the firm due to negative violation valence. In this study, we hypothesize that if employees' expectations of their organization's CSR activities are negatively violated, they will become alert and evaluate the violator (i.e., organization) more negatively.

2.1.2. Uncertainty

"Uncertainty" refers to a state of limited knowledge about existing states, future outcomes, or multiple possible outcomes [28]. Scholars have argued that violations have different effects on uncertainty, in that inconsistent negative violations increase uncertainty, whereas consistent violations (both positive and negative) lead to a decline in uncertainty [29]. As individuals' expectations are based on organizations' communications, media presence, and interactions with third parties, they expect certain kinds of behavior from an organization [30].

2.1.3. CSR Cynicism

Davis [31] defined CSR as a company's concern and responsibility for issues that involve duties beyond its legal, economic, and technical purposes. Story et al. [32] classified CSR as either internal or external. Internal CSR refers to the company's responsibilities to internal stakeholders, such as improving working conditions [33]. External CSR is an organization's responsibilities to stakeholders outside its organizational boundaries, such as the government, clients, local communities, business partners, and society [33]. Both internal and external CSR may induce cynicism from stakeholders [34]. CSR cynicism was conceptualized as "a stable individual characteristic of general disillusionment or apathy toward CSR across contexts" [35] (p. 219). According to Kuokkanen and Sun [36], even if external stakeholders have a positive attitude toward a hotel, its use of CSR for self-promotion can still induce skepticism from frequent travelers and elderly people. High levels of CSR cynicism occur when there is an incongruence between high external CSR and low internal CSR [37]. Cynicism occurs in both the internal and external business environment, and should be studied from a broader perspective covering all stakeholders.

2.1.4. Employee Distrust

Trust is defined as "the willingness of a party to be vulnerable to the actions of another party based on the expectation that the other will perform a particular action important to the trustor" [38] (p. 712). Govier [39] defined distrust as the expectation that other individuals will not act in one's best interests or will even engage in harmful behavior towards oneself. According to Cheng and Shen [40] (p. 2), stakeholders' distrust toward an organization means "their fear of and perception of sinister intentions of the organization's conduct related to the crisis".

2.1.5. Turnover Intention

Contrary to actual turnover, turnover intention refers to employees' subjective attitudes about leaving the company or their perceived likelihood to change jobs in the near future [41]. Intention here means "a statement about a specific behavior of interests" [42] (p. 2760). Turnover intention has additionally been defined as "the extent to which an employee plans to leave the organization" [43] (p. 228), and serves as a major precursor of employee turnover. According to Ranjan and Yadav [44], employees' turnover intention is affected by their cynicism, work engagement [45], work environment [46], quality of work experience [47], and organizational justice [48]. Researchers have studied turnover intention in various cultural contexts (e.g., individualistic and collectivistic cultures) and industries (e.g., hospitality and manufacturing) [49], as it is considered an effective warning indicator for problematic human resource management.

2.2. *Development of Hypotheses*

2.2.1. Negative Violation Valence and CSR Uncertainty

The relationship between violation behavior and uncertainty has been explored by communication and management scholars. Smith [50] suggested that during a job hunt, a thank-you letter from the company could be seen as a positive violation of expectations as it can reduce uncertainty. Park et al. [51] documented that negative expectancy violation (e.g., a company's violating customers' higher CSR expectancy) leads to less positive attitudes and supportive behavioral intentions. According to Kim [11], a negative violation valence for an organization in crisis can increase uncertainty about its future performance. More specifically, people with more negative violation valence about BP had higher uncertainty about its future performance, placed more blame on BP for the oil spill, and perceived BP more negatively [11]. EVT indicates that negative violation leads to more negative evaluations of a violator and its future behavior [51]. Considering that CSR is an expectation that the public sets for large organizations [52], we argue that a large organization's negative violation of its employees' expectations about its CSR activities results in their uncertainty about these activities. Thus, we propose the following:

Hypothesis (H1). *Negative violation valence is positively related to uncertainty about CSR activities.*

2.2.2. CSR Uncertainty and Cynicism

Scholars have examined the antecedents of employee cynicism. For example, Andersson [53] found that employee cynicism was influenced by employees' self-esteem and locus of control. Employee perceptions of CSR may reduce their cynicism in the workplace [54]. In particular, employee skepticism about CSR is related to cynicism [55]. According to Pfrombeck et al. [56], social exchange theory can help explain organizational cynicism in a business setting. Social exchange includes employees' uncertainty about the future actions of their organization, and may induce cynicism [56]. Therefore, if employees feel uncertain about their organization's CSR activities, they are more likely to be cynical about these activities. Thus, we propose the following:

Hypothesis (H2). *Employees' uncertainty about CSR activities is positively related to their CSR cynicism.*

2.2.3. CSR Uncertainty and Distrust

Researchers have explored the relationship between CSR and trust/distrust. Lee [57] argued that internal CSR activities create a communal environment among employees, which improves their relationship with their organization, including trust. According to Lepoutre et al. [58], when there are uncertainties about CSR content and activities, employees become cynical about CSR. Employees' feelings of uncertainty lead to indifference, which may affect their trust in the organization. Similarly, Jiang et al. [59] argued that when employees feel that CSR activities are hypocritical, this affects their trust in management. Thus, if employees feel uncertain about their organization's CSR activities, they may distrust the organization. Therefore, we propose the following hypothesis:

Hypothesis (H3). *Employees' uncertainty about their organization's CSR activities is positively related to their distrust in the organization.*

2.2.4. CSR Cynicism and Distrust

In addition to uncertainty, CSR cynicism may influence employee trust/distrust. Employees may have negative responses to CSR [35]. For example, employees may consider their organization's CSR practice to be cynical and inauthentic [60]. Tourigny et al. [61] examined Chinese employees' CSR perceptions and found that these perceptions affect their trust in their organization. According to Abraham [62], employees' organizational cynicism leads to their mistrust. Similarly, we argue that employees who perceive their organization's CSR efforts as cynical are more likely to distrust it. Thus, we propose the following hypothesis:

Hypothesis (H4). *Employees' CSR cynicism is positively related to their distrust in their organization.*

2.2.5. CSR Cynicism and Turnover Intention

Employees' CSR perceptions may influence their turnover intention [63]. Positive internal CSR can help employees increase their employability [44], which may reduce their intention to leave their organization. Furthermore, Ranjan and Yadav [44] documented that employees are less willing to quit their organization if it has strong internal CSR performance, because an organization's internal CSR reflects its welfare practices and procedural justice and therefore enhances its attractiveness, which negatively influences its employees' turnover intention. Specifically, in a Chinese society, scholars found that CSR and ethical leadership demonstrate the value of organizations and further affect employees' turnover intention [64]. In contrast, if employees perceive their organization's lowly involvement with CSR activities or consider their firms' CSR practice to be cynical, they may develop the idea of leaving their organization [64]. Therefore, we propose the following hypothesis:

Hypothesis (H5). *Employees' CSR cynicism is positively related to their turnover intention.*

2.2.6. Distrust and Turnover Intention

In addition to CSR cynicism, employees' trust in their organization may be connected to turnover intention. Zeffane and Melhem [65] examined the factors that influenced employee turnover intention and found that employees' trust had a negative effect on their turnover intention. Employees' distrust triggers their negative feelings about their organization, which leads them to consider leaving as a way of decreasing these negative feelings [65]. Similarly, we argue that employees who distrust their organization may consider quitting. Thus, we propose the following hypothesis:

Hypothesis (H6). *Employees' distrust in their organization is positively related to their turnover intention.*

3. Method

3.1. Data Collection

To test our hypotheses (see Figure 1), we conducted an online survey study. To enroll employees from large organizations (with more than 250 employees) [66] located in China, the researchers made use of the professional survey company Sojump, whose national panel contains 2 million members [67]. Upon approval from the ethics committee, we conducted a pretest in early February 2020 with 133 employees working in large organizations. The researchers then reviewed the dataset and calculated the reliability and validity of each measure. Cronbach's α for the scale of each key variable ranged from 0.86 to

0.93. Consequently, we kept the original items and continued the process of data collection. At the beginning of the questionnaire, the respondents were provided with a detailed description of CSR activities. Several examples were presented, including offering supplies such as masks, paper towels, medicine, or food to those in need, providing cash donations to the people affected, and supporting employees affected by crises by providing short-term financial relief or paid vacations. In the survey section, attention-check items such as "if you are paying attention, kindly please choose 'strongly agree' to pass" were employed to ensure the quality of the online survey. From February to March 2020, 466 participants volunteered to join this study and completed the questionnaire. The data were collected for final analysis.

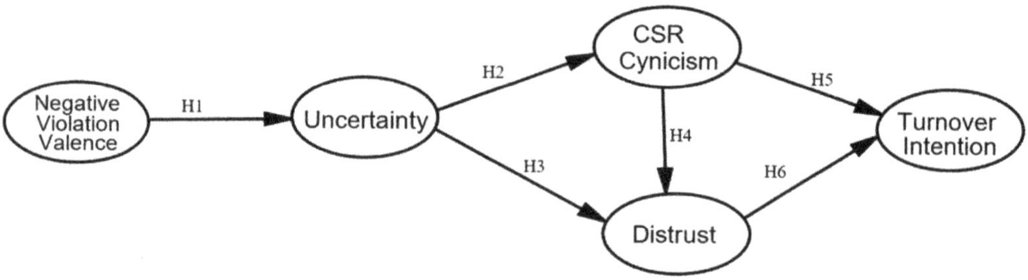

Figure 1. The conceptual model.

3.2. Participants

In the sample, the gender ratio was 51.5% female (n = 240) versus 48.5% male (n = 226). In terms of age, 81.5% (n = 380) of the respondents fell into the range from 25 to 39, 9.4% (n = 44) from 28 to 24, and 9% (n = 42) from 40 to 74. Among the 466 participants, 40.8% (n = 190) were in lower level management positions, followed by 26.6% (n = 124) in non-management positions, 29.6% (n = 138) in middle management positions, and 3% (n = 14) in top management positions. The average tenure of the respondents at their current company was approximately 4.3 years (SD = 3.5). Over one fifth of the participants (20.4%, n = 95) worked in manufacturing corporations, followed by information technology (19.7%, n = 92) and education companies (7.5%, n = 35).

3.3. Measures

All of the key variables were measured with a 5-point Likert scale ranging from "1" (strongly disagree) to "5" (strongly agree).

3.3.1. Negative Violation Valence

This construct was gauged by adopting Kim's [11] measures. Four items were used: "My organization's CSR activities during the COVID-19 crisis makes me feel a lot worse about it", "My organization's CSR activities during the COVID-19 crisis make me feel it does not care about the society/community/environment", "My organization's CSR activities during the COVID-19 crisis makes me feel negatively about it", and "My organization's CSR activities during the COVID-19 crisis makes me feel very disappointed in it" (Cronbach's $\alpha = 0.94$).

3.3.2. Uncertainty

To measure employees' uncertainty about their organizations' CSR activities, this paper adopted Kim's [11] scale. Three items were included: "I feel a lot less confident about my organization's CSR commitment", "I feel a lot less confident about my organization's social-friendly performance", and "I become much less able to predict my organization's commitment to society" (Cronbach's $\alpha = 0.90$).

3.3.3. CSR Cynicism

Following the literature about CSR cynicism [68], we adopted three items to measure employees' level of cynicism about their organization's CSR activities: "I doubt that my organization's CSR tries to solve social problems", "I doubt that my organization's CSR is actually socially responsible", and "I doubt that my organization's CSR follows the ethical responsibility to help society". The level of reliability was 0.73.

3.3.4. Distrust

To measure this construct, we applied the scale from Cheng and Chen [69] and utilized three items: "I feel that my organization will exploit my vulnerability given the chance", "I feel that the way my organization is run is irresponsible and unreliable", and "I feel that my organization cannot be trusted" (Cronbach's $\alpha = 0.81$).

3.3.5. Turnover Intention

Following Lapointe et al. [70], we adopted three items to measure employees' turnover intention: "I often think about leaving my organization", "I am actively searching for a job at another organization", and "If I could choose again, I would choose to work for another organization" (Cronbach's $\alpha = 0.87$).

3.3.6. Control Variables

The literature has shown that the working experience of employees and perceived CSR fit influence participants' CSR cynicism, distrust, and turnover intention [71–73]. Consequently, we controlled these variables in the final structural model. Work experience was measured by asking participants how many years they had worked in their organization. To measure CSR fit, we followed the scales of Moreno and Kang [71] and applied four items: "the CSR activities match our business goals", "the CSR activities are relevant to the business goals", "the CSR activities are a good fit for the business goals", and "the CSR activities are compatible with the business goals".

3.4. Statistical Procedures for Data Analysis

To test the six hypotheses, we performed correlation analysis and structural equation modeling (SEM).

4. Results

4.1. Descriptive Statistics and Correlation Analysis

To demonstrate the mean and standard deviation of each construct, we adopted the Likert scale, using "low" (1.00–1.99)", "moderately low" (2.00–2.99), "neutral" (3), "moderately high" (3.01–3.99), and "high" (4.00–5.00) as the standard. The data indicated that respondents reported moderately low levels of negative violation valence ($M = 2.60$, $SD = 1.26$) and uncertainty about their organizations' CSR activities ($M = 2.82$, $SD = 1.24$). In addition, employees reported a low level of agreement with distrust toward organizations ($M = 1.99$, $SD = 0.88$), CSR cynicism ($M = 1.78$, $SD = 0.64$), and turnover intention ($M = 1.99$, $SD = 0.98$). As shown in Table 1, these main constructs showed significant correlations to each other. The values of the inter-correlation coefficient between the constructs and the square root of average variance extracted (AVE) ranged from 0.08 to 0.88.

Table 1. Inter-correlation between the Constructs and the Square Root of AVEs (Fornell–Larcker Criterion).

Constructs	Negative Violence Valence	Uncertainty	CSR Cynicism	Distrust	Turnover Intention
Negative Violence Valence	**0.88**				
Uncertainty	0.80 **	**0.87**			
CSR Cynicism	0.11 **	0.08	**0.71**		
Distrust	0.27 **	0.18 **	0.45 **	**0.76**	
Turnover Intention	0.25 **	0.24 **	0.49 **	0.64 **	**0.83**

Note. ** Correlation is significant at the 0.01 level (2-tailed). CSR refers to corporate social responsibility; AVE refers to average variance extracted. Values in the diagonal bolded are the square root of AVE while the off-diagonals are correlations.

4.2. The Measurement Model

Before testing the hypotheses, we conducted a confirmatory factor analysis (CFA). The most conservative joint model testing criteria, according to Hu and Bentler [74], are as follows: the comparative fit index (CFI) is equal to or larger than 0.96 and the standardized root mean square residual (SRMR) is equal to or smaller than 0.10, the root mean square error of approximation (RMSEA) is equal to or smaller than 0.06, and SRMR is equal to or smaller than 0.10. The results of CFA analysis turned out to be satisfactory: $\chi^2 = 134.55$, $df = 94$, $p < 0.001$, $\chi^2/df = 1.431$, CFI = 0.992, TLI = 0.989, IFI = 0.992, SRMR = 0.031, RMSEA = 0.026 (90% CI = 0.018 − 0.042). The factor loadings of all items ranged from 0.64 to 0.91. According to Fornell and Larcker's [75] criteria, if the value of composite reliability (CR) is 0.70 or larger and that of AVE is 0.50 or larger, the reliability of CR and AVE are considered to be acceptable. Our results suggested that the values of CR ranged from 0.73 to 0.94, and the scores of AVE ranged from 0.51 to 0.78, which indicated acceptable reliability. Furthermore, Fornell and Larcker's [75] approach was employed to assess the discriminant validity of the measurement model. The square root of the AVE of each latent variable ranged from 0.71 to 0.88, higher than the correlations of any other latent variables (as shown in Table 1). Thus, discriminant validity was established and the data supported the reliability and validity of the applied measures.

4.3. Hypothesis Testing

To test the hypotheses, we employed a structural equation model for data analysis. The results indicated an excellent model fit: $\chi^2 = 192.678$, $df = 123$, $p < 0.001$, $\chi^2/df = 1.566$, CFI = 0.986, TLI = 0.980, IFI = 0.986, SRMR = 0.043, RMSEA = 0.035 (90% CI = 0.025 − 0.044). All of the path coefficients of the structural model are shown in Figure 2.

Specifically, H1 predicted a positive relationship between negative violation valence and uncertainty. The results showed that negative violation valence had a significant and positive impact on uncertainty about CSR ($\beta = 0.87$, $p < 0.001$), supporting H1. H2 further predicted that uncertainty exerts a positive impact on CSR cynicism, which was supported by the results ($\beta = 0.11$, $p < 0.05$). Uncertainty significantly positively influenced employees' perceived distrust toward their organization ($\beta = 0.17$, $p < 0.001$), which means that a higher level of uncertainty about the organization's CSR activity during the pandemic would lead to increased distrust from internal employees. Thus, H3 was supported. Hypothesis 4 posited that CSR cynicism is positively related to distrust. The data demonstrated that a significant and positive impact flow existed between CSR cynicism and distrust ($\beta = 0.57$, $p < 0.001$), supporting H4. In addition, the results showed that CSR cynicism significantly positively affects turnover intention ($\beta = 0.28$, $p < 0.001$). Thus, H5 was supported. Finally, employees' distrust led to their intention to quit their job ($\beta = 0.59$, $p < 0.001$), supporting H6.

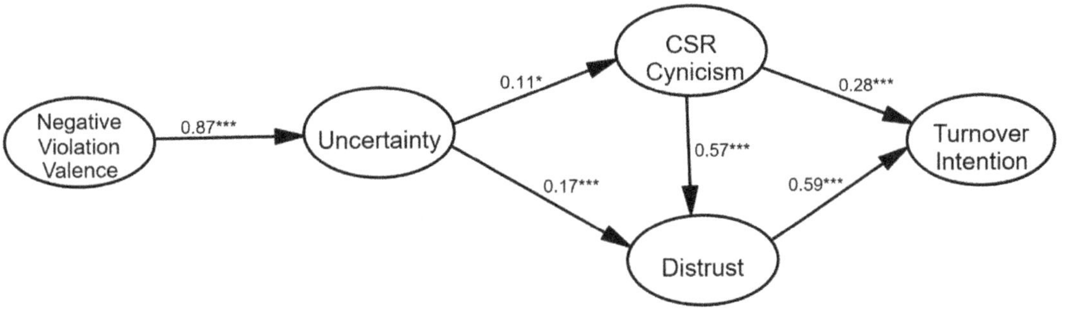

Figure 2. Results from the structural model. *Note.* Control variables in this model include the CSR fit and employees' working experience. CSR refers to corporate social responsibility. *** $p < 0.001$. * $p < 0.05$.

Indirect effects in the current model were estimated through a bootstrapping procedure (N = 5,000 samples) via Amos 20. Negative violation valence had a significant and positive indirect effect on CSR cynicism through the mediation of uncertainty ($\beta = 0.11$, $p = 0.040$, BC 95% CI: 0.01 to 0.21). Uncertainty significantly mediated the relationship between negative violation valence and distrust ($\beta = 0.23$, $p < 0.001$, BC 95% CI: 0.13 to 0.32). Negative violation valence had a positive indirect effect on turnover intention through the serial mediation of uncertainty, CSR cynicism, and distrust ($\beta = 0.17$, $p = 0.001$, BC 95% CI: 0.09 to 0.25). Moreover, uncertainty had a positive indirect effect on turnover intention through the channel of distrust and CSR cynicism ($\beta = 0.19$, $p = 0.001$, BC 95% CI: 0.10 to 0.28).

5. Discussion

The prolonged COVID-19 pandemic has created tremendous challenges for organizations' CSR practices and their relationships with employees. This study surveyed 466 employees working in large organizations in China. It found that employees' negative violation valence increased their uncertainty about CSR activities, which fostered their cynicism about CSR and distrust in their organization. Employees' CSR cynicism strengthened their distrust toward their organization, which increased their turnover intention. In this section, we discuss the theoretical and practical implications of these findings.

First, the results of this study indicate that expectancy violation theory is a useful theoretical framework for explaining employees' CSR attitudes toward organizations during a crisis. This theory provides a new understanding of the effectiveness of CSR communication in a pandemic. One of the major findings of this study is that employees' negative violation valence increases their uncertainty about their organization's CSR activities, which is consistent with previous research [11]. If employees are unsatisfied with their organization's CSR activities during the COVID-19 pandemic, they are more likely to feel uncertain about the organization's commitment to CSR and society. Thus, large organizations should make more efforts to improve their CSR activities and satisfy employee expectations during a public health crisis so that they can retain their employees' confidence in their commitment to CSR and society. Although scholars have investigated the general public's and consumers' perceptions of organizational CSR practices [11,51], they have seldom examined the perceptions of internal stakeholders such as employees. Thus, our findings fill this gap by focusing on employees' perceptions of organizational CSR practices and their consequences.

Second, as trust is considered to be a dimension of employee–organization relationships [76], this study is one of the few studies to integrate the CSR perspective with the relational perspective by documenting the effects of CSR uncertainty and cynicism on distrust. It thus advances the literature on CSR and employee–organization relationships. One important finding is that employees' uncertainty about their organization's CSR activities results in CSR cynicism and distrust in their organization. If employees feel less confident about their organization's CSR commitment, they are more likely to doubt that their organization's CSR is actually socially responsible or addresses social problems, and will consequently develop distrust in their organization [77]. Furthermore, this study found that employees' CSR cynicism positively influenced their distrust in their organization. As previous literature has indicated, CSR activities reflect company ethics and values and help organizations to act as "trustees" for the interests of employees [78] (p. 10). With the implementation of CSR activities, employees can fulfill their own social needs and become enthusiastic toward their work, as CSR helps to reach goal congruence and a common identity between employees and their organization [64]. Consequently, if employees develop their own cynicism toward their organizations' CSR, the most proximate outcome would be distrustful perceptions. Thus, large organizations should therefore promote their CSR activities to their employees and demonstrate their CSR commitment, which can induce their employees to trust them.

Third, the findings of this study contribute to the business literature by shedding light on the influence of public relations practices on organizations. The results demonstrate that employees' cynicism about their organization's CSR activities and distrust in the organization increases their turnover intention; these findings are similar to those in previous research [44]. If employees doubt that their organization's CSR helps society or solves social problems, they are more likely to consider leaving the organization. Therefore, this study advances the CSR literature by identifying employee CSR uncertainty as a new factor that may influence turnover intention. Moreover, employees who distrust their organization are more likely to leave it to work for another organization. This finding is critical, especially during the COVID-19 pandemic, because this global crisis has brought challenges to organizational management in terms of maintaining employees' trust in their organization [79]. Thus, large organizations could strengthen their CSR efforts (e.g., delegating a specific division for CSR practices, offering paid hours for employees' CSR engagement, or enhancing CSR fit with their strategic goals) to maintain their employees' trust, which can help with employee retention.

Practically, the results of this study provide important managerial implications for large organizations. The proposed model can be used to measure the effectiveness of organizational CSR practice. The COVID-19 pandemic has significantly impacted stakeholders in organizations, such as employees. Managers can apply this tool to focus on employees' perceptions of CSR communication in order to examine their expectations concerning current CSR activities and evaluate whether their activities will have a negative or positive valence. The model suggests that if CSR activities do not satisfy employees' expectations during a pandemic, then CSR cynicism and distrust toward organizations could occur, leading to increased turnover. Consequently, examining and monitoring employees' perceptions of CSR activities is beneficial for human resource management and internal crisis communication. Large companies might develop adequate measures or structures to ensure that their employees can help the companies to perform CSR work in a positive and mentally comfortable manner rather than forcing them to complete CSR activities. Leaders in firms should listen to employees and carry their interests in mind when they encourage and conduct CSR activities. An ethical and healthy leadership style and "goal congruence" between a firm and its employees can reduce employees' turnover intention [64].

In addition, this study shows that positive relationship management with internal employees might reduce employee turnover costs. During a crisis, relationships between organizations and employees are threatened [80]. If corporations ensure that their CSR activities are perceived as beneficial, ethical, and supportive during a crisis, employees will be confident about such activities and trust their organization, which will significantly reduce turnover intention.

Limitations and Directions for Future Research

Although this study contributes to the literature on CSR and internal employee management during the COVID-19 pandemic, several limitations must be stated here. First, this study only focused on internal communication within big Chinese organizations. Future studies could employ comparative methods to further validate the proposed hypotheses and explore cultural or contextual factors that might influence employees' perceptions of CSR during crises and the impact on turnover intention. For example, they could examine whether the types of companies (i.e., state-owned enterprises and private companies) might influence the relationship between employees' CSR perceptions and their distrust and turnover intention. Second, as the magnitude of violation valence might influence perceived uncertainty, future scholarship could continue to explore how employees' reactions to a violator, such as the organization during a crisis, might influence their trust in organizations and work performance. Third, employees' individual differences might influence their perceptions of an organization during a crisis. Future work could investigate how CSR involvement or value orientations [81] predict distrust and CSR cynicism.

6. Conclusions

This paper presented a timely study on CSR perceptions, distrust, and turnover intention of employees in crises of contemporary Chinese society. It contributed to the body of knowledge on CSR in building trust and shed light on the application of ethical CSR in crisis communication of China. This study also built on the most up-to-date literature and addressed an important issue on CSR practice in China from an internal employee's perspective.

Author Contributions: Conceptualization, Y.C.; methodology, Y.C.; formal analysis, Y.C.; investigation, Y.C. and Y.W.; data curation, Y.W.; writing—original draft preparation, Y.C., Y.W. and F.P.; writing—review and editing, Y.C. and Y.W.; project administration, Y.W.; funding acquisition, Y.W. All authors have read and agreed to the published version of the manuscript.

Funding: This research was funded by City University of Hong Kong (Projects No. 7200615 and No. 7005704).

Institutional Review Board Statement: The study was conducted in accordance with the Declaration of Helsinki, and approved by the Human Subjects Ethics Sub-Committee of City University of Hong Kong (reference number: 2-4-201810-03; date of approval: 6 November 2018).

Informed Consent Statement: Informed consent was obtained from all subjects involved in the study.

Data Availability Statement: The data are not publicly available due to privacy or ethical restrictions.

Conflicts of Interest: The authors declare no conflict of interest.

References

1. Murrell, J.A.; Jones, R.; Zhao, X.-P. Special Issue "Ethics, Social Responsibility and Quality of Life in Times of Crisis". *Int. J. Environ. Res. Public Health* **2021**. Available online: https://www.mdpi.com/journal/ijerph/special_issues/Times_of_Crisis (accessed on 1 May 2022).
2. Lee, S.; Singal, M. Does Corporate Social Responsibility Matter During Crises? *Boston Hosp. Rev.* **2021**. Available online: https://www.bu.edu/bhr/2021/10/29/does-corporate-social-responsibility-matter-during-crises/ (accessed on 1 May 2022).
3. Kramer, R.M. Coronavirus is Putting Corporate Social Responsibility to the Test. *Harv. Bus. Rev.* **2020**. Available online: https://hbr.org/2020/04/coronavirus-is-putting-corporate-social-responsibility-to-the-test (accessed on 1 May 2022).
4. Center for China and Globalization. Research Report on Corporate Social Responsibility (CSR) of Multinational Enterprises in China (2020–2021). Available online: http://wanghuiyao.com/archives/1727 (accessed on 2 July 2022).
5. Textor, C. Share of Companies that Engaged in CSR Actions during COVID-19 in China 2020. *Statista*, 19 April 2022. Available online: https://www.statista.com/statistics/1112861/china-corporate-social-responsibility-csr-initiatives-during-the-COVID-19-outbreak-2020/#statisticContainer (accessed on 2 July 2022).
6. Zhang, K. 61 State-Owned Enterprises Donated Over 2 Billion to Fight Against the Epidemic. *Yicai*, 31 January 2020. Available online: https://m.yicai.com/news/100484618.html (accessed on 2 July 2022).
7. Almeida, M.D.G.M.C.; Coelho, A.F.M. The antecedents of corporate reputation and image and their impacts on employee commitment and performance: The moderating role of CSR. *Corp. Repu. Rev.* **2019**, *22*, 10–25. [CrossRef]

8. Loor-Zambrano, H.Y.; Santos-Roldán, L.; Palacios-Florencio, B. Relationship CSR and employee commitment: Mediating effects of internal motivation and trust. *Eur. Res. Manag. Bus. Econ.* **2022**, *28*, 100185. [CrossRef]
9. OECD. Enterprises by Business Size (Indicator). 2022. Available online: https://data.oecd.org/entrepreneur/enterprises-by-business-size.htm (accessed on 1 July 2022).
10. Bennett, L.K.; Scruggs, X.; Woods, J.M. Surprise, hurt, and anger as emotional responses to expectancy violations following feedback messages. *Commun. Res. Rep.* **2020**, *37*, 22–33. [CrossRef]
11. Kim, S. The role of prior expectancies and relational satisfaction in crisis. *J. Mass Commun. Q.* **2014**, *91*, 139–158. [CrossRef]
12. Cheng, Y.; Hung-Baesecke, F.C.-J.; Chen, Y.-R. Social media influencer effects on CSR communication: The role of influencer leadership in opinion and taste. *Int. J. Bus. Commun.* **2021**. [CrossRef]
13. Kim, Y. Organizational resilience and employee work-role performance after a crisis situation: Exploring the effects of organizational resilience on internal crisis communication. *J. Public Relat. Res.* **2020**, *32*, 47–75. [CrossRef]
14. Tang, L.; Gallagher, C.C.; Bie, B. Corporate social responsibility communication through corporate websites: A comparison of leading corporations in the U.S. and China. *Int. J. Bus. Commun.* **2015**, *52*, 205–227. [CrossRef]
15. Tang, L.; Li, H. Corporate social responsibility communication of Chinese and global corporations in China. *Public Relat. Rev.* **2009**, *35*, 199–212. [CrossRef]
16. Chu, S.-C.; Lin, J.S. Consumers' perception of corporate social responsibility in the United States and China: A study of female cosmetics consumers. *Int. J. Strategic Commun.* **2013**, *7*, 43–64. [CrossRef]
17. Hung-Baesecke, F.C.-J.; Stacks, D.; Coombs, T.; Chen, R.Y.-R. The effects of corporate social responsibility and creating shared value on public trust, and public supportive behavior: A comparison study. In Proceedings of the 19th International Public Relations Research Conference, Miami, FL, USA, 2–5 March 2016; pp. 169–191.
18. Kim, R.C.; Moon, J. Dynamics of corporate social responsibility in Asia: Knowledge and norms. *Asian Bus. Manag.* **2015**, *14*, 349–382. [CrossRef]
19. Marquis, C.; Yang, Z. Embracing shared value in China. *China Policy Rev.* **2014**, *7*, 115–116.
20. Burgoon, J.K.; Jones, S.B. Toward a theory of personal space expectations and their violations. *Hum. Commun. Res.* **1976**, *2*, 131–146. [CrossRef]
21. Tao, W.; Lee, Y.; Sun, R.; Li, J.-Y.; He, M. Enhancing employee engagement via leaders' motivational Language in times of crisis: Perspectives from the COVID-19 outbreak. *Public Relat. Rev.* **2022**, *48*, 102133. [CrossRef]
22. Burgoon, J.K.; Hale, J.L. Nonverbal expectancy violations: Model elaboration and application to immediacy behaviors. *Commun. Monogr.* **1988**, *55*, 58–79. [CrossRef]
23. Burgoon, J.K. Interpersonal expectations, expectation violations, and emotional communication. *J. Lang. Soc. Psychol.* **1993**, *12*, 30–48. [CrossRef]
24. Afifi, W.A.; Metts, S. Characteristics and consequences of expectation violations in close relationships. *J. Soc. Pers. Relat.* **1998**, *15*, 365–392. [CrossRef]
25. Sohn, Y.J.; Lariscy, R.W. A "buffer" or "boomerang?"—The role of corporate reputation in bad times. *Commun. Res.* **2015**, *42*, 237–259. [CrossRef]
26. Helm, S.; Tolsdorf, J. How does corporate reputation affect customer loyalty in a corporate crisis? *J. Conting Crisis Man.* **2013**, *21*, 144–152. [CrossRef]
27. Guerrero, L.K.; Burgoon, J.K. Attachment styles and reactions to nonverbal involvement change in romantic dyads: Patterns of reciprocity and compensation. *Hum. Commun. Res.* **1996**, *22*, 335–370. [CrossRef]
28. Hubbard, D.W. *How to Measure Anything Workbook: Finding the Value of "Intangibles" in Business, 3rd ed*; Wiley: Hoboken, NJ, USA, 2014.
29. Afifi, W.A.; Burgoon, J.K. The impact of violations on uncertainty and the consequences for attractiveness. *Hum. Commun. Res.* **2000**, *26*, 203–233. [CrossRef]
30. Fediuk, T.A.; Coombs, W.T.; Botero, L.C. Exploring crisis from a receiver perspective: Understanding stakeholder reactions during crisis events. In *The Handbook of Crisis Communication*; Coombs, W.T., Holladay, S.J., Eds.; Wiley Blackwell: Hoboken, NJ, USA, 2010; pp. 635–656.
31. Davis, K. The case for and against business assumption of social responsibilities. *Acad. Manag. J.* **1973**, *16*, 312–322.
32. Story, J.; Castanheira, F.; Hartig, S. Corporate social responsibility and organizational attractiveness: Implications for talent management. *Soc. Respons. J.* **2016**, *12*, 484–505. [CrossRef]
33. Turker, D. Measuring corporate social responsibility: A scale development study. *J. Bus. Ethics* **2009**, *85*, 411–427. [CrossRef]
34. Basil, D.Z.; Erlandson, J. Corporate social responsibility website representations: A longitudinal study of internal and external self-presentations. *J. Marketing Commun.* **2008**, *14*, 125–137. [CrossRef]
35. Willness, C.R. Understanding stakeholders' negative responses to corporate social responsibility. In *The Oxford Handbook of Corporate Social Responsibility: Psychological and Organizational Perspectives*; Abagail, M., Deborah, E.R., Donald, S.S., Günter, K.S., Waldman, A.D., Eds.; Oxford University Press: Oxford, UK, 2019; pp. 207–238.
36. Kuokkanen, H.; Sun, W. Social desirability and cynicism biases in CSR surveys: An empirical study of hotels. *J. Hosp. Tou. Ins.* **2020**, *3*, 567–588. [CrossRef]
37. Li, Z.; Wang, F.; Yang, L. Looking in and looking out: Effects of (in) congruent corporate social responsibility on organizational cynicism. *Soc. Behav. Personal.* **2021**, *49*, 1–15. [CrossRef]

38. Mayer, R.C.; Davis, J.H.; Schoorman, F.D. An integrative model of organizational trust. *Acad. Manag. Rev.* **1995**, *20*, 709–734. [CrossRef]
39. Govier, T. Is it a jungle out there? Trust, distrust, and the construction of social reality. *Dialogue–Can. Philos. Rev.* **1994**, *33*, 237–252. [CrossRef]
40. Cheng, Y.; Shen, H.M. United airlines crisis from the stakeholder perspective: Exploring customers' ethical judgment, trust and distrust, and behavioral intentions. *Public Relat. Rev.* **2020**, *46*, 101908. [CrossRef]
41. Egan, T.; Yang, B.; Bartlett, K. The effects of organizational learning culture and job satisfaction on motivation to transfer learning and turnover intention. *Hum. Resour. Dev. Q.* **2004**, *15*, 279–301. [CrossRef]
42. Ngo-Henha, P.E. A review of existing turnover intention theories. *Int. J. Econ. Manag. En.* **2017**, *11*, 2751–2758.
43. Lacity, M.C.; Iyer, V.V.; Rudramuniyaiah, P.S. Turnover intentions of Indian IS professionals. *Inform. Syst. Front.* **2008**, *10*, 225–241. [CrossRef]
44. Ranjan, S.; Yadav, R.S. Uncovering the role of internal CSR on organizational attractiveness and turnover intention: The effect of procedural justice and extraversion. *Asian Soc. Sci.* **2018**, *14*, 76–85. [CrossRef]
45. Liu, H.L.; Lo, V.-H. An integrated model of workload, autonomy, burnout, job satisfaction, and turnover intention among Taiwanese reporters. *Asian J. Commun.* **2018**, *28*, 153–169. [CrossRef]
46. Smith, T.D. An assessment of safety climate, job satisfaction and turnover intention relationships using a national sample of workers from the USA. *Int. J. Occup. Saf. Ergo.* **2018**, *24*, 27–34. [CrossRef]
47. Zhao, X.; Sun, T.; Cao, Q.; Li, C.; Duan, X.; Fan, L.; Liu, Y. The impact of quality of work life on job embeddedness and affective commitment and their co-effect on turnover intention of nurses. *J. Clin. Nurs.* **2013**, *22*, 780–788. [CrossRef]
48. Harris, C.M.; Lavelle, J.J.; McMahan, G.C. The effects of internal and external sources of justice on employee turnover intention and organizational citizenship behavior toward clients and workgroup members. *Int. J. Hum. Resour. Man.* **2020**, *31*, 2141–2164. [CrossRef]
49. Park, J.; Min, H.K. Turnover intention in the hospitality industry: A meta-analysis. *Int. J. Hosp. Manag.* **2020**, *90*, 102599. [CrossRef]
50. Smith, S.A. The Job Searching and Career Expectations of Recent College Graduates: An Application of the Expectancy Violations Theory of Communication. Ph.D. Dissertation, The University of Arizona, Tucson, AZ, USA, 2015.
51. Park, S.-Y.; Cho, M.; Kim, S. The effect of CSR expectancy violation: Value from expectancy violation theory and confirmation bias. *J. Mark. Commun.* **2021**, *27*, 365–388. [CrossRef]
52. Lin-Hi, N.; Blumberg, I. The link between (not) practicing CSR and corporate reputation: Psychological foundations and managerial implications. *J. Bus. Ethics* **2018**, *150*, 185–198. [CrossRef]
53. Andersson, L. Employee cynicism: An examination using a contract violation framework. *Hum. Relat.* **1996**, *49*, 1395–1418. [CrossRef]
54. Serrano Archimi, C.; Reynaud, E.; Yasin, H.M.; Bhatti, Z.A. How perceived corporate social responsibility affects employee cynicism: The mediating role of organizational trust. *J. Bus. Ethics* **2018**, *151*, 907–921. [CrossRef]
55. Latif, B.; Ong, T.S.; Meero, A.; Abdul Rahman, A.A.; Ali, M. Employee-perceived corporate social responsibility (CSR) and employee pro-environmental behavior (PEB): The moderating role of CSR skepticism and CSR authenticity. *Sustainability* **2022**, *14*, 1380. [CrossRef]
56. Pfrombeck, J.; Doden, W.; Grote, G.; Feierabend, A. A study of organizational cynicism and how it is affected by social exchange relationships at work. *J. Occup. Organ. Psych.* **2020**, *93*, 578–604. [CrossRef]
57. Lee, Y. Toward a communality with employees: The role of CSR types and internal reputation. *Corp. Repu. Rev.* **2020**, *23*, 13–23. [CrossRef]
58. Lepoutre, J.; Dentchev, N.A.; Heene, A. Dealing with uncertainties when governing CSR policies. *J. Bus. Ethics* **2007**, *73*, 391–408. [CrossRef]
59. Jiang, H.; Cheng, Y.; Park, K.; Zhu, W. Linking CSR communication to corporate reputation: Understanding hypocrisy, employees' social media engagement and CSR-related work engagement. *Sustainability* **2022**, *14*, 2359. [CrossRef]
60. Onkila, T. Pride or embarrassment? Employees' emotions and corporate social responsibility. *Corp. Soc. Resp. Env. Ma.* **2015**, *22*, 222–236. [CrossRef]
61. Tourigny, L.; Han, J.; Baba, V.V.; Pan, P. Ethical leadership and corporate social responsibility in China: A multilevel study of their effects on trust and organizational citizenship behavior. *J. Bus. Ethics* **2019**, *158*, 427–440. [CrossRef]
62. Abraham, R. Organizational cynicism: Bases and consequences. *Genet. Soc. Gen. Psychol. Monogr.* **2000**, *126*, 269–292.
63. Low, M.P.; Ong, S.F.; Tan, P.M. Would internal corporate social responsibility make a difference in professional service industry employees' turnover intention? A two-stage approach using PLS-SEM. *Glo. Bus. Manag. Res.* **2017**, *9*, 24–41.
64. Lin, C.-P.; Liu, M.-L. Examining the effects of corporate social responsibility and ethical leadership on turnover intention. *Pers. Rev.* **2017**, *46*, 526–550. [CrossRef]
65. Zeffane, R.; Melhem, S.B. Do feelings of trust/distrust affect employees' turnover intentions? An exploratory study in the United Arab Emirates. *Middle East J. Manag.* **2018**, *5*, 385–408. [CrossRef]
66. Carim, L.A.R.A.; Warwick, C. Use of social media for corporate communications by research-funding organizations in the UK. *Public Relat. Rev.* **2013**, *39*, 521–525. [CrossRef]

67. Luo, Y.; Cheng, Y. The presumed influence of COVID-19 misinformation on social media: Survey research from two countries in the global health crisis. *Int. J. Environ. Res. Public Health* **2021**, *18*, 5505. [CrossRef]
68. Ji, S.; Jan, I. The impact of perceived corporate social responsibility on frontline employee's emotional labor strategies. *Sustainability* **2019**, *11*, 1780. [CrossRef]
69. Cheng, Y.; Chen, Z.F. Encountering misinformation online: Antecedents of trust and distrust and their impact on the intensity of Facebook use. *Online Inform. Rev.* **2021**, *45*, 372–388. [CrossRef]
70. Lapointe, E.; Vandenberghe, C.; Mignonac, K.; Panaccio, A.; Schwarz, G.; Richebe, N.; Roussel, P. Development and validation of a commitment to organizational career scale: At the crossroads of individuals' career aspirations and organizations' needs. *J. Occup. Organ. Psych.* **2019**, *92*, 897–930. [CrossRef]
71. Moreno, F.; Kang, J. How to alleviate consumer skepticism concerning corporate responsibility: The role of content and delivery in CSR communications. *Corp. Soc. Resp. Env. Ma.* **2020**, *27*, 2477–2490. [CrossRef]
72. Valentine, S.; Godkin, L. Banking employees' perceptions of corporate social responsibility, value-fit commitment, and turnover intentions: Ethics as social glue and attachment. *Emp. Resp. Rig. J.* **2017**, *29*, 51–71. [CrossRef]
73. Wei, L.; Kim, N. Attenuating public skepticism: Effects of pre-crisis corporate engagement and post-crisis CSR initiatives on corporate evaluations. *Public Relat. Rev.* **2021**, *47*, 101999. [CrossRef]
74. Hu, L.; Bentler, P.M. Cut off criteria for fit indexes in covariance structure analysis: Conventional criteria versus new alternatives. *Struct. Equ. Modeling* **1999**, *6*, 1–55. [CrossRef]
75. Fornell, C.; Larcker, D.F. Evaluating structural equation models with unobservable variables and measurement error. *J. Marketing Res.* **1981**, *18*, 39–50. [CrossRef]
76. Wang, Y. When relationships meet situations: Exploring the antecedents of employee communication behaviors on social media. *Soc. Sci. Comput. Rev.* **2022**, *40*, 77–94. [CrossRef]
77. Hansen, S.D.; Dunford, B.B.; Boss, A.D.; Boss, R.W.; Angermeier, I. Corporate social responsibility and the benefits of employee trust: A cross-disciplinary perspective. *J. Bus. Ethics* **2011**, *102*, 29–45. [CrossRef]
78. Balmer, J.M.T.; Fukukawa, K.; Gray, E.R. The nature and management of ethical corporate identity: A commentary on corporate identity, corporate social responsibility and ethics. *J. Bus. Ethics* **2007**, *76*, 7–15. [CrossRef]
79. Men, L.R.; Qin, Y.S.; Jin, J. Fostering employee trust via effective supervisory communication during the COVID-19 pandemic: Through the lens of motivating language theory. *Int. J. Bus. Commun.* **2022**, *59*, 193–218. [CrossRef]
80. Cheng, Y.; Shen, H.; Jiang, Q. Corporate dialogue in crises of China: Examining dialogic strategies and communicative outcomes in a child abuse scandal. *Public Relat. Rev.* **2020**, *46*, 101816. [CrossRef]
81. Oo, E.Y.; Jung, H.; Park, I. Psychological factors linking perceived CSR to OCB: The role of organizational pride, collectivism, and person–organization fit. *Sustainability* **2018**, *10*, 2481. [CrossRef]

International Journal of
Environmental Research and Public Health

MDPI

Article

The Effect of Self-Sacrificial Leadership on Employees' Organisational Citizenship Behaviour for the Environment: A Moderated Mediation Model

Yiying Qu [1], Zhenting Xu [2,*], Hong Sun [1] and Qingsheng Li [3]

1 Business School, East China University of Political Science and Law, Shanghai 200042, China; sdlzqyy@hotmail.com (Y.Q.); sunhong_ifrs@163.com (H.S.)
2 Business School, Qingdao University of Technology, Qingdao 266525, China
3 School of Business, Linyi University, Linyi 276000, China; liqingsheng@lyu.edu.cn
* Correspondence: tjphd11@126.com

Abstract: In the face of increasing environmental pressures, environmentally friendly behaviour can help companies achieve truly sustainable growth. The issue of how to promote environmental behaviour among employees is a new challenge for leaders. However, studies do not systematically reveal the mechanisms of the effects of self-sacrificial leadership on employees' organisational citizenship behaviour for the environment (OCBE). Based on social learning theory and the attitude–behaviour–context model, we investigated the impact of self-sacrificial leadership on employees' OCBE by focusing on the mediating role of the corporate social responsibility (CSR) as perceived by employees, and the moderating role of the pro-environmental organisational climate (PEOC). The results of a field survey of 461 employees (small- and medium-sized enterprises) in China indicate that self-sacrificial leadership was positively related to employees' OCBE; this relationship was partially mediated by employees' perception of CSR. Moreover, PEOC strengthened the effect of employees' perceived CSR on OCBE, and the mediating effect of employees' perceived CSR on the relationship between self-sacrificial leadership and OCBE. Our findings not only help scholars understand the mechanism of the effect of self-sacrificial leadership on employees' OCBE, but also provide insights for recommending integrated management models, social responsibility, and environmental protection.

Keywords: self-sacrificial leadership; corporate social responsibility; pro-environmental organisational climate; organisational citizenship behaviour for the environment

1. Introduction

Faced with the spread of COVID-19, extreme weather events, and economic turbulence, environmental protection and resource conservation have become important goals so that China can achieve sustainable development. As the primary mover in economic development, enterprises have assumed responsibility for environmental protection and resource conservation, implementing a series of formal regulations and measures, such as environmental industry codes and enterprise environmental regulations [1,2]. To effectively complement the environmental behaviours required by formal rules and regulations, Boiral et al. [3] developed the concept of organisational citizenship behaviour for the environment (OCBE), defining it as the spontaneous and proactive environmental behaviour of individual employees in enterprises that both contributes to the implementation of environmental initiatives facilitated by the company, and enhances its environmental performance. OCBE has become an important research issue in the Chinese context [2,4]. Environmental citizenship behaviours, such as employees voluntarily suggesting reduced energy consumption, separating waste, and using environmentally friendly items, not only contribute to the organisation's sustainable development, but also promote ecological environmental civilisation. Thus, we explore the important theoretical and practical significance of the influence factor of OCBE.

According to social learning theory, individuals learn through observation of role models to provide specific guidance for their behaviour [5]. Organisational leaders have provided an important imitation model for employees to use when adjusting their behaviours [6]. In other words, leadership has played a critical role in shaping employees' environmental behaviours [6–8]. Accordingly, our research purpose is to explore the influence mechanism of OCBE from the perspective of leadership. Self-sacrificial leadership has attracted the attention of theoretical scholars during crises caused by epidemics and environmental problems [9,10]. Self-sacrificial leadership refers to leaders who voluntarily forgo their personal interests in an effort to maximise the collective welfare [11]. The self-sacrificial leader acts in a manner that demonstrates a high level of ethical responsibilities and duties [9,11], which encourages employees to see them as role models worthy of imitation. As suggested by social learning theory, employees are more likely to learn to "put everything on the line" for others from the leader, high in self-sacrifice, which, in turn, motivates extra-role behaviour, such as organisational citizenship behaviour (OCB) [10,12]. Whereas the research has explained the role of self-sacrificial leadership in OCB, it has neglected the empirical evidence of the influence of self-sacrificial leadership on OCBE. As specific types of OCB [13], both OCBE and OCB emphasise employee-initiated behaviours within organisations that are voluntary and not required by formal reward systems or rules and regulations, and that contribute to organisational effectiveness [3]. However, unlike OCB, with its two dimensions of organisational and interpersonal relationships, OCBE involves environmentally oriented, proactive individual behaviour that complements formal corporate environmental practices [3,14]. For this reason, we examine the effect of self-sacrificial leadership on OCBE.

Why does self-sacrificial leadership enhance employees' OCBE? To answer this question, we uncover the mediating mechanism of this phenomenon. We explain the relationship between self-sacrificial leadership and employees' OCBE based on social learning theory, which suggests that employees learn from and imitate leaders' behaviours, which, in turn, affects their attitudes and behaviours [5,15]. We argue that employees are motivated to engage in OCBE by perceiving the CSR displayed by leaders through the self-sacrificial behaviour in favour of the collective and their followers. Accordingly, we empirically test the mediating effect of employees' perceived CSR on the relationship between self-sacrificial leadership and OCBE.

The attitude–behaviour–context model suggests that attitudes do not necessarily lead to a behaviour that is difficult or costly to achieve, but instead the process is also influenced by the moderating effect of situational factors [16,17]. Not all employees transform their perceptions of CSR into practical OCBE, because the motivation for their behaviour may require boundary conditions. Therefore, we also explore the moderating role of organisational situational factors in the process through which self-sacrificial leaders influence employees' OCBE. PEOC, defined as employees' shared perception of organisational policies or norms that support environmental sustainability in the workplace, has been shown to be positively related to environmental behaviours [1]. Therefore, we identify PEOC as a moderator, examining the moderating effects of PEOC on the relationship between perceived CSR and self-sacrificial leadership with employees' OCBE.

We seek to make three theoretical contributions. First, we extend both the leadership and OCBE literature by theoretically building and empirically examining a model to link self-sacrificial leadership and employees' OCBE in the Chinese context, which can direct scholars to further discuss the effect of leaders' behaviour on OCBE, and guide managers to understand the environmental effect of self-sacrificial leadership. Second, we explore the mediating effects of employees' perceived CSR on the self-sacrificial leadership–OCBE relationship, thereby expanding further knowledge of how self-sacrificial leadership encourages employees to achieve OCBE. Third, we demonstrate the moderating effect of PEOC to test a comprehensive picture of when perceived CSR and its mediating role will be enacted and yield higher OCBE among employees. We present the conceptual model in Figure 1.

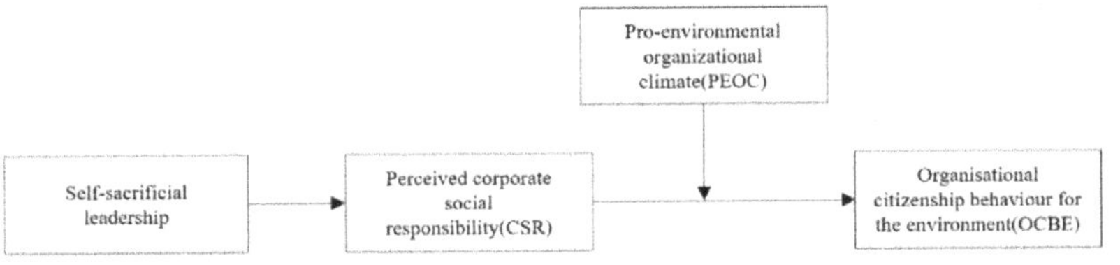

Figure 1. The conceptual model.

2. Theories and Hypotheses

2.1. Self-Sacrificial Leadership and OCBE

OCBE is defined as "individual and discretionary social behaviours that are not explicitly recognized by the formal reward system and that contribute to a more effective environmental management by organizations" [18] (p. 223). Similar to OCB, OCBE emphasises employee-initiated environmental behaviours within an organisation that are voluntary and not required by the rules and regulations of any formal reward system. Employees' OCBE can effectively complement an organisation's formal environmental system and reflect the diffusion of environmental awareness and behaviours from daily life to the organisation's internal environment [19]. Studies have demonstrated that leadership is an important predictor of OCBE [4,20]. These studies have primarily focused on the relationship among ethical leadership [15,21,22], pro-environmental transformational leadership [2], and OCBE; however, they have ignored the relationship between self-sacrificial leadership and employee OCBE. Given the importance of leadership in Chinese collective-oriented contexts, self-sacrificial leadership brings positive outcomes to organisations [9], and its modelling of high moral standards and group-oriented behaviours may positively influence employees' OCBE.

Self-sacrificial leadership is referred to as "the total/partial abandonment, and/or permanent/temporary postponement of personal interests, privileges, and welfare in the (a) division of labour, (b) distribution of rewards, and/or (c) exercise of power" [11] (p. 479). Self-sacrificial leadership involves volunteering for the benefit of the collective at the expense of one's personal resources [9,23]. The essential characteristics of self-sacrificial leaders are manifested in proactive responsibility, a collectivist orientation, and service to organisations and employees, all of which positively influence employee reciprocal behaviour [24], pro-social behaviour [23], and OCB [12,23]. For the reasons set forth below, we argue that self-sacrificial leadership influences OCBE.

First, social learning theory suggests that employees who see their leaders as role models, imitating and learning from their virtues, increase their moral responsibility and exhibit a variety of positive behaviours [25,26]. Leaders become role models for employees by demonstrating high ethical standards and maximising the collective welfare at the expense of their own, such as by voluntarily surrendering their power to benefit the collective, thus motivating employees to learn through imitation. Motivated by self-sacrificial leaders' high ethical standards and sense of responsibility, employees may consider the potential benefits they can provide to the organisation by engaging in pro-environmental behaviours. The OCBE concept includes a strong ethical component [27]; in other words, employees who engage in OCBE learn from their leaders' organisation-oriented self-sacrifice. Recent studies have provided evidence that leaders' ethical behaviour promotes employees' OCBE [3,22].

Second, unlike ethical, transformational, and charismatic leaders, one important characteristic of self-sacrificial leadership is the leader's self-sacrificial behaviour on behalf of the collective, indicating that organisational goals and welfare are rendered both salient to employees and worthy of their individual, dedicated efforts [28]. Employees are motivated to exceed the obligations of their role to volunteer to engage in environmental protection behaviour in the workplace, such as separating waste, using environmentally friendly products, and recycling old items. Although such behaviour is not required by formal organisational systems and cannot be formally rewarded [13], employees imitate their leaders' principles of doing what is needed for others and the organisation, thus demonstrating environmental citizenship behaviours. In support of our argument, research has revealed that self-sacrificial leadership is positively related to employees' OCB [12,29,30], and the concepts underlying OCB and OCBE emphasise employees' pro-organisational out-role behaviour [21,22]. Thus, we propose the following hypothesis:

Hypothesis 1 (H1). *Self-sacrificial leadership is positively related to employees' OCBE.*

2.2. Employees' Perceived CSR as a Mediator

CSR is conceptualised as "corporate behaviours which aim to affect stakeholders positively and go beyond its economic interest" [31] (p. 191). In terms of employees as stakeholders, employees' perceived CSR has been referred to as a subjective perception of CSR [31–33]. Whereas CSR is an organisational-level concept, employees' perceived CSR is an individual-level concept from the employee's perspective. Employees evaluate the social responsibility of their leader or organisation as a concern for the collective welfare or employees' interests [31]. Social learning theory proposes that leaders as role models, who are learnt from and imitated by employees, often influence employees' perception and behaviours [5]. It is more likely that employees perceive the organisation's social responsibility based on the leader's high standard of moral behaviours [34,35]. Self-sacrificial leaders with superb charisma and dedication pay more attention to the welfare of the collective or others than to their own, becoming high-level ethical role models, causing employees to perceive CSR, and stimulating positive altruistic behaviours [36], such as OCBE. When employees perceive that organisations act in a manner that is consistent with social responsibility, they demonstrate more altruism and responsibility, and people with a good sense of social responsibility are more likely to engage in pro-social behaviours, care for the environment and conserve resources, and adopt environmentally friendly citizenship behaviour. Thus, we suggest that employees' perceived CSR may affect employees' OCBE.

First, self-sacrificial leadership may facilitate employees' perception of social responsibility. According to social learning theory, people observe, learn, and imitate their role models' behaviours [5,8], which suggests that employees can imitate their self-sacrificial leaders' behaviours. Self-sacrificial leadership demonstrates the moral quality of temporarily or permanently forgoing one's own interests in favour of the collective, for example, by taking responsibility, putting the interests of the collective first, caring for employees, and assisting in career development [11]. The moral standards of self-sacrificing behaviours are perceived as CSR by employees. Thus, employees believe that leaders and their organisations go the extra mile for them or other stakeholders [34], including by working to protect the environment. Furthermore, they are likely to learn from their leaders' self-sacrificial behaviours, and are willing to actively take responsibility and make an effort for the sake of both the collective and others. Thus, self-sacrificial leadership can facilitate the CSR perceived by employees.

Second, employees' perceived CSR may positively affect their OCBE, which is framed as a spontaneous extra-role behaviour [13]. CSR perceived by employees who believe their organisation will do what is morally right for the sake of the collective is particularly important in improving those employees' OCBE. According to social learning theory, if employees recognise that corporate behaviours are praiseworthy, they tend to imitate altruistic behaviours in their own work. The more CSR is recognised by employees, the more social responsibility-driven citizenship behaviours they engage in, such as suggesting improved corporate environmental policies, and sorting and recycling office waste. Recent studies have provided evidence that CSR is related to both OCB [35–37] and green behaviour [38]. Integrating the above arguments with those supporting the positive link between self-sacrificial leadership and employees' perceived CSR discussed earlier, we propose the following hypothesis:

Hypothesis 2 (H2). *Employees' perceived CSR mediates the relationship between self-sacrificial leadership and employees' OCBE.*

2.3. PEOC as a Moderator

The attitude–behaviour–scenario model based on field theory illustrates that employees' behavioural decisions are influenced not only by their own attitudes [16], but also by organisational situational factors [17]. Organisational situational factors affect employee behaviours by creating the organisational climate [39]. Organisational climate is considered an important environmental situational factor affecting employee behaviour [40–42]. Employees integrate their own cognition and situational factors to make decisions. Therefore, we introduce PEOC, as a specific context of organisational climate in terms of environmental protection [43], to explain the moderating effect of differences in environmental climate in organisations on the impact of employees' perceived CSR on employees' OCBE.

PEOC is characterised as employees' common perception of environmental sustainability policies, norms, and practices in organisations, including support for not only an organisation's formal green system, but also its environmental requirements and values [43]. We find that PEOC is the specific organisational climate formed by a series of pro-environmental policies that promotes positive environmental values to employees, and facilitates the implementation of environmental behaviours. As an environment-oriented climate, PEOC has increased the encouragement of and support for employees' environmental behaviours, enabling employees to engage in those behaviours, such as saving resources and making environmental suggestions [1,21]. Most scholars have suggested that PEOC, or employees' perceptions of the pro-environmental facet of the organisational climate (including a range of pro-environmental concepts, procedures, and practices, along with support from their colleagues), can positively influence employee green behaviour [1,39]. We consider PEOC as a moderator that determines the extent to which employees can convert perceived CSR into positive OCBE.

Although individuals with a strong sense of social responsibility may exhibit more altruistic or citizenship behaviours [36], not all such individuals necessarily exhibit pro-environmental behaviours. Employees who have a sense of CSR need to be in an environmentally friendly atmosphere to implement individual behaviour geared towards caring for the environment and saving resources [34,35]. The pro-environmental climate represents the extent to which organisations pay attention to environmental issues, adopt formal green policies in different business processes, and support sustainable activities. Such pro-environmental norms motivate employees to implement their pro-environmental intentions (i.e., to translate their sense of social responsibility to the company into pro-environmental behaviour, such as environmental citizenship). In the workplace, employees exposed to a strong PEOC in which they can facilitate the organisation's daily work practices to support environmental goals and values are more likely to perceive that their organisation encourages them to accomplish their tasks in an eco-friendly way, facilitating environmental citizenship behaviour. Therefore, employees perceive the organisation as pro-environmental, and strongly identify with the organisation to undertake CSR to achieve its sustainable development. In contrast, employees working in a poor environmental climate may find it difficult to perceive the organisation's environmental strategy, and thus, they are more likely to engage in more organisation- or interpersonal-oriented citizenship behaviour motivated by high CSR [44], but not to engage in environmental behaviour. Thus, PEOC catalyses eco-friendly behaviours facilitated by employees with CSR, strengthening the relationship between employees' perceived CSR and OCBE. Therefore, we propose the following hypothesis:

Hypothesis 3 (H3). *PEOC positively moderates the relationship between employees' perceived CSR and OCBE such that the relationship is stronger for employees with higher levels of PEOC.*

Considering H2 and H3 and their related studies, we propose that by strengthening the positive relationship between employees' perceived CSR and OCBE, high PEOC will strengthen the indirect relationship between self-sacrificial leadership and employees' OCBE via perceived CSR. When the PEOC is high, employees are more likely to adopt the CSR they perceive from self-sacrificial leaders, and are encouraged to engage in more OCBE. In contrast, in the absence of PEOC, even if employees perceive CSR expressed by self-sacrificing leaders, they may not transform their enhanced sense of responsibility into OCBE, instead engaging in other types of performance outcomes. Taken together, we propose the following hypothesis:

Hypothesis 4 (H4). *PEOC positively moderates the mediating effect of employees' perceived CSR between self-sacrificial leadership and employees' OCBE.*

3. Methods

3.1. Procedures and Sample

The manufacturing industry has a greater impact on the environment in production and management activities, and thus, there is an urgent need for manufacturing enterprises to strengthen technological innovation and adopt clean production processes in China [18,45]. Employees in the manufacturing industry should also take environmental responsibility and implement spontaneous environmental behaviours [46]. In view of this, the survey sample of employees was collected from 16 small- and medium-sized manufacturing enterprises in the Yangtze River Delta region in China. We had good research communication with the target companies, and the survey was supported by both the persons in charge and the respondents. Before collecting the data, we gave the persons in charge advance notice, enabling them to understand the purpose of the study and what we expected them to do in the survey. A web-based research packet, containing cover letters, the questionnaire, and a confidentiality agreement, was sent via a web link. To alleviate concerns about common method bias [47], we follow the extant research to collect data during May–September 2021 in two phases [48–50]. In the first wave (time 1), the respondents were asked about their personal backgrounds, self-sacrificial leadership, and PEOC. In the second (time 2), conducted one month after time 1, they were asked about perceived CSR and OCBE. In the first round of data collection, a total of 700 questionnaires were distributed and 582 were collected; in the second round, 492 questionnaires were completed by respondents in the previous round. After eliminating invalid questionnaires, 461 valid questionnaires remained, with a valid response rate of 65.9%.

Of the respondents, 210 (45.6%) were male. The seven age cohorts were below 25 (6.9%), 25–30 (23.9%), 31–35 (27.8%), 36–40 (19.7%), 41–45 (12.1%), 46–50 (6.9%), and over 50 (2.7%) years old; educational attainment was concentrated at the college degree (19.7%) and Bachelor's degree (56.4%) levels. The average job tenure was 4.15 years (SD = 1.16).

3.2. Measures

All of the scales used in this study were originally developed in the West and applied in Chinese settings in previous studies, as shown in Table A1. We obtained the Chinese version of self-sacrificial leadership and OCBE measurements directly from Chinese scholars, and we tested a Chinese version of PEOC and perceived CSR by following Brislin's [51] translation–back–translation procedure. We invited a management professor to translate the English scale into Chinese, and then invited another management professor to translate it back. In addition, we invited bilingual management professors to check both translations to continuously revise the scale validation. Except for the control variables, all of the core variables were measured by the participants' responses to questions on a 5-point Likert-type scale ranging from "strongly disagree" to "strongly agree".

Self-sacrificial leadership: a 5-item scale developed by De Cremer and van Knippenberg [24], and later applied in Chinese settings [9], was used to measure self-sacrificial leadership. One sample item was "My supervisor is willing to make personal sacrifices in the organisation's interest". Cronbach's alpha for this measure was 0.913.

Organisational citizenship behaviour for the environment (OCBE): a 10-item scale developed by Boiral and Paillé [52], and later applied by [20] in China, was used to measure OCBE. One sample item was "I encourage my colleagues to adopt more environmentally conscious behaviours". Cronbach's alpha for this measure was 0.934.

Pro-environmental organisational climate (PEOC): a Chinese translation of the four-item scale developed by Norton et al. [43] was used to measure PEOC. Based on the purpose of the study, the four items of this scale corresponded to the organisational level. One sample item was "I encourage my colleagues to adopt more environmentally conscious behaviours". Cronbach's alpha for this measure was 0.766.

Employees' perceived corporate social responsibility (CSR): six items developed by Turkey [33] were used to measure how employees perceive CSR. One sample item was "Encourages its employees to participate in voluntary activities". Cronbach's alpha for this measure was 0.798.

Control variables: given our concern about the effects of demographic variables on OCBE [2,19,22], we controlled for employees' demographic variables, including gender (coded 1 = male and 2 = female), age (coded 1 = below 25 years, 2 = 25–30 years, 3 = 31–35 years, 4 = 36–40 years, 5 = 41–45 years, 6 = 46–50 years, and 7 = more than 50 years), and job tenure (coded 1 = below 1 year, 2 = 1–3 years, 3 = 3–5 years, 4 = 5–10 years, and 5 = more than 10 years). Education levels were hierarchically coded as 1 = high school graduate or below, 2 = college degree, 3 = Bachelor's degree, and 4 = Master's degree or above.

3.3. Analytical Strategy

We used the SPSS22.0, AMOS22.0, and PROCESS3.3 macro programs for our statistical analysis of the data. First, a set of confirmatory factor analyses (CFAs) was conducted using AMOS22.0 to test the discriminant validity among four latent variables (i.e., self-sacrificial leadership, PEOC, and employees' perceived CSR and OCBE). Next, descriptive statistical analysis and correlation analysis methods were conducted using SPSS22.0 to examine the relationships between the variables. PROCESS3.3 was used to test the moderated mediation effect in the second stage.

4. Results

4.1. Confirmatory Factor Analysis

The CFA results are shown in Table 1. The four-factor model achieved a good fit to the data: χ^2/df = 2.069, GFI = 0.914, CFI = 0.931, NFI = 0.922, and RMSEA = 0.061. We then confirmed the discriminant validity of the four-factor model by testing alternative models (three-factor, two-factor, and one-factor models). As suggested by [53], χ^2/df took values between 1 and 5; CFI, GFI, and NFI were greater than 0.9; and RMSEA was less than 0.08, indicating that the model had a good fit. As presented in Table 1, the four-factor model provided a significantly better fit than the alternative models, indicating satisfactory construct validity in the Chinese context.

Table 1. Confirmatory factor analysis.

Model	χ^2/df (*df*)	GFI	CFI	NFI	RMSEA
Four-factor model	2.069 (268)	0.914	0.931	0.922	0.061
Three-factor model					
SSL and employees' perceived CSR were combined	5.697 (271)	0.846	0.860	0.857	0.082
Two-factor model					
SSL, and employees' perceived CSR and PEOC were combined	8.126 (274)	0.721	0.739	0.730	0.103
One-factor model	11.247 (275)	0.664	0.682	0.674	0.116

Note: SSL represents self-sacrificial leadership, CSR represents corporate social responsibility, PEOC represents pro-environmental organisational climate, and OCBE represents organisational citizenship behaviour for the environment.

4.2. Common Method Bias

To effectively mitigate the common method bias arising from the same subjects or data sources, we first adopted a two-stage data collection approach while ensuring the authenticity of data acquisition through anonymity and confidentiality measures during the collection process. Second, CFA also showed that the four-factor model had a good fit, and these variables had good discriminant validity, further indicating that the common method bias in this study was not serious. Finally, the total variance explained cumulatively by the four factors extracted from the common method factors was 71.27%, and the maximum value of the variance explained by the factors was 24.98%, which was in accordance with the recommended value of the statistical test, and did not exceed 50% of the total variance. Therefore, common method bias did not affect the relationship between the variables to be tested.

4.3. Descriptive Analysis

Table 2 shows the mean, standard deviations, and correlations for the study variables. As the table shows, self-sacrificial leadership was positively related to both employee OCBE ($\beta = 0.38$, $p < 0.01$) and employees' perceived CSR ($\beta = 0.22$, $p < 0.01$). Employees' perceived CSR was positively related to employee OCBE ($\beta = 0.46$, $p < 0.01$). Therefore, these results primarily supported the proposed hypotheses, and provided the necessary preconditions for the mediating effect test.

Table 2. Means, standard deviations, and correlations.

Variables	Mean	SD	1	2	3	4	5	6	7	8
1. Gender	1.53	0.50								
2. Age	3.53	1.45	0.11							
3. Job tenure	4.15	1.16	0.07	0.18						
4. Education level	2.84	0.80	0.07	0.11	0.08					
5. SSL	3.28	0.77	−0.06	0.05	0.13	0.06	0.913			
6. Employees' perceived CSR	3.92	0.48	0.06	0.04	0.10	0.02	0.22 **	0.798		
7. PEOC	4.00	0.51	0.02	0.08	0.06	0.04	0.30 **	0.43 **	0.766	
8. OCBE	3.98	0.49	0.03	0.07	0.07	0.04	0.38 **	0.46 **	0.31 **	0.934

Note: N = 461, ** $p < 0.01$. SD = standard deviation. Reliabilities are on the diagonal parentheses. Gender is coded 1 = male and 2 = female; Age is coded 1 = below 25 years, 2 = 25–30 years, 3 = 31–35 years, 4 = 36–40 years, 5 = 41–45 years, 6 = 46–50 years, and 7 = more than 50 years; Job tenure is coded 1 = below 1 year, 2 = 1–3 years, 3 = 3–5 years, 4 = 5–10 years, 5 = more than 10 years; Education level is coded 1 = high school graduate or below, 2 = college degree, 3 = Bachelor's degree, 4 = Master's or above. SSL represents self-sacrificial leadership, CSR represents corporate social responsibility, PEOC represents pro-environmental organisational climate, and OCBE represents organisational citizenship behaviour for the environment.

4.4. Hypotheses Testing

Main effect: H1 proposes the main effect of self-sacrificial leadership on employee OCBE. Table 3 shows the hierarchical regression results. Self-sacrificial leadership was positively related to employees' perceived CSR ($\beta = 0.20$, $p < 0.01$; Model 2) and positively related to employee OCBE ($\beta = 0.29$, $p < 0.01$; Model 4), thus supporting H1.

Mediating effect: H2 predicts that employees' perceived CSR mediates the relationship between self-sacrificial leadership and employees' OCBE. We followed Baron and Kenny's [54] study to test this mediation. First, the results in Table 3 show that self-sacrificial leadership was positively related to employees' perceived CSR ($\beta = 0.20$, $p < 0.01$; Model 2). Second, as indicated in H1, self-sacrificial leadership was significantly and positively related to employees' OCBE ($\beta = 0.29$, $p < 0.01$; Model 4). Third, compared to the result shown in Model 2 in Table 3, the coefficient of the relationship between self-sacrificial leadership and employees' OCBE ($\beta = 0.19$, $p < 0.01$; Model 5) was diminished when employees' perceived CSR was included in the model, whereas employees' perceived CSR was positively related to employees' OCBE ($\beta = 0.48$, $p < 0.01$; Model 5). This indicates that employees' perceived CSR acted as a partial mediator of the relationship between self-sacrificial leadership and employees' OCBE. Thus, these results initially support H2 [54]. We used a parameter bootstrapping procedure to further verify the mediation relationship [55]. Based on a sample size of 5000, the bootstrap results show that the indirect relationship between self-sacrificial leadership and OCBE via employees' perceived CSR was significant (β = 0.55, 95% CI = (0.03, 0.10)), providing further support for H2.

Table 3. Hierarchical regression analysis results of variables.

Variables	Perceived CSR		OCBE				
	Model 1	Model 2	Model 3	Model 4	Model 5	Model 6	Model 7
Control variables							
Gender	−0.11	−0.09	−0.04	−0.04	0.04	−0.02	−0.02
Age	0.05	0.06	0.00	0.02	−0.01	0.01	0.01
Job tenure	−0.01	−0.00	−0.04	−0.02	−0.02	−0.02	−0.02
Education level	−0.01	−0.00	0.03	0.03	0.04	0.01	0.01
Independent variables							
SSL		0.20 **		0.29 **	0.19 **		
Mediator							
Employees' perceived CSR					0.48 **	0.05 **	0.04 **
Moderator							
PEOC						0.47 **	0.45 **
Interaction effect							
PEOC× Employees' perceived CSR							0.04 **
R^2	0.03	0.12	0.01	0.18	0.38	0.83	0.87
ΔR^2	—	0.09 **	—	0.17 **	0.20 **	[a] 0.82 **	0.04 **

Note: ** $p < 0.01$. [a] compared to model 3. SSL represents self-sacrificial leadership, CSR represents corporate social responsibility, PEOC represents pro-environmental organisational climate, and OCBE represents organisational citizenship behaviour for the environment.

Moderated mediation: H3 proposes that PEOC positively moderates the relationship between employees' perceived CSR and employee OCBE such that the relationship is stronger for employees with higher levels of PEOC. We first standardised employees' perceived CSR and PEOC to set the interaction term, which was entered into the regression model. As shown in Table 3, the interaction term of employees' perceived CSR and PEOC was significantly and positively related to employees' OCBE (β = 0.04, $p < 0.01$, Model 7), indicating that PEOC played a positive moderating role in the relationship between employees' perceived CSR and OCBE. Thus, H3 is supported. The interaction effects are depicted in Figure 2. H4 indicates that PEOC positively moderates the mediating effect of employees' perceived CSR between self-sacrificial leadership and employees' OCBE. We conducted PROCESS3.3 to test the second-stage moderated mediation. As shown in Table 4, the value of the index of moderated mediation was 0.0141 (95% CI = (0.0043, 0.0276)), which was significant. Then, we further tested the indirect effect of self-sacrificial leadership on employees' OCBE via employees' perceived CSR at different levels of PEOC (one SD below the mean, the mean, and one SD above the mean). As shown in Table 4, the conditional indirect effect of self-sacrificial leadership via employees' perceived CSR on OCBE was significant at the low level (95% CI = (0.0052, 0.0155)) and at the high level (95% CI = (0.0075, 0.0330)), with the estimated value of the indirect effect increasing from 0.0046 to 0.0187. Therefore, H4 is supported. The results of the hypothesized model are shown in Figure 3.

Table 4. The moderated mediation effect in the second stage.

	Effect	SE	Boot LLCI	Boot ULCI
Low PEOC	0.0046	0.0052	0.0052	0.0155
Medium PEOC	0.0117	0.0050	0.0034	0.0229
High PEOC	0.0187	0.0064	0.0075	0.0330
	Index	**SE**	**Boot LLCI**	**Boot ULCI**
Perceived CSR	0.0141	0.0059	0.0043	0.0276

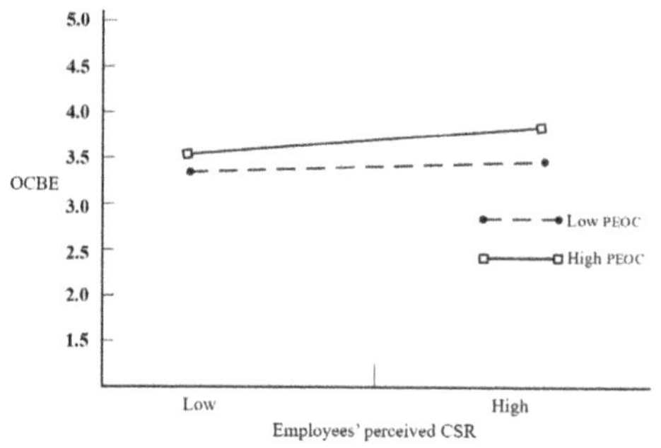

Figure 2. The interaction effect of PEOC on the relationship between employees' perceived CSR and OCBE.

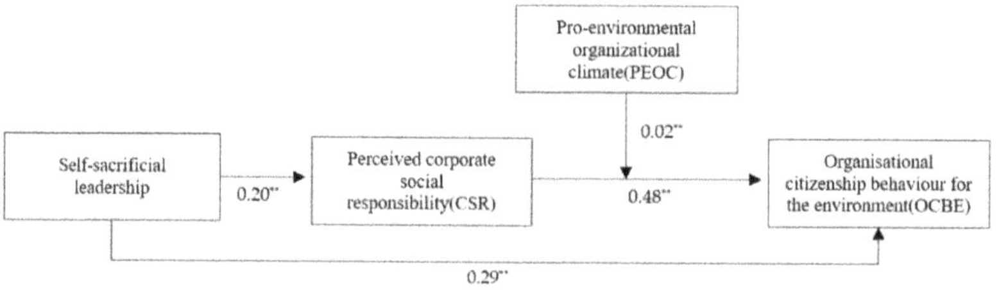

Figure 3. Result of the hypothesised model. Note: ** $p < 0.01$.

5. Discussion

5.1. Theoretical Implications

First, we theoretically establish and empirically examine a conceptual model that integrates leadership with employee OCBE theory. Our results empirically demonstrate, for the first time, that self-sacrificial leadership promotes employees' OCBE. Among the leadership theories that influence employees' OCBE, some studies have focused on transformational leadership [8] and ethical leadership [20], but none have examined the relationship between self-sacrificial leadership and employees' OCBE. In addition, we respond to the call from Lamm et al. [14] to apply a theoretical model to verify the influence of various types of leadership on OCBE, expanding the antecedents of employees' OCBE. In the field of leadership research, scholars have focused on employee performance-related outcomes of self-sacrificial leadership, such as job performance and employee creativity, ignoring the impact of self-sacrificial leadership on environmental behaviours [12]. Thus, we also answer the call from Daily et al. [13] and Zhang et al. [15] to empirically examine the environmental effect of self-sacrificial leadership. Accordingly, we not only respond to future research directions proposed by theoretical scholars, but also fill research gaps in the literature and enrich the theories of self-sacrificial leadership and OCBE.

Second, based on social learning theory, we find that employees' perceived CSR partially mediates the relationship between self-sacrificial leadership and OCBE, thus providing a new theoretical framework for understanding the influence process of self-sacrificial leadership on employees' OCBE. Self-sacrificial leaders are concerned about the collective welfare, and exhibit responsibility and dedication, both of which are perceived by employees as demonstrating the responsibility of the enterprise [9,24]. Employees then tend to exceed their formal job requirements and spontaneously devote themselves to environmental behaviours that are beneficial to the organisation's image. The results may encourage future scholars to address the impact of leadership on employees' pro-environment consequences by focusing on the employee ethical factors, including environmental self-accountability [56], prosocial motivation [57], and environmental beliefs [58].

Thus, we provide a clear theoretical framework for the influence of self-sacrificial leadership on employees' OCBE.

Third, organisational citizenship behaviour theory suggests that the study of employees' OCBE considers not only individual-level factors, but also situational factors in which individuals are placed so that the situational characteristics of individual factors affecting employees' OCBE can be clarified [39]. Therefore, we incorporate PEOC into the relationship between self-sacrificial leadership, perceived CSR, and employees' OCBE. As discussed previously, employees in a strong pro-environmental climate are likely to be motivated to engage in OCBE by perceived CSR from self-sacrificial leadership. This demonstrates the boundary conditions of employees' OCBE, and enriches PEOC theory to address new features and attributes arising from the interaction of individual and situational factors on OCBE, thus providing new perspectives for future research.

5.2. Practical Implications

To achieve sustainable development, enterprises should not only implement formal green policies in management activities, but also encourage employees' daily environmental citizenship behaviour.

First, our findings show that self-sacrificial leaders are regarded as a key for organisations' green development in the workplace. Self-sacrificial leaders can set ethical and moral examples and inspire helpfulness on the part of employees in various situations [9,39], which can enhance communication between colleagues, identification with the organisation, and the implementation of environmental protection beliefs. Thus, our work suggests that organisations can cultivate employee CSR and OCBE through enhancing self-sacrificial leadership practice in the Chinese context. When recruiting or selecting leaders, organisations strengthen the moral practices of collective benefits of leaders and guide them to adopt self-sacrificial leadership to undertake responsibility for sustainable development. Besides, more leadership training and development programs can be developed to support self-sacrificial activities to exhibit social responsibility, such as instructing leaders on how to articulate an environmental vision to employees for the collective welfare.

In addition, it may be difficult to implement formal environmental policies in all aspects of enterprise practice, so it is necessary to complement employees' spontaneous environmental behaviours [59]. Our findings show that employees in a strong pro-environmental climate are more likely to learn CSR from self-sacrificial leaders, thereby engaging in more OCBE. Therefore, while engaging in environmental management practices, leaders who forgo one's own interests in favour of the collective can encourage employees to better understand CSR, and thus to go beyond their personal interests to protect the environment for the sake of the organization and society.

5.3. Limitations and Future Research Directions

Although our study has a certain theoretical and practical value, some limitations remain. First, we adopt a self-reported measurement method that cannot completely avoid common method bias. As the variables measured refer to employees' perceptions of CSR and leadership, it is difficult to obtain assessments from others. Future research can use colleagues to assess employees' OCBE and explore the impact of the different perceptions of employees and their colleagues on employees' OCBE. Second, we use a cross-sectional design, which cannot rigorously test the causal relationship between variables. Future research can use a multiple time-point longitudinal design to enhance the validity of the causal relationship between variables. Third, the findings of this study are limited to the Chinese manufacturing context, and the sampled respondents are from a few enterprises with different pro-environmental degrees. The convenience samples of this study may be biased, which leads to a constraint on the generalisability of the findings [60]. It may be that the variance of the impact of self-sacrificial leadership on employees' OCBE exists in other industries, and thus, the scope of the study can be further expanded to a multi-industry and even cross-country context. Last, we only examine the moderating effect of PEOC among environmental factors. Future research can investigate the effects of other environmental differences, such as green human resource management [44].

6. Conclusions

We integrated research on leadership and pro-environmental behaviour to examine the links between self-sacrificial leadership and employees' OCBE. Integrating social learning theory and the attitude–behaviour–context model, we extended employees' perceived CSR to represent a mediating mechanism between self-sacrificial leadership and employee OCBE, and found that PEOC strengthens the effects of employees' perceived CSR on employee OCBE, and positively moderates the mediating role of perceived CSR between self-sacrificial leadership and employees' OCBE.

Author Contributions: Conceptualisation, Y.Q. and Z.X.; methodology, Y.Q. and Z.X.; formal analysis, Y.Q. and Z.X.; investigation, H.S. and Q.L.; writing—original draft preparation, Y.Q. and Z.X.; writing—review and editing, Y.Q and H.S.; funding acquisition, Y.Q. and Z.X. All authors have read and agreed to the published version of the manuscript.

Funding: This research was funded by the Humanities and Social Sciences General Research Program of the Ministry of Education of China, grant number 19C10276025; and Science Research Program of the East China University of Political Science and Law, grant number 20HZK017.

Institutional Review Board Statement: Not applicable.

Informed Consent Statement: Not applicable.

Data Availability Statement: The data that support the findings of this study are available from the authors upon reasonable request.

Conflicts of Interest: The authors declare no conflict of interest.

Appendix A

Table A1. Measurement items of key variables.

Variables		Items	Source
Organisational citizenship behaviour for the environment (OCBE)	1	In my work, I weigh the consequences of my actions before doing something that could affect the environment 我在开展工作之前会权衡自己的行为是否有利于环境保护	Boiral and Paillé (2012) [52]; Zhang et al. (2018) [20]
	2	I voluntarily carry out environmental actions and initiatives in my daily work activities 在我的日常工作中, 我自愿开展环保行为和举措	
	3	I make suggestions to my colleagues about ways to protect the environment more effectively, even when it is not my direct responsibility 我会给同事提出保护环境的建议, 即使这不是我的责任	
	4	I actively participate in environmental events organised in and/or by my company 我积极参与企业组织的环保活动	
	5	I stay informed of my company's environmental initiatives 我保持了解我企业的环保措施	
	6	I undertake environmental actions that contribute positively to the image of my organisation 我从事有利于企业积极形象的环保行动	
	7	I volunteer for projects, endeavours, or events that address environmental issues in my organisation 我自愿承担我企业有关环境问题的各种项目	
	8	I spontaneously give my time to help my colleagues take the environment into account in everything they do at work 我不由自主地帮助同事在工作中考虑环境问题	
	9	I encourage my colleagues to adopt more environmentally conscious behaviour 我鼓励我的同事采用更有环境意识的行为	
	10	I encourage my colleagues to express their ideas and opinions on environmental issues 我鼓励我的同事表达他们对环境问题的想法和意见	

Table A1. *Cont.*

Variables		Items	Source
Self-sacrificial leadership	1	My team leader is willing to make personal sacrifices in the team's interest 我的领导愿意为团队的利益做出个人牺牲	De Cremer and van Knippenberg (2004) [24]; Qu et al. (2021) [9]
	2	My supervisor is willing to stand up for the team members' interests, even when it is at the expense of his/her own interests 我的领导即使个人利益受损,也愿意维护组织成员利益	
	3	My team leader is always among the first to sacrifice free time, privileges, or comfort if that is important 我的领导在工作中愿意牺牲个人特权、舒适和享受	
	4	I can always count on my supervisor to help me in times of trouble, even if it is at a cost to him/her 在遇到困难的时候,我总是能指望我的领导帮助我,即使帮助我会使领导个人利益受损。	
	5	My supervisor is willing to risk his/her position if he/she believes the goals of the team can be reached that way 我的领导在实现组织目标的过程中,会作出自我牺牲	
Employees' perceived corporate social responsibility (CSR)	1	Our company encourages its employees to participate in voluntarily activities 我们公司鼓励其员工参加自愿性活动	Turker (2009a) [33]
	2	Our company policies encourage the employees to develop their skills and careers 我们公司的政策鼓励员工发展他们的技能和职业	
	3	The management of our company is primarily concerned with employees' needs and wants 我们公司的管理层主要关注员工的需求	
	4	Our company implements flexible policies to provide a good work and life balance for its employees 我们公司实施灵活的政策,为员工提供一个良好的工作和生活平衡	
	5	The managerial decisions related with the employees are usually fair 与雇员有关的管理决策通常是公平的	
	6	Our company supports employees who want to acquire additional education 我们公司支持希望获得额外教育的员工	
Pro-environmental organisational climate (PEOC)	1	Our company is worried about its environmental impact 我们公司关注自身对环境的影响	Norton et al. (2014) [43]
	2	Our company is interested in supporting environmental causes 我们公司致力于支持环保事业	
	3	Our company believes it is important to protect the environment 我们公司认为保护环境很重要	
	4	Our company is concerned with becoming more environmentally friendly 我们公司热衷于进一步的环境友好发展	

References

1. Norton, T.A.; Zacher, H.; Ashkanasy, N.M. Pro-environmental organizational culture and climate. In *The Psychology of Green Organizations*; Robertson, J.L., Barling, J., Eds.; Oxford University Press: New York, NY, USA, 2015; pp. 322–348.
2. Peng, J.; Hou, N.; Fu, B. The impact of pro-environment transformational leadership on employees' citizenship behavior for environment protection: An ability-motivation-opportunity theory perspective. *Contemp. Financ. Econ.* **2020**, *4*, 77–87. [CrossRef]
3. Boiral, O.; Talbot, D.; Paillé, P. Leading by example: A model of organizational citizenship behavior for the environment. *Bus. Strateg. Environ.* **2015**, *24*, 532–550. [CrossRef]
4. Omarova, L.; Jo, S.J. Employee pro-environmental behavior: The impact of environmental transformational leadership and GHRM. *Sustainability* **2022**, *14*, 2046. [CrossRef]
5. Bandura, A. *Social Foundations of Thought and Action*; Prentice Hall: Englewood Cliffs, NJ, USA, 1986.
6. Mulder, L.B.; Nelissen, R.M.A. When rules really make a difference: The effect of cooperation rules and self-sacrificing leadership on moral norms in social dilemmas. *J. Bus. Ethics.* **2010**, *95*, 57–72. [CrossRef]
7. Norton, T.A.; Parker, S.L.; Zacher, H.; Ashkanasy, N.M. Employee green behavior: A theoretical framework, multilevel review, and future research agenda. *Organ. Environ.* **2015**, *28*, 103–125. [CrossRef]
8. Mi, L.; Gan, X.; Xu, T.; Long, R.; Qiao, L.; Zhu, H. A new perspective to promote organizational citizenship behavior for the environment: The role of transformational leadership. *J. Clean. Prod.* **2019**, *239*, 118002. [CrossRef]
9. Qu, Y.; Xu, Z.; Yan, J. The Impact of self-sacrificial leadership on employees' work-family balance: A chain mediating model and the moderating effect of collectivism orientation. *Manag. Rev.* **2021**, *33*, 272–283. [CrossRef]
10. Mostafa, A.M.S.; Bottomley, P.A. Self-Sacrificial leadership and employee behaviours: An examination of the role of organizational social capital. *J. Bus. Ethics.* **2020**, *161*, 641–652. [CrossRef]
11. Choi, Y.; Mai-Dalton, R.R. On the leadership function of self-sacrifice. *Leadership. Quart.* **1998**, *9*, 475–501. [CrossRef]

12. He, W.; Zhou, R.; Long, L.; Huang, X.; Hao, P. Self-sacrificial leadership and followers' affiliative and challenging citizenship behaviors: A relational self-concept based study in China. *Manag. Organ. Rev.* **2018**, *14*, 105–133. [CrossRef]
13. Daily, B.F.; Bishop, J.W.; Govindarajulu, N. A conceptual model for organizational citizenship behavior directed toward the environment. *Bus. Soc.* **2009**, *48*, 243–256. [CrossRef]
14. Lamm, E.; Tosti-Kharas, J.; King, C.E. Empowering employee sustainability: Perceived organizational support toward the environment. *J. Bus. Ethics.* **2015**, *128*, 207–220. [CrossRef]
15. Zhang, J.; Chen, Y.; Liu, J. Ethical leadership and OCBE: The influence of prosocial motivation and self accountability. In *Academy of Management Annual Meeting Proceedings*; Academy of Management: Briarcliff Manor, NY, USA, 2016; p. 15588.
16. Guagnano, G.A.; Stern, P.C.; Dietz, T. Influences on attitude-behavior relationships: A natural experiment with curbside recycling. *Environ. Behav.* **1995**, *27*, 699–718. [CrossRef]
17. Xu, X.; Maki, A.; Chen, C.; Dong, B.; Day, J.K. Investigating willingness to save energy and communication about energy use in the American workplace with the attitude-behavior-context model. *Energy Res. Soc. Sci.* **2017**, *32*, 13–22. [CrossRef]
18. Boiral, O. Greening the corporation through organizational citizenship behaviors. *J. Bus. Ethics.* **2009**, *87*, 221–236. [CrossRef]
19. Ali, M.; Akhtar, N.; Anwar, F.; Usman, M. Spiritual leadership and organizational citizenship behavior for the environment. In *Academy of Management Annual Meeting Proceedings*; Academy of Management: Briarcliff Manor, NY, USA, 2020; p. 21062.
20. Zhang, J.; Yuan, Y.; Liu, J. The effect of ethical leadership on employees' organizational citizenship behavior for the environment. *Hum. Resou. Dev. China* **2018**, *35*, 19–29. [CrossRef]
21. Ahmad, S.; Islam, T.; Sadiq, M.; Kaleem, A. Promoting green behavior through ethical leadership: A model of green human resource management and environmental knowledge. *Leadersh. Org. Dev. J.* **2021**, *42*, 531–547. [CrossRef]
22. Khan, M.A.S.; Du, J.; Ali, M.; Saleem, S.; Usman, M. Interrelations between ethical leadership, green psychological climate, and organizational environmental citizenship behavior: A moderated mediation model. *Front. Psychol.* **2019**, *10*, 01977. [CrossRef]
23. Choi, Y.; Mai-Dalton, R.R. The model of followers' responses to self-sacrificial leadership: An empirical test. *Leadersh. Quart.* **1999**, *10*, 397–421. [CrossRef]
24. De Cremer, D.; van Knippenberg, D. Leader self-sacrifice and leadership effectiveness: The moderating role of leader self-confidence. *Organ. Behav. Hum. Dec.* **2004**, *95*, 140–155. [CrossRef]
25. Choi, Y.; Yoon, J. Effects of leaders' self-sacrificial behavior and competency on followers' attribution of charismatic leadership among Americans and Koreans. *Curr. Res. Soc. Psychol.* **2005**, *11*, 51–69.
26. Anser, M.K.; Shafique, S.; Usman, M.; Akhtar, N.; Ali, M. Spiritual leadership and organizational citizenship behavior for the environment: An intervening and interactional analysis. *J. Environ. Plann. Man.* **2021**, *64*, 1496–1514. [CrossRef]
27. Yam, K.C.; Klotz, A.C.; He, W.; Reynolds, S.J. From good soldiers to psychologically entitled: Examining when and why citizenship behavior leads to deviance. *Acad. Manag. J.* **2017**, *60*, 373–396. [CrossRef]
28. Halverson, S.K.; Holladay, C.L.; Kazama, S.M.; Quiñones, M.A. Self-sacrificial behavior in crisis situations: The competing roles of behavioral and situational factors. *Leadersh. Quart.* **2004**, *15*, 263–275. [CrossRef]
29. De Cremer, D.; van Knippenberg, D. Leader self-sacrifice and leadership effectiveness: The moderating role of leader prototypicality. *J. Appl. Psychol.* **2005**, *90*, 25–37. [CrossRef]
30. De Cremer, D.; Mayer, D.M.; van Dijke, M.; Schouten, B.C. When does self-sacrificial leadership motivate prosocial behavior? It depends on followers' prevention focus. *J. Appl. Psychol.* **2009**, *94*, 887–899. [CrossRef]
31. Turker, D. How corporate social responsibility influences organizational commitment. *J. Bus. Ethics* **2009**, *89*, 189–204. [CrossRef]
32. Roeck, K.D.; Delobbe, N. Do environmental CSR initiatives serve organizations' legitimacy in the oil industry? Exploring employees' reactions through organizational identification theory. *J. Bus. Ethics* **2012**, *110*, 397–412. [CrossRef]
33. Turker, D. Measuring corporate social responsibility: A scale development study. *J. Bus. Ethics* **2009**, *85*, 411–427. [CrossRef]
34. Luu, T.T. CSR and organizational citizenship behavior for the environment in hotel industry: The moderating roles of corporate entrepreneurship and employee attachment style. *Int. J. Contemp. Hosp. M.* **2017**, *29*, 2867–2900. [CrossRef]
35. Ong, M.; Mayer, D.M.; Tost, L.P.; Wellman, N. When corporate social responsibility motivates employee citizenship behavior: The sensitizing role of task significance. *Organ. Behav. Hum. Dec.* **2018**, *144*, 44–59. [CrossRef]
36. Wang, W.; Fu, Y.; Qiu, H.; Moore, J.H.; Wang, Z. Corporate social responsibility and employee outcomes: A moderated mediation model of organizational identification and moral identity. *Front. Psychol.* **2017**, *8*, 1906. [CrossRef] [PubMed]
37. Rupp, D.E.; Mallory, D.B. Corporate social responsibility: Psychological, person-centric, and progressing. *Annu. Rev. Organ. Psych.* **2015**, *2*, 211–236. [CrossRef]
38. Zhang, N.; Zhang, J.; Tian, H. Effects of corporate social responsibility characters on employee green behavior: Mechanism model based on ethical decision making. *Hum. Resou. Dev. China* **2021**, *38*, 33–47. [CrossRef]
39. Naz, S.; Jamshed, S.; Nisar, Q.A.; Nasir, N. Green HRM, psychological green climate and pro-environmental behaviors: An efficacious drive towards environmental performance in China. *Curr. Psychol.* **2021**, *40*, 1–16. [CrossRef]
40. Das, A.K.; Biswas, S.R.; Jilani, M.M.A.K.; Uddin, M. Corporate environmental strategy and voluntary environmental behavior—Mediating effect of psychological green climate. *Sustainability* **2019**, *11*, 3123. [CrossRef]
41. Dumont, J.; Shen, J.; Deng, X. Effects of green HRM practices on employee workplace green behavior: The role of psychological green climate and employee green values. *Hum. Resour. Manag.* **2017**, *56*, 613–627. [CrossRef]
42. Pham, N.T.; Thanh, T.V.; Tučková, Z.; Thuy, V.T.N. The role of green human resource management in driving hotel's environmental performance: Interaction and mediation analysis. *Int. J. Hosp. Manag.* **2020**, *88*, 102392. [CrossRef]

43. Norton, T.A.; Zacher, H.; Ashkanasy, N.M. Organizational sustainability policies and employee green behavior: The mediating role of work climate perceptions. *J. Environ. Psychol.* **2014**, *38*, 49–54. [CrossRef]
44. Zhang, J.; Liu, J. Organizational citizenship behavior for the environment: A Literature review and prospects. *Foreign Econ. Manag.* **2016**, *38*, 35–48. [CrossRef]
45. Tian, H.; Tian, J. Influence of environmentally-specific transformational leadership on employees' pro-environmental behavior. *J. Nanjing Tech. Univ. Soc. Sci. Ed.* **2020**, *19*, 76–89.
46. Reginal, L.; Rüdiger, H. Corporate greening beyond formal programs, initiatives, and systems: A conceptual model for voluntary pro-environmental behavior of employees. *Eur. Manag. Rev.* **2013**, *10*, 83–98.
47. Doty, D.H.; Glick, W.H. Common methods bias: Does common methods variance really bias results? *Organ. Res. Methods* **1998**, *1*, 374–406. [CrossRef]
48. Bledow, R.; Kühnel, J.; Jin, M.; Kuhl, J. Breaking the chains: The inverted-U-shaped relationship between action-state orientation and creativity under low job autonomy. *J. Manag.* **2022**, *48*, 905–935. [CrossRef]
49. Jiang, Z.; Hu, X.; Wang, Z.; Jiang, X. Knowledge hiding as a barrier to thriving: The mediating role of psychological safety and moderating role of organizational cynicism. *J. Organ. Behav.* **2019**, *40*, 800–818. [CrossRef]
50. Podsakoff, P.M.; MacKenzie, S.B.; Lee, J.Y.; Podsakoff, N.P. Common method biases in behavioral research: A critical review of the literature and recommended remedies. *J. Appl. Psychol.* **2003**, *88*, 879–903. [CrossRef]
51. Brislin, R.W. Back-translation for cross-cultural research. *J. Cross. Cult. Psychol.* **1970**, *1*, 185–216. [CrossRef]
52. Boiral, O.; Paillé, P. Organizational citizenship behavior for the environment: Measurement and validation. *J. Bus. Ethics* **2012**, *109*, 431–445. [CrossRef]
53. Hu, L.; Bentler, P.M. Cutoff criteria for fit indexes in covariance structure analysis: Conventional criteria versus new alternatives. *Struct. Equ. Modeling.* **1999**, *6*, 1–55. [CrossRef]
54. Baron, R.M.; Kenny, D.A. The moderator-mediator variable distinction in social psychological research: Conceptual, strategic, and statistical considerations. *J. Pers. Soc. Psychol.* **1986**, *51*, 1173–1182. [CrossRef]
55. Preacher, K.J.; Zyphur, M.J.; Zhang, Z. A general multilevel SEM framework for assessing multilevel mediation. *Psychol. Methods* **2010**, *15*, 209–233. [CrossRef] [PubMed]
56. Peloza, J.; White, K.; Shang, J. Good and guilt-free: The role of self-accountability in influencing preferences for products with ethical attributes. *J. Mark.* **2013**, *77*, 104–119. [CrossRef]
57. Grant, A.M.; Rothbard, N.P. When in doubt, seize the day? Security values, prosocial values, and proactivity under ambiguity. *J. Appl. Psychol.* **2013**, *98*, 810–819. [CrossRef] [PubMed]
58. Raineri, N.; Paille, P. Linking corporate policy and supervisory support with environmental citizenship behaviors: The role of employee environmental beliefs and commitment. *J. Bus. Ethics* **2016**, *137*, 129–148. [CrossRef]
59. Mansoor, A.; Farrukh, M.; Jahan, S.; Lee, J.K.; Wahab, S.A. Promoting green performance through green human resource practices and green servant leadership. *Asia. Pac. J. Hum. Resour.* **2021**, *59*. [CrossRef]
60. Kwan, K.H.; Chen, H.; Chiu, R.K. Effects of empowering leadership on followers' work-family interface. *Int. J. Hum. Resour. Man.* **2022**, *33*, 1403–1436. [CrossRef]

International Journal of
Environmental Research and Public Health

MDPI

Article

Investigating the Relationships between COVID-19 Quality of Life, Loneliness, Happiness, and Internet Addiction among K-12 Teachers and School Administrators—A Structural Equation Modeling Approach

Turgut Karakose [1], Tuncay Yavuz Ozdemir [2], Stamatios Papadakis [3,*], Ramazan Yirci [4], Secil Eda Ozkayran [5] and Hakan Polat [2]

1 Department of Educational Sciences, Faculty of Education, Kutahya Dumlupinar University, Kutahya 43100, Turkey; turgut.karakose@dpu.edu.tr
2 Department of Educational Sciences, Faculty of Education, Firat University, Elazig 23119, Turkey; tyavuz23@gmail.com (T.Y.O.); hakanpolat@firat.edu.tr (H.P.)
3 Department of Education, University of Crete, 74100 Rethymno, Greece
4 Department of Educational Sciences, Faculty of Education, Sutcuimam University, Kahramanmaras 46050, Turkey; yirci@ksu.edu.tr
5 Department of Educational Sciences, Faculty of Education, Bartin University, Bartin 74100, Turkey; sekartal@bartin.edu.tr
* Correspondence: stpapadakis@uoc.gr

Abstract: It is well acknowledged that the roles of both school administrators and teachers have changed due to the global education crisis caused by COVID-19. During this challenging and critical period, it is essential to investigate how those working in the education sector who undertake strategic tasks for sustainable education are affected by the new conditions brought about by the COVID-19 pandemic. This study investigates the interrelationships between COVID-19 quality of life, loneliness, happiness, and Internet addiction. The research was designed according to the relational survey model, was conducted with 432 school administrators and teachers working in K-12 schools. The research data was collected through online questionnaires, and structural equation modelling (SEM) was used to test and analyze proposed hypotheses. The study's results revealed a positive relationship between the COVID-19 related quality of life and loneliness, and that loneliness significantly positively predicts Internet addiction. In this context, due to the impact of COVID-19 on the life quality, the participants' loneliness levels significantly increased, and this increase in loneliness caused them to become addicted to using the Internet. Interestingly, it was also determined that a positive relationship exists between loneliness and happiness and that as the loneliness of individuals increased, their level of happiness also increased. In many studies conducted prior to the COVID-19 pandemic, a negative relationship was revealed between loneliness and happiness. In the current study conducted during the pandemic, the relationship between the two variables was positive. SEM results revealed that COVID-19 directly affects the quality of life, Internet addiction, loneliness, and happiness of school administrators and teachers. Furthermore, it was determined that Internet addiction indirectly affects the relationship between loneliness and happiness.

Keywords: COVID-19; pandemic; COVID-19 quality of life; loneliness; Internet addiction; happiness; school administrator; teacher; K-12 education; structural equation modelling

1. Introduction

Humankind has faced many pandemics of different types from the past to the present, and significant numbers of people have lost their lives during these times. Successive plagues related to the Black Death (c. 1347–1351) saw humanity left practically helpless and powerless, as did the Spanish flu, which resulted in the death of millions of people worldwide [1]. These pandemics, which emerged suddenly and spread rapidly, brought radical societal changes. Today, humanity is again struggling with a deadly pandemic, COVID-19, and the psychosocial and economic effects of this pandemic have affected practically every aspect of modern-day human life, and as such, have been profoundly and widely felt on a global scale.

The COVID-19 disease, which first appeared in Wuhan in China's Hubei province in December 2019, was soon declared a global pandemic by the World Health Organization (WHO) in March 2020. It led to an unprecedented worldwide public health crisis [2–5] in just a short time. Most governments reacted similarly, if not together, against the spread and effect of the virus, recognizing that if its spread were left uncontrolled, the ensuing loss of life would be devastating. As a result, degrees of quarantine were imposed worldwide via government mandate and local regulation, albeit with varying degrees of scope and strictness of application [6].

As a result, the adverse effects of the pandemic suppressed many areas of human social life, such as health, education, the economy, sports, and religious activities, which effectively impacted practically everyone's lives and harmed the daily operations of most companies and institutions in some way. From this perspective, the COVID-19 global pandemic has impacted the social dimensions of life more than the individual. Therefore, it was perhaps inevitable that COVID-19 would soon become a field of significant research activity for many disciplines [7]. Since the beginning of the COVID-19 pandemic, it has been observed that human behaviours and habits, shaped from hundreds of years of experience, underwent a rapid and radical change in just a brief period. The situation that emerged due to these changes was the "new normal" [8]. People unprepared for the chaos caused by the pandemic were directly affected in terms of their health and economic and sociocultural aspects [4,9–13]. The global infectious diseases of such pandemics negatively affect the physical, social, and psychological functions of both individuals and societies as a whole and thereby result in a widespread impact of significant and essential consequences [13,14]. In addition, during such pandemics, it becomes essential to understand the reflections of people's psychological states [15].

This study's primary focus is to examine the interrelationships between COVID-19 quality of life, loneliness, happiness, and Internet addiction among school administrators and teachers. The spread of the epidemic, schools' closure and the transition to distance education started a new process for students, teachers, and school administrators [16]. Uncertainty brought by the pandemic has caused some crises in education, and school administrators and teachers have been negatively affected by this crisis. Dealing with many problems such as the deterioration of work-life balance, psychological disorders, and the negative impact on the quality of life with COVID-19 has also affected teachers' and school administrators' happiness levels. When the academic databases are examined, it is seen that very few of them have a positive perspective on the effects of the pandemic. It also seems that there are a few studies in positive education during the pandemic [17]. Another problem is that scientific literature mainly focuses on clinical the effects of the COVID-19 rather than the psychosocial effects. It is undeniable that if the psychological aspect of the fight against the epidemic is neglected, the struggle will be incomplete.

Teachers and school administrators, who ensured the continuation of educational activities throughout the epidemic, have undertaken essential responsibilities. It has been considered essential to examine the relationships between the quality of life, happiness levels, loneliness, and Internet addiction levels of teachers and school administrators, who have continued their responsibilities such as being a source of motivation for students, leading and being a role model during the pandemic period [18]. When the COVID-19 literature is examined, it has been seen that there are very few studies focusing on the psychological state of school administrators and teachers during the epidemic. This specific research is the outcome of a modest effort to fill this gap in the field.

2. Literature Review

In 1948, the World Health Organization defined health as "not merely the absence of disease but a state of complete physical, mental and social well-being" [19]. It was also emphasized that people's lives are meaningful and should be experienced at a certain level of "life quality". The World Health Organization has conducted or supported many studies since the 1980s to measure and evaluate the quality of life [20]. The restrictions concerning the COVID-19 pandemic, to which people were previously largely unaccustomed, undoubtedly harmed their quality of life.

The concept of quality of life dates back to ancient times in sociology and medicine. Plato's "Republic" (427–347 BC) and Aristotle's "Nicomachus Ethics" (384–322 BC), both written in ancient times, include serious discussion on the quality of life and shows how the concept has long existed from our distant past right through until today [21]. The World Health Organization defines the quality of life as the standard of living that individuals perceive in line with their culture, values, goals, and expectations from life [22]. In addition, quality of life is seen as a comprehensive health outcome that reflects individuals' perceptions of physical and mental health, social relationships, and general well-being [23,24]. In the related literature, it has been suggested that quality of life is an essential predictor of the permanence of overall health and well-being [19]. Despite the perceived importance of quality of life in health and medicine, there is an ongoing conceptual and methodological debate about its true meaning and what it should measure [25].

The quarantine, lockdown, and curfew practices introduced during the COVID-19 pandemic effectively cut off or dramatically curtailed most forms of direct contact between people not of the same household. This situation exacerbated feelings of loneliness considerably more during the pandemic [26–28]. Although loneliness is a universal problem, the relevant literature contains numerous studies that have been conducted on the topic of loneliness in recent years. In the foundation of this feeling, a more intense perception of loneliness exists connected to sociocultural structure and dynamics [29]. Sigmund Freud first used the term loneliness in 1939 to describe a person's internal structure, which can change completely after the experience of loneliness. Years later, Sullivan detailed Freud's definition of loneliness, arguing that humans are social animals that need contact and that loneliness is considered the result of this need going unmet [30]. Individuals can experience inadequate relationships and social lives that are not perceived as individually satisfactory can profoundly affect their lives. This situation has caused individuals to isolate themselves from society further and thereby experience profound loneliness [31,32].

Although loneliness is a known human emotion, it is also considered a complex situation experienced differently by each individual, and therefore cannot be explained with a single reason. Measures and practices that aim to eliminate the feelings of loneliness may differ according to the individual [33]. The definition of loneliness is a situation in which interpersonal relationships deteriorate, social participation decreases, and an individual can feel lonely and misunderstood [34]. The changing living conditions can exemplify this due to mandatory social restrictions introduced during the COVID-19 pandemic. During this process, individuals became isolated within closed areas, and the increasing amount of time they spent being inactive also directly affected their quality of life [35]. Among the measures implemented during the pandemic, the most common was social isolation, a measure that dramatically changed the lifestyle and habits of many individuals worldwide [36]. As a result, social relations decreased, and loneliness increased due to this enforced period of extended isolation [37]. Studies have shown that high-level restrictions can result in loneliness due to quarantine measures and that loneliness is associated with higher psychosocial distress and lower life satisfaction [38].

Another behavioural change observed in people during the COVID-19 pandemic was digital media usage. With people primarily forced to stay in their homes during the pandemic, many started to spend more time using the Internet [39–41]; however, in utilizing the Internet, many borders and barriers between people were effectively removed, or at least circumnavigated. In addition, with the speed of today's Internet-based communication, the medium has helped make people's lives easier and, as such, has become a tool associated with an increased quality of life. With its various functionality and ubiquitous spread, digital media has become a phenomenon that needs to be considered sociologically, psychologically, and socially [42].

The 2020 World Internet Usage and Social Media Statistics report published by We Are Social stated that the number of people using the Internet worldwide had increased by 7% (298 million new users) compared to data reported in only January 2019, reaching a new total of 4.54 billion global users. The average Internet user spends 6 h and 43 min online every day, which is 3 min less than in the previous year but equal more than 100 days of connected time per Internet user per year. Considering that an average person has about 8 h of sleep every 24, their Internet usage now constitutes more than 40% of each person's waking time [43].

In the related literature, Internet addiction has been defined as an impulse control disorder unrelated to using intoxicating substances [44]. It has been stated that people addicted to using the Internet cannot control their usage and experience feelings of anxiety when they are unable to do so. In addition, it is known that even if they make efforts to reduce their Internet usage, they may fail in that endeavour and subsequently try to hide their continued usage [45]. It became inevitable that irregular use of the Internet, at more moderate and controlled levels, has fast become a thing of the past, and that has been especially notable during the COVID-19 pandemic period [46]. However, during this period, people have been essentially forced to spend more time at home and conduct most of their work remotely using online tools, and a need for increased social usage has significantly increased many people's daily Internet usage. The researches on the relationship between internet addiction, happiness and loneliness have different results in different samples. For instance, Alqahtani et al. [47] found that there is no relationship between internet addiction, loneliness and life satisfaction ($p > 0.01$) in the Saudi population; however, Erol and Cirak [48] found a significant correlation between loneliness and Internet addiction in the Turkish context. Ansari et al. [49] found that participants' happiness scores were statistically significantly associated with internet addiction.

Various research has demonstrated that the COVID-19 pandemic has deeply affected people's moods and that this effect has been primarily negative [50–52]. The negative emotional states experienced by people during the pandemic have also reduced their happiness levels [53–55]. One of the most basic human needs is happiness, as when individuals are happy, they feel more prosperous and more secure. Happiness has the potential to make every moment of life different [56]. In essence, an individual experiences more positive emotions than negative, and the more satisfied they are with their life in general, the greater the level of happiness they will likely experience. However, the negative impact of living with a contagious and pandemic disease on happiness is undeniable [57,58]. Therefore, it has been stated that experiencing fear of COVID-19 can directly reduce happiness amongst individuals and negatively affect their mental health [59]. Curfews and lockdowns imposed at the national and/or local level, especially in Europe and the United States, have led to significant increases in searches on topics such as boredom, loneliness, anxiety, and sadness in the Google search engine [60].

During the COVID-19 pandemic, people in many countries worldwide experienced some form of negative emotional experience. The concept of "new normal" that emerged with COVID-19 has dramatically affected the individuals' life quality, and therefore their perception of loneliness. At the same time, with the temporary (and some permanent) closure of businesses and services experienced during the pandemic period, an inevitable rise in Internet addiction amongst individuals has been seen to increase. As such, their happiness expectations have also significantly changed.

3. Materials and Methods

3.1. Purpose of the Study and Hypotheses

The current study examined the interrelationships between COVID-19 quality of life, loneliness, happiness, and Internet addiction among school administrators and teachers. The Structural Equation Model (SEM) was selected, a comprehensive method that discovers and confirms causality between various variables and combines different analyses such as multiple regression, path analysis, and factor analysis [61]. In this context, the hypotheses developed in line with the general purpose of the current research are as follows:

Hypothesis 1 (H1): *COVID-19′s impact on quality of life is positively associated with loneliness.*

Hypothesis 2 (H2): *Loneliness is positively related to Internet addiction.*

Hypothesis 3 (H3): *Loneliness is negatively related to happiness.*

Hypothesis 4 (H4): *Internet addiction is negatively related to happiness.*

Hypothesis 5 (H5): *Internet addiction indirectly affects the relationship between loneliness and happiness.*

Figure 1 presents a hypothetical model for the relationships between the variables examined in the study.

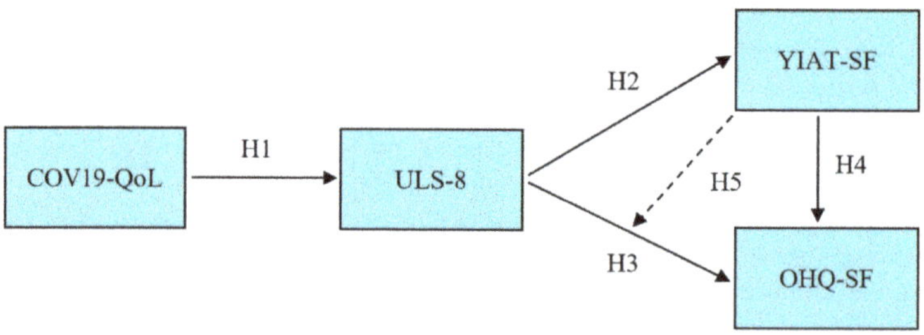

Figure 1. Hypothesized relationships of the research model [COV19-QoL = COVID-19 Quality of Life; ULS-8 = Loneliness; YIAT-SF = Internet Addiction; OHQ-SF = Happiness].

3.2. Study Design

The research is a relational study that examines the COVID-19 related quality of life and the relationships between loneliness, happiness, and Internet addiction levels amongst teachers and school administrators. A relational study was selected to examine relationships between variables [62,63]. Within the scope of the current research, a multifactorial predictive correlational design was employed. This design analyzed direct and indirect causal relationships between independent and dependent variables [61,64]. In this context, the study examines in detail the effect of COVID-19 as experienced by school administrators and teachers on their quality of life and examines the direct and indirect relationships between loneliness, happiness, and Internet addiction.

3.3. Participants

This study, conducted using Structural Equation Modeling (SEM), was deemed appropriate to determine the sample size required by structural modelling, as SEM tests are sensitive to sample size [65]. In this context, it has been stated that it is appropriate for the sample size to be ten times the number of items (variables) [66]. Accordingly, a sample size of at least 320 participants was deemed sufficient for the current study, considering its total of 32 variables (items). It was also considered possible that some participants may complete the data collection instrument incompletely or incorrectly, and therefore the scale was applied to a more significant number of participants to reach a sufficient sample of acceptable data.

Using simple random sampling, 454 people were determined and included. According to the Ministry of Education statistics, 7.452 teachers work at 581 Kutahya province (Turkey) schools. The researchers defined the 88 schools randomly and contacted the principals via email and telephone. The research purpose was explained, and they were kindly requested to participate in the research. The scales were submitted electronically via Google Forms. As a result of the initial data analysis, 22 were excluded from the dataset due to extreme values. Therefore, the research was conducted with 432 school administrators and teachers working in K-12 schools during the 2021-2022 academic year in Kutahya. The sociodemographic characteristics of the participants are presented in Table 1.

Table 1. Sociodemographic profile of the respondents.

Variables	Description	*f* (*N* = 432)	(%)
Gender	Male	182	42.1
	Female	250	57.9
Age (years)	20–30	36	8.3
	31–40	276	63.9
	41+	120	27.8
Occupation	Teacher	210	48.6
	Vice-principal	134	31.0
	Principal	88	20.4
Seniority (service years)	0–5	20	4.6
	6–10	106	24.5
	11–15	136	31.5
	16–20	102	23.6
	21+	68	15.7
COVID-19 infected (self)	Yes	104	24.1
	No	328	75.9
COVID-19 vaccinated (self)	Yes	398	92.1
	No	34	7.9
Daily Internet usage (hours)	1–2	56	13.0
	2–3	150	34.7
	3–4	118	27.3
	4–5	64	14.8
	5+	44	10.2

When the summary data in Table 1 are examined, it can be seen that the ratio of male and female participants is close to each other. Additionally, the rate of teachers and administrators infected with COVID-19 was low (7.9%). This situation may be explained by the high "vaccination" rates, also shown in Table 1. According to data from the Turkish Ministry of National Education, the rate of teachers having received two doses of a COVID-19 vaccine has reached 86%. According to the national data, as of 8 November 2021, the entire Turkish population's vaccination rate was 79.25% [67]. Therefore, the rate of teachers having received a double vaccine dose is higher than that of the general population. Another interesting aspect of the data shown in Table 1 is that the rate of participants whose daily Internet usage was 5 h or more was 10.2%.

3.4. Data Collection and Data Analysis

3.4.1. Measurements

Within the scope of the research, the study's data were collected using the COVID-19 Quality of Life Scale (COV19-QoL), the Oxford Happiness Questionnaire Short Form (OHQ-SF), the Short-form UCLA Loneliness Scale (ULS-8), the Short form of Young's Internet Addiction Test (YIAT-SF), as well as a Personal Information Form developed by the researchers for the study.

The scales used in the study were reviewed and their application approved by the Kutahya Governorship and Provincial Directorate of National Education, with legal permission granted for the study to be performed with K-12 teachers and school administrators (Permit: 53490996-44-E.7646169).

COVID-19 Quality of Life Scale (COV19-QoL)

The original COV19-QoL scale was developed by Repišti et al. [68], and Sümen and Adibelli [69] subsequently conducted a Turkish validity and reliability study. The Turkish version (COV19-QoLTR) consists of six items covering mental health's leading quality of life areas. The scale is a five-point, Likert type (1 = *Strongly disagree* to 5 = *Strongly agree*) instrument that aims to evaluate the feelings and thoughts of individuals during the past seven days. There are no reverse-coded items on the scale. The scale's score is calculated by dividing the total score by the number of items. A higher score indicates a more significant impact of the pandemic on the individual's quality of life. The Cronbach's alpha coefficient of the COV19-QoLTR scale was 0.910 for the data obtained from the general population [69].

Oxford Happiness Questionnaire Short Form (OHQ-SF)

The OHQ-SF scale, which was developed initially by Hills and Argyle [70] to measure an individual's level of happiness, was adapted to the Turkish context by Dogan and Cotok [71]. The scale consists of seven items formed as a five-point, Likert-type instrument, and both Item 1 and Item 7 are reverse-coded. High scores achieved from the scale indicate a high level of happiness. The internal consistency coefficient of the one-dimensional scale was calculated as 0.74, and the test-retest reliability coefficient was 0.85.

Short-Form UCLA Loneliness Scale (ULS-8)

The ULS-8 scale was originally developed by Hays and DiMatteo [72] and later adapted to the Turkish context by Yıldız and Duy [73]. The scale consists of seven items as a five-point, Likert-type instrument scale, with Item 5 being reverse-coded. As a result of Exploratory Factor Analysis, the scale consisted of a single dimension. Confirmatory Factor Analysis revealed that the unidimensional structure showed a good fit ($\chi^2 = 27.12$, $SD = 14$, $\chi^2/SD = 1.94$, RMSEA = 0.06, RMR = 0.03, SRMR = 0.04, GFI = 0.97, AGFI = 0.95, CFI = 0.98), NFI = 0.96, NNFI = 0.97). A low score from the ULS-8 scale indicates a low feeling of loneliness, while a high score indicates increased loneliness. The internal consistency coefficient of the scale was calculated as 0.74, with a test-retest reliability coefficient of 0.84.

Short-Form of Young's Internet Addiction Test (YIAT-SF)

The YIAT-SF scale was adapted to Turkish by Kutlu et al. [74]. The scale is constructed as a five-point, Likert type (1 = *Never* to 5 = *Always*) instrument with 12 items formed within a single dimension. There are no reverse-coded items in the YIAT-SF scale. The combined score obtainable from the scale can vary between the lowest score of 12 and the highest of 60, with a higher score indicating a higher level of Internet addiction. The Cronbach's alpha coefficient of the scale was calculated as 0.91 for university students and 0.86 for adolescents.

3.4.2. Data Analysis

After obtaining the necessary permissions to conduct the research, the data collection instruments were sent to the participants online. The obtained data were then analyzed using IBM's SPSS package program, with the Maximum Likelihood method applied using the SPSS Amos module. Sample size, multicollinearity problem, normality, and extreme values were also examined as prerequisites for applying the Structural Equation Model (SEM) [75]. First, the Z-score values of the variables were excluded from the dataset, with 22 data outliers found not between −1 and +1. Next, correlation analysis was performed to determine multicollinearity problems among the variables. Where correlation values are below 0.90, it may be said that no multicollinearity problem exists [75]. In the analysis performed in the current study, correlations between the variables were examined, and it was determined that the correlation coefficients between the variables were all below the 0.90 value (see Table 2). In line with this data finding, it was determined that no multicollinearity problem was found to exist between the variables. To determine the multicollinearity problem, the VIF and tolerance values of the independent variables were examined, and it was determined that the values did not cause any multicollinearity problems (see Table 3). Another prerequisite for SEM analysis is that the data exhibits normal distribution. The analysis examined the kurtosis and skewness values of the variables, and it was determined that the dataset was normally distributed (see Table 4).

Table 2. Correlation values between scales.

Scale	COV19-QoL	OHQ-SF	ULS-8	YIAT-SF
COVID-19 Quality of Life Scale (COV19-QoL)	1	0.160	−0.221	−0.096
Oxford Happiness Questionnaire Short Form (OHQ-SF)		1	−0.279	−0.094
Short-Form UCLA Loneliness Scale (ULS-8)			1	0.149
Short form of Young's Internet Addiction Test (YIAT-SF)				1

Table 3. VIF and Tolerance values of independent variables.

Scale	VIF	Tolerance
COVID-19 Quality of Life Scale (COV19-QoL)	1.033	0.968
Oxford Happiness Questionnaire Short Form (OHQ-SF)	1.033	0.968
Short-Form UCLA Loneliness Scale (ULS-8)	1.016	0.984

Table 4. Mean, standard deviation, skewness, and kurtosis values of the scales ($N = 432$).

Scale	Min	Max	$\bar{X}$	*SD*	Skewness	Kurtosis
COV19-QoL	1.00	4.00	1.5139	0.7645	0.933	0.867
OHQ-SF	1.00	5.00	2.4074	1.132	0.520	−0.628
ULS-8	1.00	5.00	3.2963	0.9849	−0.124	−0.549
YIAT-SF	1.00	5.00	3.2130	1.119	0.051	−0.863

Therefore, it was taken into account that the data obtained within the scope of the research showed normal distribution, that the sample size was sufficient, and that neither linearity nor multicollinearity problems were present. The covariance matrix and the Maximum Likelihood methods were applied to test the measurement and structural models. In analyzing the data, the impact of COVID-19 on quality of life and the measurement models of the variables of happiness, loneliness, and Internet addiction were tested with Confirmatory Factor Analysis (CFA). Whether or not the measurement models were validated was examined using the Chi-square $(\chi^2)/SD$, GFI, AGFI, CFI, RMSEA, IFI, and TLI (NNFI) fit indices. Finally, whether or not the proposed hypothetical model was confirmed was then examined according to the specified fit indices. Diagrams were created using Flowchart Maker & Online Diagram Software [76].

4. Results

The findings obtained from the correlation analysis of the data collection tools applied in the study are presented in Table 2.

Table 2 shows that the COVID-19 related quality of life had a positive relationship with happiness ($r = 0.160$, $p < 0.01$), whereas loneliness had a negative relationship with COVID-19 related quality of life ($r = -0.221$, $p < 0.01$), and Internet addiction had a significant negative relationship with COVID-19 related quality of life ($r = -0.096$, $p < 0.01$). In addition, negative relationships were revealed between happiness and loneliness ($r = -0.279$, $p < 0.01$), and between happiness and Internet addiction ($r = -0.094$, $p < 0.01$). Finally, the relationship between loneliness and Internet addiction was positive ($r = 0.0149$, $p < 0.01$) at a significant level. When these findings were evaluated, the correlations between the variables ranged from −0.279 and 0.149. These values also show that no multicollinearity problem existed between the study variables.

Table 3 presents the VIF and tolerance values for the independent variables in the measurement model.

Cokluk et al. [75] emphasized that VIF values should be less than ten and tolerance values greater than 0.10. Accordingly, when Table 3 is examined, it can be seen that no multicollinearity or multicollinearity problems were found between the variables examined in the current study.

In Table 4, the mean, standard deviation, skewness, and kurtosis values of the measurement model variables.

Finally, the data were examined in order to determine whether or not it was normally distributed. According to Table 4, the skewness value was 0.933, and the kurtosis value was 0.867 for the Impact of COVID-19 on Quality of Life. For the Oxford Happiness Scale Short Form, the skewness value was 0.520, and the kurtosis value was −0.628. For the UCLA Loneliness Scale Short Form, the skewness value was −0.124, and the kurtosis value was −0.549. For the Short form of Young's Internet Addiction Scale, the skewness value was 0.051, and the kurtosis value was −0.863. In light of these results, it may be said that the skewness coefficients of the variables were found to be within acceptable limits and that the data exhibited a normal distribution.

When Table 4 is examined, the scores obtained from the COVID-19 Quality of Life Scale on the impact of the pandemic on the quality of life can be seen to vary between 1 and 4. The participants' opinions presented an average score of $\overline{X} = 1.1539$ ($SD = 0.7645$), which may be interpreted as the pandemic having impacted little on the participants' quality of life. The scores obtained from the Oxford Happiness Questionnaire Short-Form scale ranged from 1 to 5, with an average value of $\overline{X} = 2.4074$ ($SD = 1.132$), which points to a moderate happiness score during the COVID-19 pandemic. Although the scores obtained from the Short-Form UCLA Loneliness Scale varied between 1 and 5, the participant opinions averaged at $\overline{X} = 3.2963$ ($SD = 0.9849$), which may be interpreted as a high level of loneliness experienced the pandemic. The scores obtained from the short form of Young's Internet Addiction Test ranged from 1 to 5, and the participants' opinions had an arithmetic mean of 3.213 ($SD = 1.119$), which are considered above the medium level. As known, the Internet addiction of individuals has increased during the COVID-19 pandemic. In addition, when the kurtosis and skewness values of the dataset were examined, it was determined that the data exhibited a normal distribution.

4.1. Assessment of Measurement Model

Before assessing the structural model, Cronbach's Alpha values of the scales were examined for construct reliability. The reliability values (Cronbach's Alpha) were 0.84, 0.89, 0.77 and 0.89 as presented by Table 6. Therefore the reliability of the scales were confirmed. In addition, we examined the validity of the scales used in the research, and confirmatory factor analysis was conducted. Confirmatory Factor Analysis of measurement tools used in SEM research should be repeated with the existing dataset. For this purpose, relevant analyses of the scales applied in the study were conducted. The fit indices of this analysis are presented in Table 5.

Table 5. Confirmatory Factor Analysis results of the scales.

Scale	χ^2/SD	GFI	AGFI	IFI	TLI	CFI	RMSEA
COV19-QoL	3.292	0.982	0.947	0.990	0.977	0.989	0.073
OHQ-SF	1.923	0.987	0.969	0.984	0.972	0.983	0.046
ULS-8	2.932	0.979	0.951	0.975	0.956	0.975	0.067
YIAT-SF	3.974	0.928	0.896	0.942	0.924	0.941	0.083

The COVID-19 Quality of Life Scale (COV19-QoL) is a one-dimensional scale of six items. The measurement model was tested with first-level CFA, and it was found that all paths related to the six items in the scale were statistically significant at the 0.01 level. According to the CFA results, the *t*-values of the scale varied between 10,041 and 13,702. Values for the COV19-QoL scale were established as $\chi^2/SD = 3.292$, GFI = 0.982, AGFI = 0.947, IFI = 0.990, TLI = 0.977, CFI = 0.989, and RMSEA = 0.073 (see Table 5). According to the CFA results, it was determined that the GFI, IFI, TLI, CFI, and RMSEA values had a good fit and that the χ^2/SD value was revealed as being in the acceptable range.

The Oxford Happiness Questionnaire Short Form (OHQ-SF) is a one-dimensional scale consisting of seven items. With CFA, all of the paths except for Item 7 in the scale were statistically significant at the 0.01 level. Since the path for Item 7 was not statistically significant, the item was excluded from the analysis. In the subsequent analysis, it was determined that the *t*-values of the scale varied between 10,041 and 13,702. In addition, the OHQ-SF scale was found to have values of $\chi^2/SD = 1.923$, GFI = 0.987, AGFI = 0.969, IFI = 0.984, TLI = 0.972, CFI = 0.983, and RMSEA = 0.046 (see Table 5), and that all of these values can be said to have a good fit.

The Short-Form UCLA Loneliness Scale (ULS-8) consists of one dimension and seven items. With CFA, it was seen that all paths related to the seven items in the scale were statistically significant at the 0.01 level. According to the CFA results, the *t*-values of the scale varied between 10,041 and 13,702. The values for the ULS-8 scale were $\chi^2/SD = 2.932$, GFI = 0.979, AGFI = 0.951, IFI = 0.975, TLI = 0.956, CFI = 0.975, and RMSEA = 0.067 (see Table 5), and all of these values can be said to have a good fit.

The Short-Form of Young's Internet Addiction Test (YIAT-SF) is a one-dimensional scale consisting of 12 items. The measurement model was tested with CFA, and all paths related to the 12 items in the scale were found to be statistically significant at the 0.01 level. According to the CFA results, the *t*-values varied between 10,041 and 13,702. The values of the YIAT-SF scale were established as being $\chi^2/SD = 3.974$, GFI = 0.928, AGFI = 0.896, IFI = 0.942, TLI = 0.924, CFI = 0.941, and RMSEA = 0.083 (see Table 5). According to the CFA results, it was determined that the χ^2/SD, GFI, IFI, TLI, and CFI values were within the acceptable range and that the RMSEA value had a good fit.

Construct validity was also examined using average variance extracted (AVE) and composite reliability (CR) in the research. Composite reliability (CR) score should exceed the acceptable value of 0.7 for all factors, and the average variance extracted (AVE) must be greater than 0.5 for all variables [77–79]. AVE and CR scores can be seen in Table 6.

Table 6. Reliability and convergent validity results.

Constructs	Cronbach's Alpha	CR	AVE
COV19-QoL	0.84	0.72	0.68
ULS-8	0.77	0.71	0.67
OHQ-SF	0.89	0.70	0.66
YIAT-SF	0.89	0.71	0.66

It can be seen in Table 6 that Cronbach's Alpha scores range from 0.77 to 0.89. AVE scores are above 0.50, and CR scores are above 0.70 for each construct, showing the constructs' consistency. In the light of these results, we can state that convergent validity was established.

4.2. Assessment of the Structural Model

For research purposes, the direct relationship of COVID-19's effect on the quality of life with loneliness and loneliness with happiness and Internet addiction were investigated according to SEM (see the hypothetical model presented in Figure 1). In addition, the mediating effect of happiness in the relationship between loneliness and Internet addiction was also examined. Testing the final model revealed that the *t*-values ranged from −14,619 to 24,824. In addition, the standardized path coefficient between the COVID-19 related quality of life and loneliness in the model was found to be 0.45, and the standardized path coefficient between loneliness and happiness was found to be 0.01. The fit indices of the hypothetical model can be seen in Table 7.

Table 7. Fit indices of the structural model.

Fit Indices	Good Fit	Acceptable Fit	Structural Model
X^2/sd	$0 \leq \chi^2/sd \leq 3$	$3 \leq \chi^2/sd \leq 5$	3.66
CFI	$0.95 \leq CFI \leq 1.00$	$0.90 \leq CFI \leq 0.95$	0.89
AGFI	$0.90 \leq AGFI \leq 1.00$	$0.85 \leq AGFI \leq 0.90$	0.89
GFI	$0.95 \leq GFI \leq 1.00$	$0.90 \leq GFI \leq 95$	0.89
TLI	$0.95 \leq TLI \leq 1.00$	$0.90 \leq TLI \leq 0.95$	0.89
IFI	$0.95 \leq IFI \leq 1.00$	$0.90 \leq IFI \leq 0.95$	0.90
RMSEA	$0.00 \leq RMSEA \leq 0.05$	$0.05 \leq RMSEA \leq 0.08$	0.08

Source: [80–85].

The fit indices of the hypothetical model were calculated as $\chi^2/SD = 3.66$. In addition, the values were determined as GFI = 0.89, AGFI = 0.89, IFI = 0.90, TLI = 0.89, CFI = 0.89, and RMSEA = 0.08. When the fit indices of the model were examined, it can be seen that all values had an acceptable fit except GFI and TLI values, however; the GFI and TLI values in the model are very close to the acceptable fit. Schermelleh-Engel & Moosbrugger [85] state that it is always possible that a model may fit the data, although one or more fit measures may suggest a bad fit. As a result, the analyses showed that the final hypothetical model outlined in the research could be said to be confirmed. In this context, the proposed SEM is presented in Figure 2.

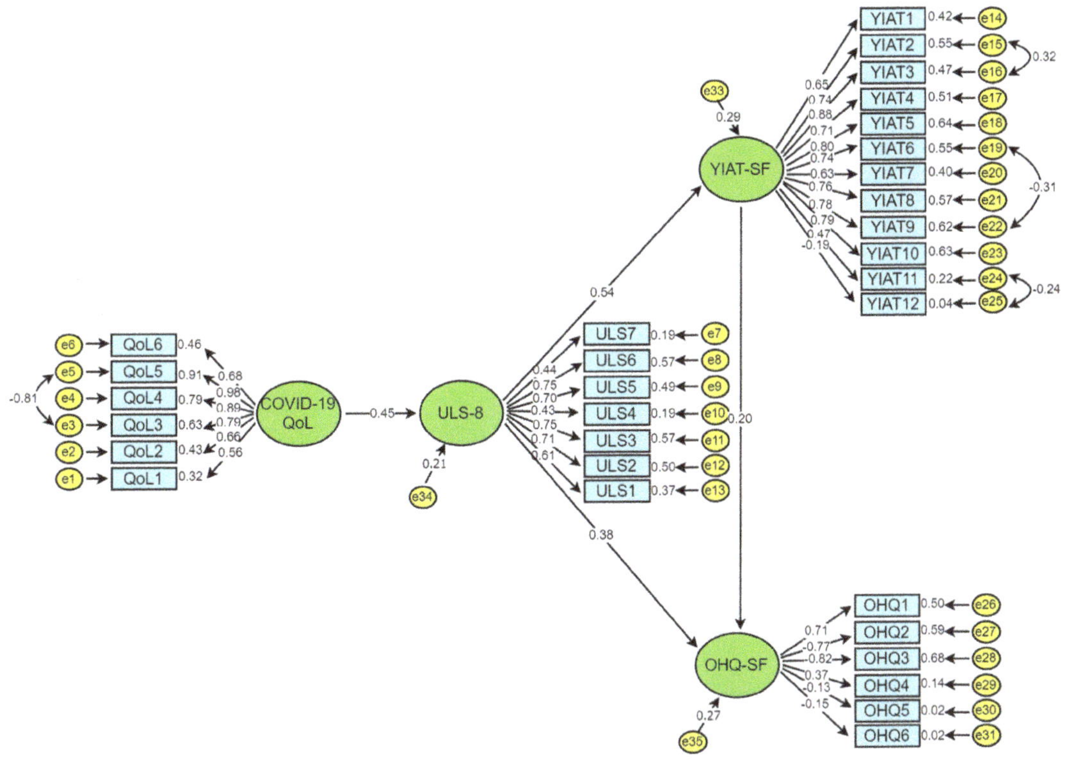

Figure 2. Final hypothesized model.

The standardized regression coefficient between the COVID-19 related quality of life and loneliness was calculated as 0.45. This value shows a positive relationship between the COVID-19 related quality of life and loneliness, which explained 47.6% of the variance of loneliness. Kline [65] stated that an effect size of around 0.10 is considered "small", whereas an effect size of around 0.30 is "medium", and an effect size of around 0.50 is described as "large". Accordingly, the standardized regression coefficient between the COVID-19 related quality of life and loneliness can have a medium effect size. This result shows that the COVID-19 related quality of life positively and significantly predicts loneliness. In other words, as the impact of COVID-19 on the quality of life of individuals increases, their level of loneliness also increases to a significant degree. This result revealed that the first hypothesis of the research (H1: "COVID-19′s impact on quality of life is positively associated with loneliness") is confirmed.

The standardized regression coefficient between loneliness and Internet addiction was 0.54. This value shows that a positive relationship exists between loneliness and Internet addiction. Loneliness was shown to explain 20.3% of the variance of Internet addiction. The standardized regression coefficient between loneliness and Internet addiction shows a large effect size, and it can therefore be said that loneliness predicts Internet addiction positively and with statistical significance. This result reveals that the second hypothesis of the research (H2: "Loneliness is positively related to Internet addiction") is confirmed.

In Figure 2, it can be seen that the standardized regression coefficient between loneliness and happiness is 0.38. This finding reveals a positive and moderate relationship between loneliness and happiness. In other words, as the loneliness of individuals increased, the level of their happiness also increased. Loneliness was shown to explain a 36.2% variance of happiness, and therefore that it has a moderate effect on the happiness levels of individuals. This result revealed that the third hypothesis of the research (H3: "Loneliness is negatively related to happiness") is rejected. While in many studies prior to the pandemic, a negative relationship was established between loneliness and happiness, in the current study conducted during the COVID-19 pandemic, the relationship between the two variables was positive. This may be explained by those individuals with increased levels of loneliness, being in isolation from their normal social life, having felt more positive regarding the effect of their loneliness, having considered that they were more protected and safer from the negative effects of the virus. In addition, the satisfaction of individuals who had the opportunity to spend more time with their families during the pandemic may have affected this result. Therefore, the positive relationship between happiness and loneliness can also be remarkable in revealing an indirect effect of the pandemic on the mood of individuals.

When Figure 2 is examined, it can be seen that the standardized regression coefficient between Internet addiction and happiness was 0.20. This finding reveals a positive relationship between Internet addiction and happiness, and Internet addiction explained a 36% variance in happiness. In light of this finding, it may be said that Internet addiction positively and significantly predicts the happiness of individuals to a statistical degree. This result reveals that the fourth hypothesis of the research (H4: "Internet addiction is negatively related to happiness") is rejected.

The increased Internet usage levels of individuals during the COVID-19 pandemic period can be interpreted as having protected individuals from some of the negative effects of the pandemic and thereby contributed positively to their happiness levels. This result reveals that the fifth hypothesis of the research (H5: "Internet addiction indirectly affects the relationship between loneliness and happiness") is confirmed. In this context, Figure 2 shows that Internet addiction (0.54 * 0.20 = 0.108) had a 10.8% indirect effect on the relationship between loneliness and happiness. In the final hypothetical model tested through SEM, it was found that the COVID-19 related quality of life predicted the loneliness level of individuals, and as the loneliness level of individuals increased, their Internet addiction and happiness levels also increased.

5. Discussion

The research findings revealed a strong positive relationship between the impact of COVID-19 on the quality of life and the loneliness level of the participants. In this context, the individuals experienced increased loneliness as the impact of COVID-19 on their quality of life increased. Due to the rapid transmission and increased mortality from COVID-19, governments worldwide soon implemented extraordinary measures in an attempt to contain the next pandemic [86–88]. The quality of life was adversely affected due to curfews, travel restrictions, and isolation measures introduced during this period [89,90]. The impact of COVID-19 on the quality of life and the increasing sense of loneliness introduced new problems and exacerbated others [91–93]. For example, the current study investigated the impact of the COVID-19 pandemic on the quality of life of school administrators and teachers, and it was psychological effects that were primarily identified.

Furthermore, it was concluded that the school administrators and teachers experienced a negative psychological effect during the pandemic period. Experiencing negative situations such as difficulty in establishing healthy communication, emotional change, difficulty in anger control, and the desire to be alone is considered an adverse effect of COVID-19 on the quality of life [94]. This current study presents similarities with research conducted in several countries, with different samples and age groups [95–97].

The current research results revealed that the loneliness level of the participants during the COVID-19 pandemic predicted their Internet addiction positively and significantly. The statistical data obtained showed that the effect size between these two variables was large. These findings also coincide with other studies in the literature that examined the relationship between two variables. Alheneidi et al. [98] emphasized that a strong relationship existed between loneliness and problematic Internet usage and that feelings of loneliness tend to increase as the time spent using the Internet increases. In a study conducted by Deutrom, Katos, and Ali [99], it was revealed that loneliness could positively predict problematic Internet use. In the pre-COVID-19 period, similar findings were reached in studies focusing on the relationship between loneliness and Internet usage. For example, Kim et al. [100] and Karakose et al. [101] determined that feelings of loneliness caused increased Internet usage, and those individuals spent more time using the Internet to compensate for the socialization lacking from their real life. However, this situation can cause individuals to move away from healthier social activities and real-life [102,103]. During the COVID-19 pandemic, many people spent significantly more time using the Internet due to quarantine measures and curfews. While students and teachers had to conduct lessons over the Internet with online tools [103], businesses of all kinds utilized tools such as Zoom to conduct meetings more frequently than before and for extended periods [99]. Therefore, individuals' increased Internet usage should not be perceived as a particularly negative or abnormal situation given the circumstances. Kraut and Burke [104] stated that positive or negative Internet usage relates to how individuals use the Internet, what they talk about with others when using the Internet, and whom they talk to. Hacker et al. [105] stated that during the COVID-19 pandemic, web-conferencing systems that utilize the Internet's infrastructure made people's everyday life easier, allowed meetings to occur that would otherwise not have happened, facilitated access to various daily activities, and provided a form of virtual "togetherness". In the studies conducted in this area, it has been frequently emphasized that the opportunities presented during the pandemic period of compulsory digitalization and the Internet's usage can also be said to have added value.

The results from the current research revealed a positive and moderate relationship between loneliness and happiness. Accordingly, it may be understood that the level of loneliness moderately affects the happiness levels of individuals. This result can be explained by individuals who spent more time with their families during the COVID 19 pandemic were satisfied overall with their situation. Working mothers, especially during the pandemic restrictions, had the opportunity to spend more time with their children. In this context, individuals who remained distant from the intensity of their everyday working life for a particular time may have been satisfied with the increased opportunity to spend time alone with their families. In a study on happiness, Petrovič et al. [106] compared happiness levels before and during the COVID 19 pandemic.

Contrary to expectations, at the end of their study, no significant change was detected in the participants' happiness levels. Individuals who stayed at home and experienced loneliness during the pandemic period may have turned this complicated process into an opportunity by organizing different activities within the confines of their own homes. However, some studies in the literature concluded that the happiness levels of individuals, especially in older people, were found to have been negatively affected during the COVID-19 period and that decreased levels of happiness triggered anxiety, tension, fatigue, and stress can cause depression [107–109]. The psychological effects caused by COVID-19 have been shown to cause different moods in different age groups and this has forced policymakers and administrators to take necessary measures regarding different age groups.

Finally, the current study's findings revealed a positive relationship between Internet addiction and happiness. Ballarotto et al. [110] determined that Internet usage was more frequently for entertainment, business, and educational activity during the COVID-19 pandemic. However, some studies conducted prior to the pandemic reported negative relationships between Internet addiction and happiness [111–115]. During the COVID-19 pandemic, Internet usage was shown to have increased dramatically across almost all age groups [116]. It may be stated that individuals use the Internet for shopping, attending online classes, managing jobs remotely and keeping in touch with people through online meetings, obtaining information or entertainment. This emerging situation is also interesting as it shows that Internet addiction has a multidimensional effect on the mood of individuals in both the pre-and post-COVID-19 pandemic.

Limitations and Directions for Future Research

Although this study provides significant findings regarding the relationships between COVID-19 quality of life, loneliness, happiness, and Internet addiction, it undoubtedly has certain limitations. The research was conducted with a sample consisting only of school administrators and teachers, whilst it is known that emotional states associated with COVID-19 may vary among individuals working in different occupational groups. In addition, it may be said that the age group in the study sample was not homogeneously distributed and that the density consisted of participants between the ages of 21 and 40 years old (63.9%). However, the effects of the COVID-19 pandemic on individuals may differ in young, middle-aged, and older age groups. For this reason, conducting further detailed studies on the effects of the COVID-19 pandemic on larger samples from different age and occupational groups may present a more comprehensive evaluation of the subject. Another limitation of the current study is the period in which the data were collected. This experimental study was based on participants' self-reports after all quarantine practices and restrictions had been lifted. In addition, when the data were collected, the number of COVID-19 cases in Turkey was low and the significance of the pandemic as a psychological threat was felt less than previously. This situation may have caused the participants to have presented a false image of their recollections. Therefore, future studies could examine the relationships between different variables in more detail using a longitudinal research approach.

6. Conclusions

In conclusion, according to Structural Equation Modelling, the current research proposed a new model from examining the relationships between the impact of COVID-19 on the quality of life, happiness, loneliness, and Internet addiction levels of teachers and school administrators. The variables observed in the proposed conceptual model were analyzed through path analysis, and the relevant model was then tested. The findings revealed that the impact of COVID-19 on the quality of life has a direct or indirect effect on the loneliness, happiness, and Internet addiction levels of the participants. As a result, it was seen that the fit values of the hypothesis model proposed within the scope of the research were at an acceptable level and that the model was confirmed.

Author Contributions: Conceptualization, T.K., R.Y. and T.Y.O.; methodology, T.K., S.P., T.Y.O. and R.Y.; formal analysis, T.K., S.P., T.Y.O., R.Y. and H.P.; data curation, T.K., H.P., S.E.O. and T.Y.O.; writing—original draft preparation, T.K., S.P., R.Y. and S.E.O.; writing, T.K., H.P., S.E.O. and R.Y.; review and editing, T.K., S.P. and R.Y.; supervision, T.K. and S.P. All authors have read and agreed to the published version of the manuscript.

Funding: This research received no external funding.

Institutional Review Board Statement: The study was conducted according to the guidelines of the Declaration of Helsinki, and approved by the Institutional Review Board of Provincial Directorate of National Education, the Republic of Turkey Kutahya Governorship (Ref: 53490996-44-E.7646169, 9 June 2020).

Informed Consent Statement: Informed consent was obtained from all subjects involved in the study.

Data Availability Statement: The data presented in this study are available on request from the corresponding author.

Conflicts of Interest: The authors declare no conflict of interest.

References

1. Shek, D.T.L. COVID-19 and quality of life: Twelve reflections. *Appl. Res. Qual. Life* **2021**, *16*, 1–11. [CrossRef]
2. Karakose, T.; Malkoc, N. Psychological impact of the COVID-19 pandemic on medical doctors in Turkey. *Soc. Behav. Pers.* **2021**, *49*, e9890. [CrossRef]
3. Ren, L.-L.; Wang, Y.-M.; Wu, Z.-Q.; Xiang, Z.-C.; Guo, L.; Xu, T.; Jiang, Y.-Z.; Xiong, Y.; Li, Y.-J.; Li, X.-W.; et al. Identification of a novel coronavirus causing severe pneumonia in human: A descriptive study. *Chin. Med. J.* **2020**, *133*, 1015–1024. [CrossRef]
4. World Health Organization. *Naming the Coronavirus Disease (COVID-19) and the Virus That Causes It*; World Health Organization: Geneva, Switzerland, 2020. Available online: https://www.who.int/emergencies/diseases/novel-coronavirus2019/technical-guidance/naming-the-coronavirus-disease-(COVİD-2019)-and-thevirus-that-causes-it (accessed on 14 November 2021).
5. Zhu, N.; Zhang, D.; Wang, W.; Li, X.; Yang, B.; Song, J.; Zhao, X.; Huang, B.; Shi, W.; Lu, R.; et al. A novel coronavirus from patients with pneumonia in China, 2019. *N. Engl. J. Med.* **2020**, *382*, 727–733. [CrossRef]
6. Greyling, T.; Rossouw, S.; Adhikari, T. A tale of three countries: What is the relationship between COVID-19, lockdown and happiness? *S. Afr. J. Econ.* **2021**, *89*, 25–43. [CrossRef] [PubMed]
7. Bozlu, B.; Guclu, S. The COVID-19 Pandemic and transformations in solo-living individaul's perception of family. *Eurasian J. Res. Soc. Econ.* **2021**, *8*, 55–75. Available online: https://dergipark.org.tr/en/pub/asead/issue/60135/854998 (accessed on 5 November 2021).
8. Karakose, T.; Yirci, R.; Papadakis, S. Exploring the Interrelationship between COVID 19 phobia, work-family conflict, family-work conflict, and life satisfaction among school administrators for advancing sustainable management. *Sustainability* **2021**, *13*, 8654. [CrossRef]
9. Huang, C.; Wang, Y.; Li, X.; Ren, L.; Xhao, J.; Hu, Y.; Cao, B. Clinical features of patients infected with 2019 novel coronavirus in Wuhan, China. *Lancet* **2020**, *395*, 497–506. [CrossRef]
10. Karakose, T. The impact of the COVID-19 epidemic on higher education: Opportunities and implications for policy and practice. *Educ. Process Int. J.* **2021**, *10*, 7–12. [CrossRef]
11. Karakose, T.; Demirkol, M. Exploring the emerging COVID-19 research trends and current status in the field of education: A bibliometric analysis and knowledge mapping. *Educ. Process Int. J.* **2021**, *10*, 7–27. [CrossRef]
12. Karakose, T.; Malkoc, N. Behavioral and interpersonal effects of the COVID-19 epidemic on frontline physicians working in Emergency Departments (EDs) and Intensive Care Units (ICUs). *Acta Med. Mediterr.* **2021**, *37*, 437–444. [CrossRef]
13. Qiu, J.; Shen, B.; Zhao, M.; Wang, Z.; Xie, B.; Xu, Y. A nationwide survey of psychological distress among Chinese people in the COVID-19 epidemic: Implications and policy recommendations. *Gen. Psychiatry* **2020**, *33*, e100213. [CrossRef]
14. Yezli, S.; Khan, A. COVID-19 social distancing in the Kingdom of Saudi Arabia: Bold measures in the face of political, economic, social and religious challenges. *Travel Med. Infect. Dis.* **2020**, *37*, 101692. [CrossRef] [PubMed]
15. Algahtani, F.D.; Hassan, S.-u.-N.; Alsaif, B.; Zrieq, R. Assessment of the Quality of Life during COVID-19 Pandemic: A Cross-Sectional Survey from the Kingdom of Saudi Arabia. *Int. J. Environ. Res. Public Health* **2021**, *18*, 847. [CrossRef] [PubMed]
16. Akbana, Y.E.; Rathert, S.; Agcam, R. Emergency remote education in foreign and second language teaching. *Turk. J. Educ.* **2021**, *10*, 97–124. [CrossRef]
17. Burke, J.; Arslan, G. Positive education and school psychology during COVID-19 pandemic. *J. Positive Sch. Psychol.* **2020**, *4*, 137–139. [CrossRef]
18. Akyavuz, E.K.; Cakin, M. Covid-19 School Administrators' Views on the Effect of Covid-19 Pandemic on Education. *Electronic Turk. Stud.* **2020**, *15*, 723–737. [CrossRef]
19. Fayers, P.M.; Machin, D. *Quality of Life: The Assessment, Analysis and Reporting of Patient-Reported Outcomes*, 3rd ed.; Wiley: Hoboken, NJ, USA, 2016.
20. Yildiz, S.; Cetinkaya, F. Obesity and Quality of Life Study in Adults. *Ahi Evran Med. J.* **2020**, *4*, 29–34. [CrossRef]
21. Edisan, Z.; Kadioglu, F. The ancient predecessors of quality of life. *Lokman Hekim J.* **2013**, *3*, 1–4. Available online: https://dergipark.org.tr/en/pub/mutftd/issue/43194/523878 (accessed on 10 November 2021).
22. The WHOQOL Group. People and health: What quality of life? *World Health Forum* **1996**, *17*, 354–356. Available online: https://apps.who.int/iris/bitstream/handle/10665/54358/WHF_1996_17%284%29_p354-356.pdf?sequence=1&isAllowed=y (accessed on 10 November 2021).
23. Kratz, A.L.; Sander, A.M.; Brickell, T.A.; Lange, R.T.; Carlozzi, N.E. Traumatic brain injury caregivers: A qualitative analysis of spouse and parent perspectives on quality of life. *Neuropsychol. Rehabil.* **2017**, *27*, 16–37. [CrossRef] [PubMed]
24. Papakostas, G.I.; Petersen, T.; Mahal, Y.; Mischoulon, D.; Nierenberg, A.A.; Fava, M. Quality of life assessments in major depressive disorder: A review of the literature. *Gen. Hosp. Psychiatry* **2004**, *26*, 13–17. [CrossRef]
25. Haraldstad, K.; Wahl, A.; Andenæs, R.; Andersen, J.R.; Andersen, M.H.; Beisland, E.; Borge, C.R.; Engebretsen, E.; Eisemann, M.; Halvorsrud, L.; et al. A systematic review of quality of life research in medicine and health sciences. *Qual. Life Res.* **2019**, *28*, 2641–2650. [CrossRef]
26. Dahlberg, L. Loneliness during the COVID-19 pandemic. *Aging Ment. Health* **2021**, *25*, 1161–1164. [CrossRef]
27. Killgore, W.D.; Cloonan, S.A.; Taylor, E.C.; Dailey, N.S. Loneliness: A signature mental health concern in the era of COVID-19. *Psychiatry Res.* **2020**, *290*, 113117. [CrossRef]
28. Luchetti, M.; Lee, J.H.; Aschwanden, D.; Sesker, A.; Strickhouser, J.E.; Terracciano, A.; Sutin, A.R. The trajectory of loneliness in response to COVID-19. *Am. Psychol.* **2020**, *75*, 897–908. [CrossRef] [PubMed]

29. Ugurlu, A. Investigating the relationship between loneliness and alienation levels of university students according to some variables. *Mediterr. J. Sport Sci.* **2021**, *4*, 308–319. [CrossRef]
30. Bekhet, A.K.; Zauszniewski, J.A.; Nakhla, W.E. Loneliness: A concept analysis. *Nurs. Forum* **2008**, *43*, 207–213. [CrossRef]
31. Bulus, M. Loneliness in university students. *Pamukkale Uni. J. Edu.* **1997**, *3*, 82–90. Available online: https://dergipark.org.tr/en/pub/pauefd/issue/11140/133271 (accessed on 10 November 2021).
32. Karakose, T.; Yirci, R.; Kocabas, I. A qualitative study of the novice principals' problems in the school management process and solutions. *Pak J. Stat.* **2014**, *30*, 1365–1378.
33. Korkut, G.; Gencturk, Z. Examining the relation between the loneliness levels and family involvement of university students. *Eurasian J. Int. Stud.* **2020**, *8*, 209–231. [CrossRef]
34. Bal, Z.; Kantar, E.C.; Ucar, T. The Relationship of Loneliness with Social Support, Breastfeeding, and Maternal Attachment. *Univ. Health Sci. J. Nurs.* **2021**, *3*, 21–28. [CrossRef]
35. Caglayan Tunc, A.; Zorba, E.; Cingoz, Y.E. The Effect of Exercise on Quality of Life in the Period of Pandemic (COVID 19). *Int. J. Contemp. Edu. Stud.* **2020**, *6*, 127–135. Available online: https://dergipark.org.tr/en/pub/intjces/issue/55238/749857 (accessed on 3 November 2021).
36. Askin, R.; Bozkurt, Y.; Zeybek, Z. COVID-19 Pandemic: Psychological Effects and Therapeutic Interventions. *Istan. Tic. Univ. J. Soc. Sci.* **2020**, *19*, 304–318. Available online: https://dergipark.org.tr/en/pub/iticusbe/issue/55168/753233 (accessed on 6 November 2021).
37. Holt-Lunstad, J. The potential public health relevance of social isolation and loneliness: Prevalence, epidemiology, and risk factors. *Public Policy Aging Rep.* **2017**, *27*, 127–130. [CrossRef]
38. Benke, C.; Autenrieth, L.K.; Asselmann, E.; Pané-Farré, C.A. Lockdown, quarantine measures, and social distancing: Associations with depression, anxiety and distress at the beginning of the COVID-19 pandemic among adults from Germany. *Psychiatry Res.* **2020**, *293*, 113462. [CrossRef] [PubMed]
39. Cellini, N.; Canale, N.; Mioni, G.; Costa, S. Changes in sleep pattern, sense of time and digital media use during COVID-19 lockdown in Italy. *J. Sleep Res.* **2020**, *29*, e13074. [CrossRef]
40. Vargo, D.; Zhu, L.; Benwell, B.; Yan, Z. Digital technology use during COVID-19 pandemic: A rapid review. *Hum. Behav. Emerg. Technol.* **2021**, *3*, 13–24. [CrossRef]
41. Wong, A.; Ho, S.; Olusanya, O.; Antonini, M.V.; Lyness, D. The use of social media and online communications in times of pandemic COVID-19. *J. Intensive Care Soc.* **2021**, *22*, 255–260. [CrossRef]
42. Ergun, G.; Meric, M. Examining the relationship, the internet use, happiness and life satisfaction of university students. *J. Anatolia Nurs. Health Sci.* **2020**, *23*, 233–240. [CrossRef]
43. We Are Social. *Digital 2020 Global Digital Overview*; We Are Social: Milan, Italy, 2020; Available online: https://wearesocial.com/digital-2020 (accessed on 4 November 2021).
44. Young, K.S. Internet addiction: The emergence of a new clinical disorder. *Cyberpsychol. Behav.* **1998**, *1*, 237–244. [CrossRef]
45. Totan, T.; Ercan, B.; Ozturk, E. The effects of happiness and self-esteem on internet addiction with loneliness. *Edu. 7 J. Yeditepe Univ. Fac. Edu.* **2019**, *8*, 20–35. Available online: https://dergipark.org.tr/en/pub/edu7/issue/51553/611381 (accessed on 13 November 2021).
46. Király, O.; Potenza, M.N.; Stein, D.J.; King, D.L.; Hodgins, D.C.; Saunders, J.B.; Demetrovics, Z. Preventing problematic internet use during the COVID-19 pandemic: Consensus guidance. *Compr. Psychiatry* **2020**, *100*, 152180. [CrossRef] [PubMed]
47. Alqahtani, A.F.; Alqarni, M.H.; Alotaibi, S.B.; Fattah, S.; Alhalawany, R.M. Relationship between Level of Internet Addiction, Loneliness and Life Satisfaction among College of Health and Rehabilitation Sciences Students' at Princess NourahBint Abdulrahman University. *Menoufia Nurs. J.* **2020**, *5*, 55–74. [CrossRef]
48. Erol, O.; Cirak, N.S. Exploring the loneliness and internet addiction level of college students based on demographic variables. *Contemp. Educ. Technol.* **2019**, *10*, 156–172. [CrossRef]
49. Ansari, H.; Ansari-Moghaddam, A.; Mohammadi, M.; Peyvand, M.; Amani, Z.; Arbabisarjou, A. Internet addiction and happiness among medical sciences students in southeastern Iran. *Health Scope* **2016**, *5*, e33600. [CrossRef]
50. Li, S.; Wang, Y.; Xue, J.; Zhao, N.; Zhu, T. The impact of COVID-19 epidemic declaration on psychological consequences: A study on active Weibo users. *Int. J. Environ. Res. Public Health* **2020**, *17*, 2032. [CrossRef] [PubMed]
51. Pandey, V.; Talan, A.; Mahendru, M.; Shahzad, U. Studying the psychology of coping negative emotions during COVID-19: A quantitative analysis from India. *Environ. Sci. Pollut. Res.* **2021**, 1–8. [CrossRef]
52. Zhu, Y.; Zhang, L.; Zhou, X.; Li, C.; Yang, D. The impact of social distancing during COVID-19: A conditional process model of negative emotions, alienation, affective disorders, and post-traumatic stress disorder. *J. Affect. Disord.* **2021**, *281*, 131–137. [CrossRef] [PubMed]
53. Peker, A.; Cengiz, S. COVID-19 fear, happiness and stress in adults: The mediating role of psychological resilience and coping with stress. *Int. J. Psychiatry Clin. Pract.* **2021**. [CrossRef]
54. Yildirim, M.; Guler, A. Positivity explains how COVID-19 perceived risk increases death distress and reduces happiness. *Pers. Individ. Differ.* **2021**, *168*, 110347. [CrossRef] [PubMed]
55. Yang, H.; Ma, J. How an epidemic outbreak impacts happiness: Factors that worsen (vs. protect) emotional well-being during the coronavirus pandemic. *Psychiatry Res.* **2020**, *289*, 113045. [CrossRef]

56. Kirik, A.M.; Sonmez, M. The examination of relationship between communication and happiness. *Inonu Univ. E-J. Faculty Commun.* **2017**, *2*, 15–26. Available online: https://dergipark.org.tr/en/pub/inifedergi/issue/27641/292862 (accessed on 8 November 2021).
57. Lau, A.L.D.; Chi, I.; Cummins, R.A.; Lee, T.M.C.; Chou, K.-L.; Chung, L.W.M. The SARS (Severe Acute Respiratory Syndrome) pandemic in Hong Kong: Effects on the subjective well-being of elderly and younger people. *Aging Ment. Health* **2008**, *12*, 746–760. [CrossRef]
58. Karakose, T. The Relationship between Medical Students' Time Management Skills and Academic Achievement. *Stud. Ethno-Med.* **2015**, *9*, 19–24. [CrossRef]
59. Satici, S.A.; Kayis, A.R.; Satici, B.; Griffiths, M.D.; Can, G. Resilience, hope, and subjective happiness among the Turkish population: Fear of COVID-19 as a mediator. *Int. J. Ment. Health* **2020**, 1–16. [CrossRef]
60. Brodeur, A.; Clark, A.E.; Fleche, S.; Powdthavee, N. Assessing the impact of the coronavirus lockdown on unhappiness, Loneliness, and boredom using Google trends. *arXiv* **2020**, arXiv:2004.12129. Available online: https://arxiv.org/abs/2004.12129 (accessed on 6 November 2021).
61. Fraenkel, J.R.; Wallen, N.E. *How to Design and Evaluate Research in Education*, 6th ed.; McGraw-Hill: New York, NY, USA, 2006.
62. Johnson, R.B.; Christensen, L. *Educational Research Quantitative, Qualitative, and Mixed Approaches*, 5th ed.; Sage: Thousand Oaks, CA, USA, 2014.
63. Sonmez, V.; Alacapinar, F.G. *Illustrated Scientific Research Methods*, 4th ed.; Ani Publishing: Ankara, Turkey, 2016.
64. Karagoz, Y. *SPSS and AMOS 23 Applied Statistical Analyses*; Nobel Publishing: Ankara, Turkey, 2016.
65. Kline, R.B. *Principles and Practice of Structural Equation Modeling*, 3rd ed.; Guilford: New York, NY, USA, 2011.
66. Kline, R.B. Book Review: Handbook of psychological assessment. *J. Psychoeduc. Assess.* **1994**, *12*, 180–185. [CrossRef]
67. Anatolia Agency. *Daily Vaccine Data*; Anatolia Agency: Ankara, Turkey, 2021; Available online: https://www.aa.com.tr/tr/p/covid-19-asi (accessed on 11 November 2021).
68. Repišti, S.; Jovanović, N.; Kuzman, M.R.; Medved, S.; Jerotić, S.; Ribić, E.; Majstorović, T.; Simoska, S.M.; Novotni, L.; Milutinović, M.; et al. How to measure the impact of the COVID-19 pandemic on quality of life: COV19-QoL–the development, reliability and validity of a new scale. *Glob. Psychiatry* **2020**, *3*, 1–10. [CrossRef]
69. Sumen, A.; Adibelli, D. Adaptation of the COV19-QoL Scale to Turkish culture: Its psychometric properties in diagnosed and undiagnosed individuals. *Death Stud.* **2021**, 1–8. [CrossRef]
70. Hills, P.; Argyle, M. The Oxford Happiness Questionnaire: A compact scale for the measurement of psychological well-being. *Pers. Individ. Differ.* **2002**, *33*, 1073–1082. [CrossRef]
71. Dogan, T.; Cotok, N.A. Adaptation of the short form of the Oxford Happiness Questionnaire into Turkish: A Validity and Reliability Study. *Turk Psychol. Counseling Guidan. J.* **2011**, *4*, 165–172.
72. Hays, R.D.; DiMatteo, M.R. A short-form measure of loneliness. *J. Pers. Assess.* **1987**, *51*, 69–81. [CrossRef]
73. Yildiz, M.A.; Duy, B. Adaptation of the short-form of the UCLA loneliness scale (ULS-8) to Turkish for the adolescents. *J. Psychiatry Neuro. Sci.* **2014**, *27*, 194–203. [CrossRef]
74. Kutlu, M.; Savci, M.; Demir, Y.; Aysan, F. Turkish adaptation of Young's Internet Addiction Test-Short Form: A reliability and validity study on university students and adolescents. *Anatolian J. Psychiatry* **2016**, *17*, 69–76. [CrossRef]
75. Cokluk, O.; Sekercioglu, G.; Buyukozturk, S. *Multivariate Statistics for Social Sciences: SPSS and LISREL Applications*; Pegem Akademy: Ankara, Turkey, 2014.
76. Flowchart Maker & Online Diagram Software. Available online: https://app.diagrams.net/ (accessed on 31 August 2021).
77. Hair, J.F.; Black, W.C.; Babin, B.J.; Anderson, R.E.; Tatham, R.L. Multivariate data analysis 6th edition. Pearson Prentice Hall. New Jersey. humans: Critique and reformulation. *J. Abnormal Psychol.* **2006**, *87*, 49–74.
78. Mendi, B.; Mendi, O. Evaluation of Validity and Reliability of the Turkish Version of the E-lifestyle Instrument. *J. Yasar Univ.* **2015**, *10*, 6624–6632. [CrossRef]
79. Yaslioglu, M.M. Factor Analysis and Validity in Social Sciences: Application of Exploratory and Confirmatory Factor Analyses. *Istanbul Univ. J. School Bus.* **2017**, *46*, 74–85.
80. Baumgartner, H.; Homburg, C. Applications of structural equation modeling in marketing and consumer research: A review. *Inter. J. Res. Market.* **1996**, *13*, 139–161. [CrossRef]
81. Bentler, P.M. Multivariate analysis with latent variables: Causal modeling. *Ann. Rev. Psych.* **1980**, *31*, 419–456. [CrossRef]
82. Browne, M.W.; Cudeck, R. Alternative ways of assessing model fit. In *Testing Structural Equation Models*; Bollen, K.A., Long, J.S., Eds.; Sage: Beverly Hills, CA, USA, 1993; pp. 136–162.
83. Hooper, D.; Coughlan, J.; Mullen, M.R. Structural Equation Modelling: Guidelines for Determining Model Fit. *Elect. J. Bus. Res. Methods* **2008**, *6*, 53–60.
84. Bentler, P.M.; Bonett, D.G. Significance tests and goodness of fit in the analysis of covariance structures. *Psych. Bull.* **1980**, *88*, 588–606. [CrossRef]
85. Schermelleh-Engel, K.; Moosbrugger, H. Evaluating the fit of structural equation models: Tests of significance and descriptive goodness-of-fit measures. *Methods Psychol. Res. Online* **2003**, *8*, 23–74.
86. Ferreira, L.N.; Pereira, L.N.; Da Fé Brás, M.; Ilchuk, K. Quality of life under the COVID-19 quarantine. *Qual. Life Res.* **2021**, *30*, 1389–1405. [CrossRef]

87. Zhang, Y.; Ma, Z.F. Impact of the COVID-19 pandemic on mental health and quality of life among local residents in Liaoning Province, China: A cross-sectional study. *Int. J. Environ. Res. Public Health* **2020**, *17*, 2381. [CrossRef] [PubMed]
88. Karakose, T.; Yirci, R.; Papadakis, S.; Ozdemir, T.Y.; Demirkol, M.; Polat, H. Science Mapping of the Global Knowledge Base on Management, Leadership, and Administration Related to COVID-19 for Promoting the Sustainability of Scientific Research. *Sustainability* **2021**, *13*, 9631. [CrossRef]
89. Dehkordi, A.H.; Aslani, M.; Ebadi, A.; Repišti, S.; Moradveisi, B.; Gheshlagh, R.G. Examination of the psychometric properties of the Persian version of the COVID-19-impact on Quality of Life Scale. *Health Qual. Life Outcomes* **2021**, *19*, 188. [CrossRef] [PubMed]
90. Rabacal, J.; Oducado, R.M.; Tamdang, K. COVID-19 impact on the quality of life of teachers: A cross-sectional study. *Asian J. Public Opin. Res.* **2020**, *8*, 478–492.
91. Cauberghe, V.; Van Wesenbeeck, I.; De Jans, S.; Hudders, L.; Ponnet, K. How adolescents use social media to cope with feelings of loneliness and anxiety during COVID-19 lockdown. *Cyberpsychol. Behav. Soc. Netw.* **2021**, *24*, 250–257. [CrossRef]
92. Grossman, E.S.; Hoffman, Y.S.; Palgi, Y.; Shrira, A. COVID-19 related loneliness and sleep problems in older adults: Worries and resilience as potential moderators. *Pers. Individ. Differ.* **2021**, *168*, 110371. [CrossRef]
93. Pai, N.; Vella, S.-L. COVID-19 and loneliness: A rapid systematic review. *Aust. New Zealand J. Psychiatry* **2021**, *55*, 1144–1156. [CrossRef]
94. Ucar, R. The views of school administrators and teachers on the quality of life during the coronavirus (COVID-19) pandemic. *Istan. Ticaret Uni. J. Soc. Sci.* **2021**, *20*, 463–486. [CrossRef]
95. Bryson, W.J. Long-term health-related quality of life concerns related to the COVID-19 pandemic: A call to action. *Quality Life Res.* **2021**, *30*, 643–645. [CrossRef]
96. Ravens-Sieberer, U.; Kaman, A.; Erhart, M.; Devine, J.; Schlack, R.; Otto, C. Impact of the COVID-19 pandemic on quality of life and mental health in children and adolescents in Germany. *Eur. Child Adolesc. Psychiatry* **2021**, 1–11. [CrossRef] [PubMed]
97. Shamblaw, A.L.; Rumas, R.L.; Best, M.W. Coping during the COVID-19 pandemic: Relations with mental health and quality of life. *Can. Psychol.* **2021**, *62*, 92–100. [CrossRef]
98. Alheneidi, H.; AlSumait, L.; AlSumait, D.; Smith, A.P. Loneliness and Problematic Internet Use during COVID-19 Lock-Down. *Behav. Sci.* **2021**, *11*, 5. [CrossRef] [PubMed]
99. Deutrom, J.; Katos, V.; Ali, R. Loneliness, life satisfaction, problematic internet use and security behaviours: Re-examining the relationships when working from home during COVID-19. *Behav. Inf. Technol.* **2021**, 1–15. [CrossRef]
100. Kim, J.; LaRose, R.; Peng, W. Loneliness as the cause and the effect of problematic Internet use: The relationship between internet use and psychological well-being. *Cyberpsychol. Behav.* **2009**, *12*, 451–455. [CrossRef] [PubMed]
101. Karakose, T.; Yirci, R.; Uygun, H.; Ozdemir, T.Y. Relationship between High School Students' Facebook Addiction and Loneliness Status. *EURASIA J Math. Sci. Tech. Ed.* **2016**, *12*, 2419–2429. [CrossRef]
102. Li, J.; Zhou, L.; Van Der Heijden, B.; Li, S.; Tao, H.; Guo, Z. Social Isolation, Loneliness and Well-Being: The Impact of WeChat Use Intensity During the COVID-19 Pandemic in China. *Front. Psychol.* **2021**, *12*, 707667. [CrossRef]
103. Ozturk, F.O.; Ayaz-Alkaya, S. Internet addiction and psychosocial problems among adolescents during the COVID-19 pandemic: A cross-sectional study. *Arch. Psychiatr. Nurs.* **2021**, *35*, 595–601. [CrossRef] [PubMed]
104. Kraut, R.; Burke, M. Internet use and psychological well-being: Effects of activity and audience. *Commun. ACM* **2015**, *58*, 94–100. [CrossRef]
105. Hacker, J.; Vom Brocke, J.; Handali, J.; Otto, M.; Schneider, J. Virtually in this together–how web-conferencing systems enabled a new virtual togetherness during the COVID-19 crisis. *Eur. J. Inf. Syst.* **2020**, *29*, 563–584. [CrossRef]
106. Petrovič, F.; Murgaš, F.; Králik, R. Happiness in Czechia during the COVID-19 pandemic. *Sustainability* **2021**, *13*, 10826. [CrossRef]
107. Gaeta, L.; Brydges, C.R. Coronavirus-related anxiety, social isolation, and loneliness in older adults in Northern California during the stay-at-home order. *J. Aging Soc. Policy* **2021**, *33*, 320–331. [CrossRef]
108. Santini, Z.I.; Jose, P.E.; Cornwell, E.Y.; Koyanagi, A.; Nielsen, L.; Hinrichsen, C.; Meilstrup, C.; Madsen, K.R.; Koushede, V. Social disconnectedness, perceived isolation, and symptoms of depression and anxiety among older Americans (NSHAP): A longitudinal mediation analysis. *Lancet Public Health* **2020**, *5*, e62–e70. [CrossRef]
109. Yildirim, H.; Isik, K.; Aylaz, R. The effect of anxiety levels of elderly people in quarantine on depression during COVID-19 pandemic. *Soc. Work in Public Health* **2021**, *36*, 194–204. [CrossRef] [PubMed]
110. Ballarotto, G.; Marzilli, E.; Cerniglia, L.; Cimino, S.; Tambelli, R. How Does Psychological Distress Due to the COVID-19 Pandemic Impact on Internet Addiction and Instagram Addiction in Emerging Adults? *Int. J. Environ. Res. Public Health* **2021**, *18*, 11382. [CrossRef] [PubMed]
111. Derin, S.; Bilge, F. Internet Addiction and The Level of Subjective Well-Being in Adolescents. *Turk Psychol. Counseling Guidan. J.* **2016**, *6*, 35–51. Available online: https://dergipark.org.tr/en/pub/tpdrd/issue/42744/515910 (accessed on 9 November 2021).
112. Ferraro, G.; Caci, B.; D'amico, A.; Blasi, M. Behavior: Internet addiction disorder: An Italian study. *Cyberpsychol. Behav.* **2006**, *10*, 170–175. [CrossRef]
113. Kitazawa, M.; Yoshimura, M.; Hitokoto, H.; Sato-Fujimoto, Y.; Murata, M.; Negishi, K.; Mimura, M.; Tsubota, K.; Kishimoto, T. Survey of the effects of internet usage on the happiness of Japanese university students. *Health Qual. Life Outcomes* **2019**, *17*, 151. [CrossRef] [PubMed]

114. Kozan, H.I.O.; Kavakli, M.; Ak, M.; Kesici, S. The associations among smartphone addiction, general belongingness and happiness: A structural equation modelling. *J. Clin. Psychiatry* **2019**, *22*, 436–444. [CrossRef]
115. Rastgar, S.; Abdollahi, M.; Shahgholian, M. Internet addiction, social intimacy and happiness in college students. *J. Iran. Psychol.* **2014**, *11*, 159–168. Available online: https://www.sid.ir/en/journal/ViewPaper.aspx?id=427145 (accessed on 5 December 2021).
116. Dong, H.; Yang, F.; Lu, X.; Hao, W. Internet addiction and related psychological factors among children and adolescents in China during the coronavirus disease 2019 (COVID-19) epidemic. *Front. Psychiatry* **2020**, *11*, 00751. [CrossRef]

International Journal of
Environmental Research and Public Health

MDPI

Article

Impact Study on Social Accounting Matrix by Intrabusiness Analysis

Monica Laura Zlati [1], Romeo-Victor Ionescu [2] and Valentin Marian Antohi [3,4,*]

[1] Department of Accounting, Audit and Finance, Stefan cel Mare University, 720229 Suceava, Romania; sorici.monica@usm.ro
[2] Department of Administrative Sciences and Regional Studies, Dunarea de Jos University, 800201 Galati, Romania; ionescu_v_romeo@yahoo.com
[3] Department of Business Administration, Dunarea de Jos University, 800001 Galati, Romania
[4] Department of Finance, Accounting and Economic Theory, Transylvania University of Brasov, 500036 Brasov, Romania
* Correspondence: valentin_antohi@yahoo.com

Abstract: According to the current concerns about social welfare and environmental protection, integrated in a model assimilated to intrabusiness relations, our research started from the analysis of the initial model SAM, which will be transformed in order to develop the SAMI model under six research objectives. The need of improving SAM matrix started to connect it directly to the regional economic systems and continued to a new approach on Input-Output Analysis. Nowadays, SAM describes the intraregional connections between regional economic actors using the role of different income categories. Moreover, SAM can quantify different regional multipliers. All deficiencies previously identified in connection to SAM model have been reviewed and resolved within the proposed SAMI model by the authors of this paper. The purpose of this research is the launch of an absolutely new mathematical model (SAMI) and its practical testing at regional level. This model is able to systematize the links between the local and regional businesses, under the matrix (SAMI) flow, for all kinds of companies and to assist the regional decision, as well. Czamanski was not able to escape from the input-output prison's approach. This is why he continued to use the linear interdependencies between the industries, economic sectors and economic actors. The income is able only to approximate the individuals and other economic actors' welfare. If the increase in the average and aggregate income is doubled by an unfair distribution of income in two countries which have the same average income, the effects on welfare vary a lot. A relatively similar effect comes from the government policy differences in income distribution and redistribution.

Keywords: social corporative responsibility; social accounting matrix; business environment; intrabusiness transactions; environment impact

1. Introduction

Regional accounting (regional accounts) was developed and put into connection to the regional development at the beginning of the '70s [1]. The model was well correlated to the input-output analysis and brought special matrix SAM (social accounting matrix), as it was defined by P. Batey and A. Rose [2].

Starting with this classic model, many pressures on the accounting system's entropy have been identified, even that it was initially built in order to satisfy the needs of internal information users [3,4]. The process developed at the same time as the globalization's increasing across the world economy.

The micro and macroeconomic diversification of the information actors and users, including EU27 and other regional organisations which developed common economic development systems, led to the entropy disturbing and pointed out the initial accounting system vulnerability in its relation to the new reporting needs. These needs were met by increasing external pressures on the system, along with external reporting regulations to which the accounting systems had to align.

Through his application, the inventor of the SAM matrix proved a visionary spirit that anticipated these entropy disturbances at the time of designing the model. The further evolution of the information exchange could not be predicted at the real level of its expansion.

The SAM matrix is current because it is based in prediction on a consistent data system which captures socio-economic interdependencies and translates them into an input-output picture which defines the socio-economic framework of interest at a given time at regional or national level. The main drawback is the yearly fluctuations of the data, which reduces the quality of the forecast. Through the punctual nature of the analysis, the method allows the development of relevant policies based on interlinked observations from several areas of economic and social interest. This is the main advantage of the method and the reason why it is current, with respect to the criteria of objective data evaluation.

The SAM approach has led to enough updates, not infrequently contradictory. The basic problem is that the model (matrix) has to operate with a multitude of information coming from different sources, including data from prior years. This introduces the concept of flexible 'cross entropy' in the definition of SAM, which allows the introduction of the errors in variables and inequality constraints [5].

Starting from these considerations, the authors of this paper have proposed to reposition the social accounting matrix in relation to the new market demands, using the objective evaluation of the previous critical proposals on this instrument and developing a new concept by incorporating a very visible component: intrabusiness transactions, which reflect globally the amplitude of the international economy.

The main aim of this research is to improve the SAM matrix approach in direct connection with the regional dimension in the context of a new approach to the input-output theory. As a result, the objectives of the study were to: identify vulnerabilities for model SAM and intrabusiness sectoral flows, defining a social accounting matrix model based on intrabusiness exchanges, testing our proposed model, disseminating test results and formulating proposals for public policies' decision makers.

The new model proposed is valid and applicable to any international region with conclusive results regarding the connections between the economic environment and the macro-environment through public policies in different sectors of activity.

In order to accurately and fluently identify the impact of inter-business transactions within the SAM matrix, the influences of technological exchanges have been marginalized, with the impact in particular on the dynamics of financial flows, which are currently the engine of the economy. These flows have faced a regress since Czamanski's conceptualization of the model to date, based on free access to information and the digitization of the economy.

The paper is structured into five sections, of which the Introductory section studies the impact of the SAM concept on the current regional reality and the ways to improve it based on the need for IT-supported decision making. Section 2 contains the literature review addressing the dynamics of the concept and the main shortcomings that can be improved in the authors' research. Section 3 presents the working methodology and design of the proposed new SAMI model, while Section 4 presents the main results of the research and discussions based on them. The last section Conclusions and policy implications presents the conclusions that the authors publicly disseminate with the research.

2. Literature Review

The social accounting represents an interesting subject for many specialists who responded to the challenge of updating the model.

In real economy, using their macroeconomic function, the companies make their contribution to the macroeconomic sector directly through the financial component (payment of taxes and fees) [6] and indirectly, through the social component (labour absorption, reduction in social disparities, regulation of the trade mechanism, etc.) [7,8].

The social accounting implies addressing cost-benefit measures on environmental issues [9], in order to limit pollution and other negative effects on the environment (reduction in biodiversity), but also complementary measures to boost the main macroeconomic indicators through the business component (GDP, total investment, reducing inflation by limiting deviations from the consumer price index [7,10].

There are social accounting studies which point out that the distributional structure of policies to mitigate disparities in social matters can be adjusted by effective measures to increase sectoral competitiveness and cost-benefit adjustment [11].

The intra-sectoral cooperation based on competitive exchanges linked to controlled excise limitation may increase the favorable impact of the competitiveness of domestic firms, including on foreign markets [12].

The budget allocation to support affected sectors and economic activity in less-favored areas is a key point for economic growth if these sectors are correctly identified and prices are adjusted according to the specific needs of the area (optimal price transmission mechanism) [13].

The Generally Calculable Balance Model (CGE) [14] develops a theory of quantitative policies for access to socio-economic effects in industries with environmental impact. The result of the model reveals the equation of reproducing the consumption behavior in a controlled economy at a given time. The model details the price transmission mechanism without identifying the influences of dynamic development processes. The model is based on social accounting matrix developed by Czamanski starting to 1970. A new model was realised 27 years later. It starts from the identifying flows between the microeconomic and macroeconomic component through actions of local authority regulations. Finally, the model realises a regional more complex input-output analysis through which disaggregation of regional interrelation multipliers, interregional feedbacks and evaluation of intra-sectoral functional components occur [15].

The social accounting model was applied in order to explain and to quantify the impact of the climate changes on Western Australia. The research covered 71 experiments focused on the winter rainfall and concluded that almost 70% of the observed trend is congruent with the SAM trend in that region. The information in the data series was not modelled stochastically as [16–18], but by means of the SAM matrix which revealed the need for new data. On the other hand, the analysis considered that "other forcing factors have to be invoked to fully account for the observed rainfall reduction" [19].

SAM was used in Spain, too. The model was able to estimate the water footprint of Huesca region. The analysis was based on the logical supposition that the water footprint covers the water needed for the production of the goods and services consumed by the inhabitants plus the direct consumption in the households. These consumptions were quantified using an open input-output model. The main result of the analysis was that the agrarian water use represented the greatest water consumer [20]. A similar approach to water resource reduction [21] uses the SAM matrix to simulate the evolution of shadow prices and agricultural output. The authors introduce the following macro indicators into the SAM matrix: macroeconomic variables including GDP, government's revenues/expenditures, households' income, and net exports. The results of the study show that the water crisis has a major impact on the agricultural economy, and that the SAM matrix can provide information for sustainable policy formulation.

The use of the SAM matrix in the income distribution analysis was carried out by M. Harun, A. Zakariah, and M. Azali [22]. For this purpose, detailed aggregation and disaggregation of accounts were used which have covered public expenditure in production sectors and household groups. The analysis highlighted the ability of the

SAM approach in highlighting chains of linkages from changes in demand to changes in production, factor incomes, household incomes and final demands.

An extension of the SAM matrix in the field of environment was carried out by O. Banerjee, M. Cicowiez, R. Vargas, and M. Horridge [23]. The authors proposed a new model (ESAM–Environmental Social Accounting Matrix), which completed the computerized picture of the interdependent relationship between the economy and the environment in a dynamic, unified and relevant way for issuing social policies on environmental protection.

Another approach to population health during the pandemic [24] was carried out using the SAM matrix. The conclusion of the study shows that based on financial flows it is possible to predict the behaviour of economic agents (social responsibility) in terms of income and expenditure related to combating the effects of the pandemic, including vaccination.

The model was developed later by adding interregional network transfers to a complex theory that presents structured flows that occur within social accounting. The matrix model was also structured and developed by other authors [25,26], who added that they applied for the calculation of sectoral productivity or the calculation of the matrix price multiplier.

The spatial economic interactions and flows patterns under Social Accounting Matrices (SAM) approach led to the conclusion that it can be used to quantify the spatial employment impacts of the Common Agricultural Policy. The SAM was extended, and its structure, assumptions and characteristics were redefined at interregional level [27].

The different methods of building regional SAMs, according to General Equilibrium Models with spatial characteristics were analysed starting from a large literature review. The final goal of this analysis consisted of analysing Colombian regions with such new models [28].

The applicability of SAM was extended to urban development, urbanization projects and urban life cycle forecasting. This is why SAM takes into consideration elements such as the following: heterogeneous land developers, housing consumers and planning agencies. The same SAM can support the solution of dividing the metropolitan areas into a multitude of sprawling cities [29].

Czamanski's approach is used even outside EU27, for improving the management in the enterprises from the food industry in Moldova, for example. The analysis realised a synthesis of the economic concepts in the energetic management from food industry. Moreover, it proposes models and systems of energetic management able to decrease the consumption of energetic resources and to improve the environment [30].

The first intermediate conclusion is that the model further raises the interest of researchers due to the need to correlate macroeconomic policies with flows made at the level of economic entities. As a result, the present analysis proposes a study on the applicability of the regional social accounting matrix on intra-business relations for the top 52 companies in the urban growth area in Galati, Romania.

3. Research Methodology

In order to develop the model SAMI, the research started from the analysis of the initial model SAM, which will be transformed according to the research objectives:

O1: Identification of the building vulnerabilities for model SAM according to the present conditions on the global market. According to the literature, there are contradictions regarding the mirroring of environmental issues in the SAM matrix [9], correlation of the matrix model with Generally Calculable Balance Model (CGE) [14], or the use of the matrix in connection with the urbanisation processes [29].

O2: Identification of the intrabusiness sectoral flows according to the social accounting criteria.

O3: The literature has taken the first steps in this area [31], highlighting that there is a correlation between intra- and interbusiness connections with implications for consumption, investment and other equilibrium economic relationships.
O4: Defining the social accounting matrix model based on intrabusiness exchanges;
O5: Testing the model for a growth pole in EU27;
O6: Dissemination of the model's results in connection to the realities in the growth pole;
O7: Evaluating the public policies' efficiency in the growth pole by using model SAMI.

According to the System of National Accounts, the initial SAM was created to quantify the regional economic transactions. There are differences related to SAM's translation from national to regional level. As a result, SAM presents the regional economy in a static manner for each year. The static approach represents a challenge for the model, which will be solved in this paper.

SAM represents a classic matrix with its rows and columns which represent the classical economic actors: households, companies, public sector and rest of world. The economic actors are analysed under their double hypostasis: buyers and sellers. As a logical result, the expenditures are quantified on the columns and the revenues from sales are pointed out on the rows.

An important advantage in using SAM matrix is that the number of columns and rows can be increased as the analysis asks [5]. The introduction of the net investment in SAM matrix was realised in 2008 [32]. As a result, the actual SAM matrix structure is that presented in Table 1 [33].

Table 1. Scheme of SAM. Source [33].

	Companies	Households	Public Sector	Other	Net Investment	Total (Revenues)
Companies		C	G_F	$(X-I)_K$	Inv	$C+G_F+(X-I)_K+I$
Households	W		G_H	$(X-I)_C$		$S+G_H+(X-I)_C$
Public sector	T_F	T_H				T_F+T_H
Other	$(X-I)_K$	$(X-I)_C$				$(X-I)_K+(X-I)_C$
Net investment		S_H	S_G			S_H+S_G
Total (expenditures)	$S+T_F+(X-I)_K$	$C+T_H+(X-I)_C+S_H$	$G_F+G_H+S_G$	$(X-I)_C+(X-I)_K$	Inv	

Where: T–taxes; S–wages; I–imports; E–exports; S–savings; Inv–investment; C–consumption; G–governmental sector. Indexes: F–firms; H–households; G–governmental sector; C–goods consumption; K–capital.

The need of improving SAM matrix started to connect it directly to the regional economic systems [34] and continued to a new approach on Input-Output Analysis [35]. Nowadays, SAM describes the intraregional connections between regional economic actors using the role of different income categories. Moreover, SAM can quantify different regional multipliers as well.

Starting with the matrix model, where consumption represents a direct function of revenues, in relation to a temporal update rate, SAMI (SAMIntrabusiness) matrix proposed in this paper is defined as:

If c_{ij}–production cost of the good i in industry j and q_{ij}–the quantity of goods i realised in industry j at a given time, then (∃) C–a consumption function defined as:

$$C = \sum_{i,j=1}^{n}\left(\gamma_{ij} + \prod_{ij=1}^{n}\left(\left(q_{ij}\right)^{(1-\alpha)} * \left(c_{ij}\right)^{(1+\beta)}\right)\right), \quad (1)$$

where α, $\beta > 0$, α, β, economic multipliers for quantitative and qualitative consumption; γ_{ij}, the impact of sectoral policies developed by authorities in favor of the business environment; $\left(q_{ij}\right)^{(1-\alpha)}$ the quantity of goods i realised in industry j and purchased by consumers at a certain point in time; and $\left(c_{ij}\right)^{(1+\beta)}$ the sale price of the good i in industry j. It can be said that C_j is in relation to R, according to the next formula:

$$R_i = \sum_{i,j=1}^{n}\left(\gamma_{ij} + \prod_{ij=1}^{n}\left(\left(q_{ij}\right)^{(1-\alpha)} * \left(c_{ij}\right)^{(1+\beta)}\right) - \prod_{ij=1}^{n}\left(\left(q_{ij}\right)^{(\alpha)} * \left(c_{ij}\right)^{(1)}\right)\right). \quad (2)$$

As a result, $C = R - \frac{R}{(1+a)^t}$, where R is the intrabusiness remuneration. Moreover, R represents the update rate in a directly proportional relationship to the impact of sectoral policies developed by authorities in favor of the business environment and t–the optimum moment for which the function produces competitiveness.

Matrix SAMI is defined using the above relations as follows:

$$SAMI = \begin{bmatrix} \frac{C_1}{R_1} & \cdots & \frac{C_1}{R_i} \\ \vdots & \ddots & \vdots \\ \frac{C_j}{R_1} & \cdots & \frac{C_j}{R_j} \end{bmatrix} = \begin{bmatrix} 1 - \frac{1}{(1+a_1)^{t_1}} & \cdots & 1 - \frac{1}{(1+a_1)^{t_i}} \\ \vdots & \ddots & \vdots \\ 1 - \frac{1}{(1+a_j)^{t_1}} & \cdots & 1 - \frac{1}{(1+a_j)^{t_i}} \end{bmatrix} \quad (3)$$

The matrix will focus, under the case study, on inter-business relationships for the 52 companies that are the subject of this study.

4. Results and Discussion

As a result of the regional analysis of the economic performance of the top 52 companies in the growth pole Galati, worrying developments regarding turnover in the region were pointed out. The first intermediate conclusion is that the regional decreased by 2.23 million € during the analysed period.

The main contributor to this decreasing is the metallurgical industry (including steel industry), which achieved an economic counterperformance regarding the turnover of about 6.38 million €, so much that the analysis took into consideration one of the greatest steel factories across the EU27. At the opposite pole, IT services, manufacturing, commerce and construction have brought annual growth in turnover of 0.85–1.06 million €. They have, on average, reduced the negative impact of the increase in turnover in the metallurgical industry (see Figure 1).

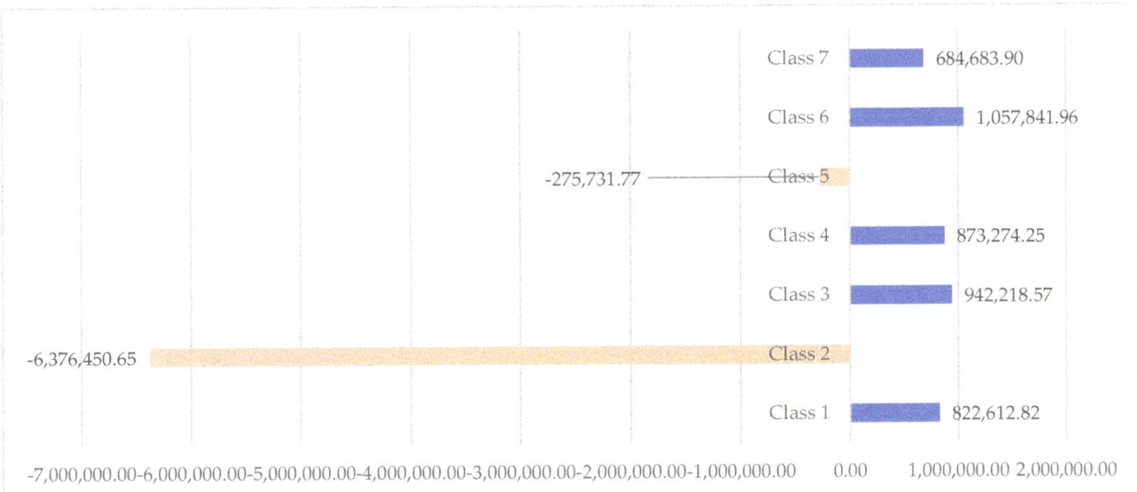

Figure 1. Histogram representation of the distribution of achievements on the Turnover of Top 50 companies in Galati (€). Source: Authors' processing based on the information provided on Topfirme.com. Accessed date: 5 June 2018.

The turnover level reveals the structural changes of the regional economy based on the general policy of the local administration, which was more conservative in terms of investment, including infrastructure, while increasing the fiscal pressure on economic agents, notably by increasing taxes. The pollution taxes applied to metallurgical operators were the biggest ones and they were finally materialized in economic branch rebound.

The general trend of profitability faces opposite evolution compared to that of the turnover. The companies from IT services (Class 6) achieved an annual gross profit accumulation of 1.91 million €

(1.6 million € net profit). The 16% difference in industry is represented by the taxation of the profit and quantifies direct contributions of micro to the macroeconomic sectors.

The metallurgical industry (Class 2) faces an average profitability of 0.51 million € and no significant difference between gross and net values. This means the withdrawal of companies from the profitability area, the accumulation of losses in the industry and the decrease in productivity. The manufacturing industry (Class 3) achieves the third rank in profitability, with an average annual value of 0.27 million €. A non-performance in terms of profitability is achieved in the transport services segment (Class 5). This industry faces a negative turnover capitalization of 0.28 million € per year and also records annual losses of 0.08 million. €.

The losses are motivated by the lack of investment in port infrastructure and the lack of interest of the authorities in the financial support of the branch, which through this measure manages to accumulate a negative trend of the employees as we shall see below (see Figure 2).

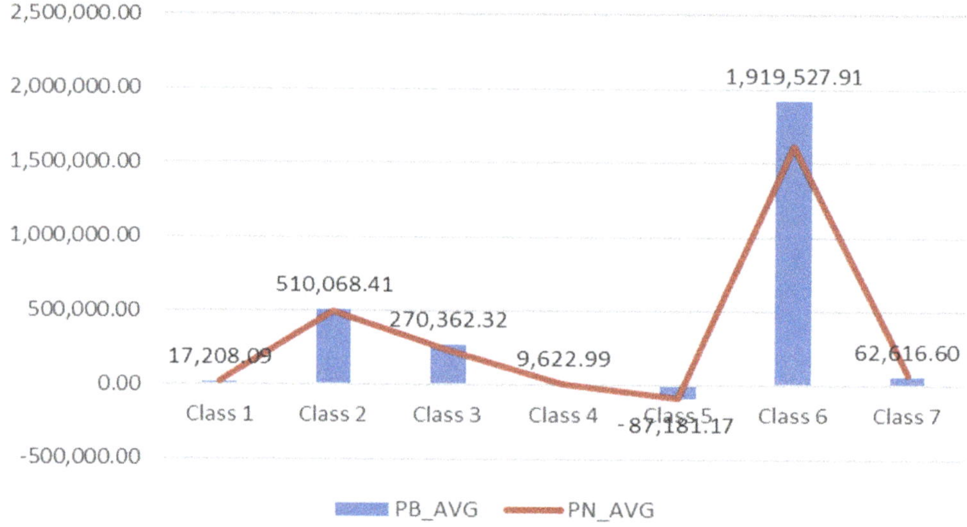

Figure 2. Regional distribution of profitability by industries during 2012–2017. Source: Authors' processing based on the information provided on Topfirme.com. Accessed date: 5 June 2018.

The company capitalization is positive on average (8.94 million € annual), but the structural differences are significant across the 7 NACE Rew.2 classes (Statistical Classification of Economic Activities in European Community). Thus, the transport services sector proved to be unprofitable and redundant. Under the turnover, the result is an average annual capitalization of 20.64 million €, which means inefficient allocation of resources and inefficient management of social accounting. A second major instability generator is the non-performance of metallurgical industry (Class 2). During 2012–2017, it has recorded an average annual reduction in the capitalization of the five companies of 15.74 million €. As a result, the capital accumulations in the transport services sector decreased. A good performance, but without the support of local authorities–bad management–is recorded by the IT services sector, which achieves an average annual capitalization of 2.13 million €. This capitalization is considered by the authors of this paper as being sustainable in relation to the other mentioned above performances (see Figure 3).

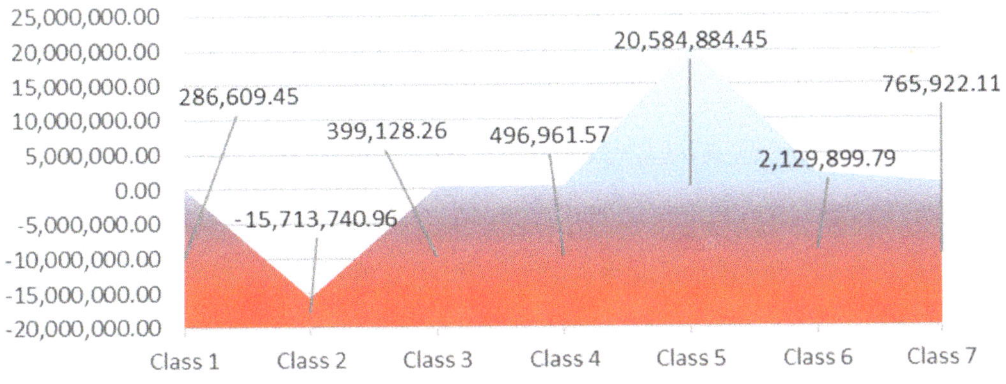

Figure 3. Regional capitalization of the companies at industry level during 2012–2017 (euros). Source: Authors' processing based on the information provided on Topfirme.com. Accessed date: 5 June 2018.

Inventory level is another indicator of bad social management reflecting, for companies in the metallurgical industry, an additional accumulation of 1.43 million €. On the transport services segment, where a capitalization of 20.64 million € was realised annually, the value of stocks increased only by 0.02 million €. Significant inventory accumulations are made in the engineering and technical consulting sector to the capitalization of enterprises (0.74 million € increase in annual inventory versus 0.77 million € increase in capitalization companies). This is unsustainable, as capitalization would be reflected in long-term investment and would be matched by growth in turnover and debt reduction. In this case, the annual debt growth on Class 7–Engineering services is similar to the increase in stocks (0.78 million € compared to 0.74 million € increase in inventories). This points out the need for a different approach to public investment, the need to re-prioritize established objectives and the import of know-how on the social accounting segment.

Low performances in terms of debt growth were recorded in the metallurgical industry, where debt grew by almost 8.19 million € annually (100% of the average annual increase). The other classes, excepting Class 5–Transport services, recorded an increase in debt service of 0.94 million € out of which 0.78 million € related to the engineering and technical consulting services. The transport services (Class 5) recorded a reduction in the debt service by using solutions to support the sector by the public segment (social accounting flows). However, these flows were not effectively managed, and generated bad management, negative profitability and turnover decreasing (see Figure 4).

The non-performance of social accounting management can be assessed at first analysis by quantifying the number of employees by activity categories. During 2012–2017, the number of employees decreased by an average of 54 employees, mainly due to the reduction in employees in the metallurgical industry (−91 people annually). In the service, engineering, food, construction and commerce sectors, the annual average growth of employees varied between 12 and 7 employees. This has diminished the negative trend of the metallurgical industry. Even if the capitalization in the transport services is significant, there is a decrease in the number of employees of six persons per year (see Figure 5).

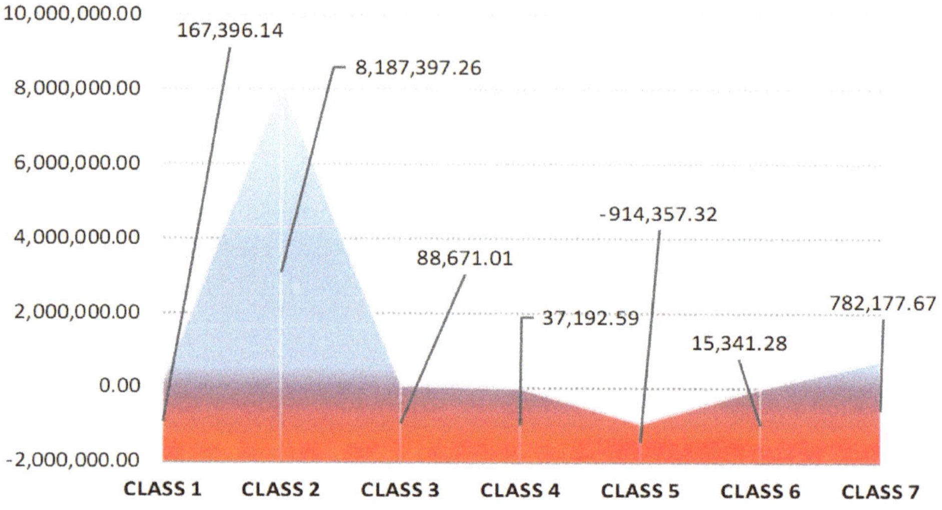

Figure 4. Evolution of average indebtedness at industry level (€). Source: Authors' processing based on the information provided on Topfirme.com. Accessed date: 5 June 2018.

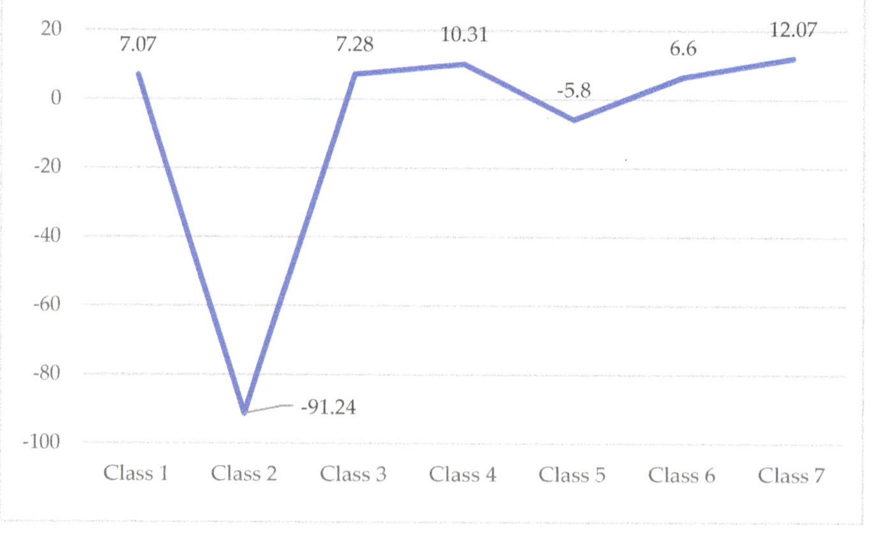

Figure 5. Annual average evolution of the number of employees per industry (persons). Source: Authors' processing based on the information provided on Topfirme.com. Accessed date: 5 June 2018.

The SAMI matrix at the branch level, calculated on the basis of the moving averages of the period 2012–2017 transposed structured by sectors of activity, in the reference region, is as follows:

$$SAMI = \begin{bmatrix} 1-\frac{1}{(1+a_1)^{t_1}} & \cdots & 1-\frac{1}{(1+a_1)^{t_i}} \\ \vdots & \ddots & \vdots \\ 1-\frac{1}{(1+a_j)^{t_1}} & \cdots & 1-\frac{1}{(1+a_j)^{t_i}} \end{bmatrix} = \begin{bmatrix} 2 & 0 & 0 & -2 \\ 0 & 2 & 4 & 0 \\ 2 & 0 & -1 & 0 \\ 2 & 0 & 0 & 0 \\ -5 & 0 & 1 & 0 \\ 2 & 0 & -4 & 0 \\ 2 & 0 & 2 & -2 \end{bmatrix} \underset{i=6;t=7}{\Leftrightarrow}$$
$$\begin{bmatrix} \frac{1}{(1+a_1)^{t_1}} & \cdots & \frac{1}{(1+a_1)^{t_i}} \\ \vdots & \ddots & \vdots \\ \frac{1}{(1+a_j)^{t_1}} & \cdots & \frac{1}{(1+a_j)^{t_i}} \end{bmatrix} = \begin{bmatrix} -1 & 1 & 1 & 3 \\ -1 & -1 & -3 & 1 \\ -1 & 1 & 2 & 1 \\ -1 & 1 & 1 & 1 \\ -4 & 1 & 0 & 1 \\ -1 & 1 & -5 & 1 \\ -1 & 1 & -1 & 3 \end{bmatrix} \underset{i=6;t=7}{\Leftrightarrow} \gamma_{ij} = \begin{bmatrix} -1 & 1 & 1 & 3 \\ 1 & -1 & -3 & 1 \\ -1 & 1 & 2 & 1 \\ -1 & 1 & 1 & 1 \\ -4 & 1 & 0 & 1 \\ -1 & 1 & -5 & 1 \\ -1 & 1 & -1 & 3 \end{bmatrix} \quad (4)$$

The data presented as a matrix flow are derived from the calculation of the moving averages over the 6 years of the study (2012–2017) for the 52 companies grouped in seven areas of interest, of which the metallurgical sector is by far the most unsatisfactory. In dynamics, the data structure is presented according to the data in Figure 6. The following notes and formulas have been used:

Class	No companie	Class	CA_AVG	PB_AVG	PN_AVG	CAP_AVG	ST_AVG	DAT_AVG	SAL_AVG
1	6	Class 1 - Food Industry	▲ 822,613	▼ 17,208	▼ 20,794	▬ 286,609	▼ 292,222	▲ 167,396	▲ 7
2	5	Class 2 - Metallurgical industry	▼ -6,376,451	▼ 510,068	▬ 498,532	▼ -15,713,741	▲ 1,433,529	▼ 8,187,397	▼ -91
3	8	Class 3 - Manufacturing industry	▲ 942,219	▼ 270,362	▼ 235,180	▬ 399,128	▼ -30,915	▲ 88,671	▲ 7
4	27	Class 4 - Construction and trade	▲ 873,274	▼ 9,623	▼ 4,568	▬ 496,962	▼ 186,974	▲ 37,193	▲ 10
5	2	Class 5 - Transportation services	▲ -275,732	▼ -87,181	▼ -80,397	▲ 20,584,884	▼ 24,568	▲ -914,357	▲ -6
6	1	Class 6 - IT	▲ 1,057,842	▲ 1,919,528	▲ 1,613,719	▬ 2,129,900	▼ 57	▲ 15,341	▲ 7
7	3	Class 7 - Engineering and technical consultancy services	▲ 684,684	▼ 62,617	▼ 72,071	▬ 765,922	▬ 739,072	▲ 782,178	▲ 12
	52	***Total***	***-2,271,551***	***2,702,225***	***2,364,467***	***8,949,665***	***2,645,508***	***8,363,819***	***-54***

Figure 6. Evolution of performance indicators highlighted by the main categories of financial and patrimonial interest for the studied entities. Source: Authors' processing based on the information provided on Topfirme.com. Accessed date: 5 June 2018.

-CA_AVG represents the average dynamic industry turnover between 2012 and 2017 and is calculated according to the formula:

$$\text{A\_AVG} = \frac{\sum_{i=1}^{7}\sum_{t=1}^{6}(CA_{it} - CA_{it-1}) * n_{it}}{\sum_{t=1}^{6} n_{it}}; \quad (5)$$

-PB_AVG represents the average dynamic industry gross profit between 2012 and 2017 and is calculated according to the formula:

$$\text{PB\_AV} = \frac{\sum_{i=1}^{7}\sum_{t=1}^{6}(PB_{it} - PB_{it-1}) * n_{it}}{\sum_{t=1}^{6} n_{it}} \quad (6)$$

-PN_AVG represents the average dynamic industry net profit between 2012 and 2017 and is calculated according to the formula:

$$\text{PN\_AVG} = \frac{\sum_{i=1}^{7}\sum_{t=1}^{6}(PN_{it} - PN_{it-1}) * n_{it}}{\sum_{t=1}^{6} n_{it}} \quad (7)$$

-CAP_AVG represents the average dynamic capitalization of companies by industry during 2012–2017 and is calculated according to the formula:

$$\text{CAP\_AVG} = \frac{\sum_{i=1}^{7}\sum_{t=1}^{6}(CAP_{it} - CAP_{it-1}) * n_{it}}{\sum_{t=1}^{6} n_{it}} \quad (8)$$

-ST_AVG represents the average stock accumulation by industries in dynamics during 2012–2017 and is calculated according to the formula:

$$\text{ST\_AVG} = \frac{\sum_{i=1}^{7}\sum_{t=1}^{6}(ST_{it} - ST_{it-1}) * n_{it}}{\sum_{t=1}^{6} n_{it}} \quad (9)$$

-DAT_AVG represents the average dynamic debt ratios per industry between 2012 and 2017 and is calculated according to the formula:

$$\text{DAT\_AVG} = \frac{\sum_{i=1}^{7}\sum_{t=1}^{6}(DAT_{it} - DAT_{it-1}) * n_{it}}{\sum_{t=1}^{6} n_{it}} \quad (10)$$

-SAL_AVG represents the average of labor dynamic absorption by industries between 2012 and 2017 and is calculated according to the formula:

$$\text{SAL\_AVG} = \frac{\sum_{i=1}^{7}\sum_{t=1}^{6}(SAL_{it} - SAL_{it-1}) * n_{it}}{\sum_{t=1}^{6} n_{it}} \quad (11)$$

The classes presented in Figure 6 are defined as follows:

(a) Class 1–Food industry;
(b) Class 2–Metallurgical industry;
(c) Class 3–Manufacturing industry
(d) Class 4–Construction and trade;
(e) Class 5–Transport services;
(f) Class 6–IT services;
(g) Class 7–Engineering and technical consultancy services.

The above presented data are interpreted according to impact indicator allocation keys (symbol of change in importance according to Figure 6). These data, through comparative study, can be structured in five major categories of socio-accounting influence, namely:

(a) Lack of efficiency or lack of public policies;
(b) Fiscal requirements;
(c) Lack of market, inefficiency of intra-business exchanges;
(d) Increasing indebtedness;
(e) Effectiveness of social policies.

This structure has highlighted some areas that need to be monitored and some areas that need to be thoroughly revised in order to reduce impact and mitigate effects.

The trends of the indicators presented in Figure 6 have been quantified as follows:

(a) Quote 1–upward trend over the average growth rate, coefficient 5;
(b) Quote 2–upward trend as the average of the indicator, coefficient 3;
(c) Quote 3–rising trend below the average growth rate of the indicator, coefficient 1;
(d) Quote 4–downward trend of the indicator, coefficient 0.

In order to quantify the effectiveness of public policies, the evolution trends of the indicators CA_AVG and CAP_AVG, coded according to quotes 1 to 4 above, have been compared. The result consists of a difference in the efficiency of public policies by classes of activity (see Table 2).

Table 2. Evaluating the effectiveness of public policies.

Class of Activity	CA_AVG	CAP_AVG	Effectiveness of Public Policies	Effectiveness Level
1-5 Class 1–Food industry;	5	3	2	Efficient
1-5 Class 2–Metallurgical industry;	0	0	0	Neutral
1-5 Class 3–Manufacturing industry	5	3	2	Efficient
1-5 Class 4–Construction and trade;	5	3	2	Efficient
1-5 Class 5–Transport services;	0	5	−5	Inefficient
1-5 Class 6–IT services;	5	3	2	Efficient
1-5 Class 7–Engineering and technical consultancy services.	5	3	2	Efficient

Red: Inefficient; Yellow: Efficient.

In order to quantify the effectiveness of the fiscal policies, the evolution trends of the indicators PB_AVG și PN_AVG, coded according to quotes 1 to 4 above have compared. The result consists of a difference in the efficiency of fiscal policies by classes of activity (see Table 3).

Table 3. Evaluating the effectiveness of fiscal policies.

Class of Activity	PB_AVG	PN_AVG	Effectiveness of Fiscal Policies	Effectiveness Level
Class 1–Food industry;	1	1	0	Neutral
1-5 Class 2–Metallurgical industry;	1	3	2	Efficient
1-5 Class 3–Manufacturing industry;	1	1	0	Neutral
Class 4–Construction and trade;	1	1	0	Neutral
Class 5–Transport services;	0	0	0	Neutral
Class 6–IT services;	5	5	0	Neutral
Class 7–Engineering and technical consultancy services.	1	1	0	Neutral

Yellow: Efficient.

The next step was to quantify the effectiveness of the intra-business exchanges, the evolution trends of the indicators ST_AVG and PB_AVG, coded according to quotes 1 to 4 above have been compared. The result consists of a difference in the efficiency of intrabusiness exchanges by classes of activity (see Table 4).

The quantifying of the microeconomic remuneration efficiency in relation to increasing indebtedness implies the analysis of the evolution trends of the DAT_AVG and CAP_AVG indicators, coded according to above quotes 1 to 4, resulting in a difference in the efficiency of microeconomic remuneration by classes of activity (see Table 5).

Table 4. Assessing the effectiveness of intra-business exchanges on sales markets by classes of activity.

Class of Activity	ST_AVG	PB_AVG	Effectiveness of Intra-Business Exchanges	Effectiveness Level
Class 1–Food industry;	1	1	0	Neutral
1-5 Class 2–Metallurgical industry;	5	1	4	Maximum Efficient
1-5 Class 3–Manufacturing industry;	0	1	−1	Inefficient
1-5 Class 4–Construction and trade;	1	1	0	Neutral
1-5 Class 5–Transport services;	1	0	1	Efficient
1-5 Class 6–IT services;	1	5	−4	Inefficient
1-5 Class 7–Engineering and technical consultancy services.	3	1	2	Efficient

Red: Inefficient; Green: Maximum Efficient; Yellow: Efficient.

Table 5. Evaluation of the efficiency of the microeconomic remuneration in relation to the increase in the indebtedness by classes of activity.

Class of Activity	DAT_AVG	CAP_AVG	Efficiency of the Microeconomic Remuneration	Efficiency Level
1-5 Class 1–Food industry;	1	3	−2	Inefficient
1-5 Class 2–Metallurgical industry;	0	0	0	Neutral
Class 3–Manufacturing industry;	3	3	0	Neutral
Class 4–Construction and trade;	3	3	0	Neutral
Class 5–Transport services;	5	5	0	Neutral
Class 6–IT services;	3	3	0	Neutral
1-5 Class 7–Engineering and technical consultancy services.	1	3	−2	Inefficient

Red: Inefficient.

Finally, in order to quantify the social policies efficiency, the analysis took into consideration the evolution trends of the SAL_AVG and CA_AVG indicators, coded according to above quotes 1 to 4, resulting in the lack of efficiency of social policies in the reference area–the growth pole l Galati, Romania (see Table 6).

Table 6. Evaluating the effectiveness of social policies.

Class of Activity	SAL_AVG	CA_AVG	Efficiency of the Social Policies	Efficiency Level
Class 1–Food industry;	5	5	0	Neutral
Class 2–Metallurgical industry;	0	0	0	Neutral
Class 3–Manufacturing industry;	5	5	0	Neutral
Class 4–Construction and trade;	5	5	0	Neutral
Class 5–Transport services;	0	0	0	Neutral
Class 6–IT services;	5	5	0	Neutral
Class 7–Engineering and technical consultancy services.	5	5	0	Neutral

The above indicators were computed by applying the impact coefficients to the annual trend of the indicator for the six categories of the SAMI matrix. The significance values of the efficiency level are shown in Figure 7:

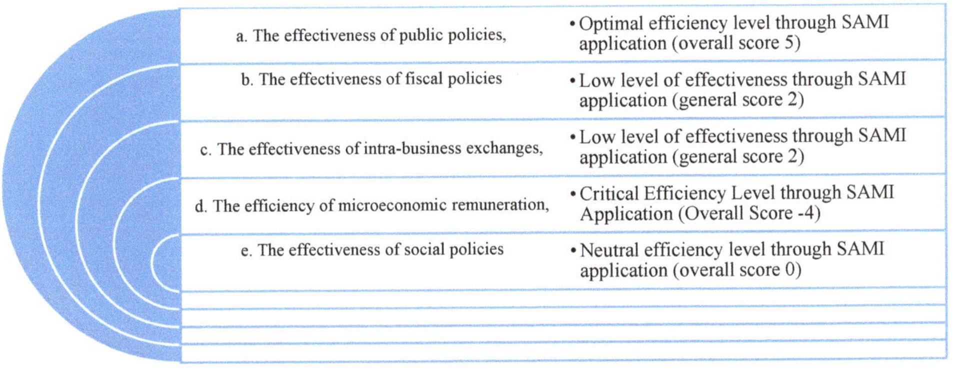

Figure 7. SAMI's scheme developed by the authors.

The model applied at the inter-business level brings real benefits to all actors involved in regional trade exchanges by assessing the regional level of social accounting development and by highlighting the critical points through which the system fails due to bureaucratic or bad management policies.

To achieve Objective 1 of the research (O1: Identification of SAM model building vulnerabilities in relation to the current global market conditions), a critical analysis of the vulnerabilities of the SAM model was developed based on the literature review.

The regional accounting model was updated 25 years later [15]. This was the result of the model inability to satisfy the quantifying of the regional development. As a result, the new one can measure the long-term potential growth of a regional economy, while the analysis takes into consideration the changes in invested capital, human capital, natural resources, infrastructure and environmental factors. The resulting SAM matrix points out the main goods and monetary flows (see Table 7).

The authors of the paper succeeded in improving the meaning of the approach in the above figure. On the other hand, the model is based on the classic SAM matrix.

A new intermediate conclusion is that Czamanski is not able to escape from the input-output prison's approach. This is why he continued to use the linear interdependencies between the industries, economic sectors and economic actors.

There are some challenges related to welfare, as well. From point of view of the authors of this paper, welfare is not dimensioned only by goods and services. Of course, it depends directly on the income level, but it does not cover only consumption, income and higher savings. There are enough elements which cannot be bought with money and have contributions to welfare. As a result, income is able only to approximate the individuals' and other economic actors' welfare.

An interesting approach is that money is able to contribute indirectly to greater happiness [36]. The economic realities presents many situations when the aggregate income's increase doesn't have correspondent in individuals' welfare (The increase in the duration and intensity of work done by each individual or the increase in the retirement age bring more money but not more wealth).

There are other outputs (weapons for example) which have no effect on the individuals' welfare even that they contribute to an increase in income (GDP). The lower quality outputs have the same effect. These two examples lead to the conclusion that welfare is directly related to consumption, not to production [37].

Table 7. SAM vs. SAMI analysis.

Indicators	Business	Households	Governments	Rest of the World	Intergenerational Transfers		Output
					Investments	Regional Endowment	
Business	Intermediate goods and services	Personal consumption	Current governmental purchases of goods and services	Net exports; Dividends and interest from rest of the world	Net domestic private investments; Public investments.	Technical progress; Depletion of non-renewable resources, renewable resources, soil resources; Degradation of the environment	*Adjusted net regional/national product (NRP)*
1-8 SAM results	International analysis without globalisation factor	Traditional consumption evaluation under the influence of international markets	Analysis of government policies in the context of the international markets' expansion	Trade agreements in the context of customs protectionism	National Strategic Investment Policies	Technical Progress analyzed from the perspective of competitive advantage	Business services aiming at territorial expansion and winning international markets
1-8 SAMI results	Strength model, including globalisation factor; Business to business analysis.	Evaluation of the global acquisition for the digitized society under the influence of the global markets	Analysis of Cohesion Policies in context of the global markets	Multinational corporative policies in the context of free movement of goods and services	The role of FDI in the context of globalization; Financing schemes at European level	Technical Progress in the global digitized society	Analysis of intra-business exchanges, quantification of financial flows and strategic development agreements on long-term for economic entities through global partnerships
1-8 Households	Wages, salaries, other labour income; Net personal interest; Proprietor's income; Rental income; Business transfers		Net interest paid by governments; Transfer payments less social security contributions			Increase in human capital	
1-8 SAM results	Labour productivity analysis by intruder Input-Output method		Assessing the success of social policies through their monetary side	SAM model does not quantify the elements of labor migration and the global change in consumer behavior under the impact of global trade	SAM model doesn't cover intergenerational transfers related to investments	SAM evaluates inter-regional transfers at the household level by increasing the value of the skilled labour.	The outputs of the SAM matrix are limited to the development of human capital in the traditional context of national markets engaged in international competitions.
1-8 SAMI results	Introduction of CSR values and staff motivation for optimizing labor productivity		Quantifying sustainable social protection efforts through social cohesion policies at European level	The elements of global trade are quantified by intrabusiness financial flows	SAMI, through its regional component, quantifies the impact of investments on households	Aspects regarding labor migration and social protection of European citizens through CBM community monitoring mechanisms are introduced in the SAMI matrix	SAMI integrates innovative concepts on social responsibility and community monitoring to assess the impact of households in social accounting

Table 7. *Cont.*

Indicators	Business	Households	Governments	Rest of the World	Intergenerational Transfers		Output
					Investments	Regional Endowment	
1-8 Governments	Corporate taxes; Social security taxes; Indirect taxes; Surplus of government enterprises less subsidies	Personal taxes; Local taxes				Increase in value of subsoil resources	
1-8 SAM results	Financing the economy through the business component is quantified through SAM exclusively through taxation.	Financing the economy through the social component is quantified through SAM exclusively through taxation.		SAM does not assess the financing of macroeconomics through external financing mechanisms (European Sector Financing Scheme, for example).	SAM does not quantify the intra-regional impact of the investments.	SAM sets the foundations for sustainable development concepts but does not assess them at the current market demands' level.	SAM carries out a fiscal quantification of the macroeconomics' remuneration through the classic components of fiscal mechanisms and does not correspond to the current requirements on the complexity of fiscal policies applied at regional level.
1-8 SAMI results	The introduction of intra-business flows strengthens the financing component by adding the multiplier effect of the economy to the commercial and investment chains.	SAMI highlights regional labor transfers as a potential development factor.		SAMI encompasses European funding schemes in the context of macro and micro financial flows.	SAMI quantifies the intra-regional impact of the investments.	SAMI quantifies the sustainability objectives mentioned in Agenda 2030.	SAMI quantifies intra-business exchanges and sustainable development components. SAMI improves the prospect of macroeconomic remuneration on the society's integrated financial flows based on interchange.
1-8 Rest of the world			Transfer payments		Net investment or disinvestment in the rest of the world		

Table 7. *Cont.*

Indicators	Business	Households	Governments	Rest of the World	Intergenerational Transfers		Output
					Investments	Regional Endowment	
1-8 SAM results	SAM does not quantify global intra-business flows.	Phenomena such as migration of qualified labour with impact on the development of a region (concrete case analyzed in the paper) are not analyzed by SAM. The impact of labour transfer through the size of goodwill elements at regional entity level is a major vulnerability of the model.	The monetary payment system, as a support to the national economy, is addressed by SAM in payments balances' equilibrium, but the global dimensions to which national monetary systems must currently face cannot be quantified.		SAM quantifies net investment as growth support. Currently, under the pressure of multinationals, the SAM model does not distinguish between national private and public net investments.	SAM does not quantify this component.	The international component is partially quantified by SAM by taking into account the transfer of payments and net investment.
1-8 SAMI results	SAMI quantifies global intra-business flows.	SAMI quantifies goodwill by identifying intra-business flows.	The efficiency of public policies quantified by the model translates precisely the need for funding based on the global trade of national economies, including up to the regional level–growth poles.		SAMI quantifies net investment as growth support. Currently, under the pressure of multinationals, the SAMI model distinguishes between private and public national net investments.	SAMI is focused on regional development, intra-business flows and the expansion of public-private entropy in the region.	The international component is quantified by SAMI at regional level by increasing system entropy and highlighting globalization in all its aspects.
1-8 Savings	Retained earnings NRP	Personal savings	Governments' surplus or deficit on current account				
1-8 SAM results	SAM quantifies performance through the Adjusted net regional/national product (NRP), calculating a global accumulation value based on Input–Output method.	SAM quantifies indirect welfare through personal savings.	SAM quantifies social welfare through the surplus or deficit of the balance of payments.	SAM does not quantify the impact of global trade on the region's welfare.		SAM doesn't quantify the regional dimension of welfare.	Welfare is calculated by extrinsic accumulation function.

Table 7. *Cont.*

Indicators	Business	Households	Governments	Rest of the World	Intergenerational Transfers		Output
					Investments	Regional Endowment	
1-8 SAMI results	SAMI quantifies the transaction performance and economic chain which gives it greater sustainability and greater entropy of the analyzed regional system.	SAMI takes into account the social policy elements introduced by international cohesion agreements and precisely quantifies welfare based on the capacity of the system to provide long-term sustainable growth.	SAMI quantifies the viability of the macro system through demand-supply interaction with the economic environment in the region, which highlights the entropy of the system.	SAMI quantifies the impact of global trade on the regional welfare.		SAMI accomplishes this by introducing into the equation the assessment of sustainable regional development.	SAMI quantifies welfare through sustainable accumulation as well as through intra-business flows.
1-8 Changes in wealth					Net increase in assets	Net increase in endowment	Net increase in wealth
1-8 SAM results	SAM does not quantify the asymptotic curves of the evolution of welfare at the level of economic agents.	SAM does not quantify changes in population welfare, this being a vulnerability of the system.	The national economic performance materialized in the medium- and long-term growth of the economy is omitted by the SAM model.	The impact of global trade on economic well-being is ignored by SAM, which is destabilized in fulfilling its function of assessing social accounting as a whole.	SAM evaluates intra-regional investment transfers through net asset growth, not highlighting the qualitative side induced by technological progress.	SAM performs a rough assessment of the endowment growth with an emphasis on environmental components, making a preliminary review of sustainable development.	SAM concretises the change of welfare by conceptualizing net growth in welfare, which represents the quintessence of the model.
1-8 SAMI results	SAMI aims at calculating the asymptotic curves for NACE Rev2 activity domains evaluating on their basis the interaction of economic policies with the business environment (see Figure 7).	SAMI, through regional dimension and intra-business flows quantification, places individuals as beneficiaries of the system and evaluates population welfare based on sustainable regional development.	These changes include macro phenomena such as inflation/deflation, unemployment, population migration, etc. and are quantified and evaluated at the level of public policy efficiency through the proposed SAMI model.	SAMI involves assessing the impact of global trade on regional sustainable development for growth poles and materializes in a multimodal complex of social accounting.	SAMI focuses on competitiveness and relates intra-regional transfers both to technological progress and to know-how.	SAMI evaluates all aspects of sustainable regional development, and through intrabusiness flow components highlights the effectiveness of sustainable development in growth poles.	SAMI emphasizes net growth in welfare through sustainable policy components and intra-business flows, potentiating their application to current market conditions.

Source: Authors' contribution.

If the increase in the average and aggregate income is doubled by an unfair distribution of income in two countries which have the same average income, the effects on welfare vary a lot. A relatively similar effect comes from the government policy differences in income distribution and redistribution.

A limit of SAM approach is that it does not take into consideration the underground economy and the fact that the output increasing is not always equal to the consumption increasing. Moreover, the SAM matrix takes into consideration the externalities only under the regional endowment.

All deficiencies previously identified have been reviewed and resolved within the proposed SAMI model. At this moment, the goals of the Objective 1 were satisfied.

The present research responds to the proposed Objective 2 (O2: Identify intrabusiness sectoral flows according to social accounting criteria) by calculating the efficiency of intra-business exchanges (see Table 3). The efficiency scoreboard was built on activity classes and allowed comparative analysis of sustainable accumulation in terms of profitability as a result of inventory dynamics by classes of activity over the period 2012–2017, the period for which full data were reported for the 52 companies included in the sample. This is because some of the companies have barely entered in the top in recent years.

The matrix model proposed in this paper was defined in the methodology section. As a result, the proposed Objective 3 (O3: Defining the social accounting matrix model based on intrabusimess exchanges) was also met.

The testing of the proposed model was carried out in steps to assess the effectiveness of public policies, fiscal policies, intra-business exchanges, assessing the efficiency of microeconomic remuneration and the effectiveness of social policies. These tests have allowed the construction of NACE Rev.2 and have demonstrated the sustainability of the model by obtaining valid results, micro, macro and regional causality correlations. As a result, the Objective 4 of the research (O4: Testing the growth model for the EU27) has been validated.

The results were disseminated and a general regional efficiency table for the growth pole was built (see Table 5). The Objective 5 of the research was also achieved (O5: Dissemination of model results in relation to market realities in the growth pole).

The final objective, Objective 6, of the research reveals the vulnerability of the public policies promoted in the growth pole (O6: Evaluation of the efficiency of public policies in the growth pole by applying the SAMI model), making a precise radiography of the government's bad management with a direct impact on the bad management of the economic agents.

The main regional deficiencies concern the poor quality of the transport infrastructure (lack of airport, lack of interconnection with the TEN-T network, administrative bureaucracy, inefficiency in the management of the free zone), factors that inhibit sustainable development in the region benefiting from the existence of the river transport infrastructure, the existence of economic agents as locomotives of the economic growth (DAMEN, ARCELOR, Mineral Port), the existence of a university center of tradition, etc.

The results of the study reflect the fact that the SAMI matrix is a forward-looking tool that addresses the shortcomings identified in Table 7 and systematizes the linkages between businesses conducted regionally for representative firms (with regional decision-making power).

The aggregate distribution function reflects the fact that relevant models can be designed based on the systematization of the decision within the SAMI matrix, eliminating vulnerabilities through distributions and redistributions leading to sustainable policy making.

The objectives achieved in this research may constitute new working hypotheses for future extended research in Ecology and environment.

5. Conclusions and Policy Implications

Through this research, the authors proposed the development of the SAMI matrix for intra-business relations. The study has a high practical applicability through easy-to-use methodology, the punctual diagnosis of intra-business flows and by identifying the vulnerabilities of the social accounting system.

The results of the study can be applied both by the representatives of the local authorities as well as by the top management and the stakeholders of economic units generating economic growth.

There is no doubt that the present approach has a strong connection to the public policies' implementation. For the beginning, this approach is based on main categories of financial and patrimonial interest for the studied entities. All these entities are elements of the public policies for sustainable development.

On the other hand, the public policies have to be efficient. As a result, the authors succeeded in quantifying the effectiveness of public policies using seven classes of activity, two indicators (CA_AVG and CAP_AVG) and dedicated values (from 0 to 5). According to these, the analysis was able to identify the Transport services as an inefficient industry which has to be a priority for the public policy (see Table 2).

A distinct analysis covers the fiscal policies. The result of this analysis is that these policies had a good impact on the Metallurgical industry (see Table 3).

Moreover, the authors of this paper proposed a new instrument (SAMI) which is able to assist the public policy decision makers in improving the implementation of specific public policies and in obtaining better performances. These performances cover the classical four economic actors (business, households, governments and rest of the world) but take into consideration the intergenerational transfers regarding Investments and Regional endowment.

The final goal of SAMI is the analysis of intra-business exchanges, quantification of financial flows and strategic development agreements in the long-term for economic entities through global partnerships (see Table 7). All of these are elements of the public policies, as well.

We can conclude that the proposed model proved to be valid by correlating the empirical demonstration with the values resulting from the applicative study, the identified problems being real and very current.

The limitations of the study consist of the small number of indicators taken into account and the relatively limited scope of data analysis, the authors proposing to deepen their current study in a future article by refining input use and broadly defining financial outputs and the ecology and environment under the impact of the COVID-19 pandemic.

Author Contributions: Conceptualization, R.-V.I. and V.M.A.; methodology, R.-V.I. and M.L.Z.; validation, R.-V.I., M.L.Z. and V.M.A.; formal analysis, V.M.A.; investigation, R.-V.I. and M.L.Z.; resources, V.M.A.; data curation, M.L.Z.; writing—original draft preparation, R.-V.I. and M.L.Z.; writing—review and editing, M.L.Z. and V.M.A.; visualization, V.M.A.; supervision, R.-V.I. All authors have read and agreed to the published version of the manuscript.

Funding: This research received no external funding.

Institutional Review Board Statement: Not applicable.

Informed Consent Statement: Not applicable.

Data Availability Statement: We used public data from Eurostat and the World Health Organization.

Conflicts of Interest: The authors declare no conflict of interest.

References

1. Czamanski, S. *Regional and Interregional Social Accounting*, 1st ed.; Lexington Books: Lanham, ID, USA, 1973.
2. Batey, P.W.J.; Rose, A.Z. Extended Input-Output Models: Progress and Potential. *Int. Reg. Sci. Rev.* **1990**, *13*, 27–49. [CrossRef]
3. Tache, F.L. Advice in electronic commerce. In Proceedings of the 2009 3rd International Workshop on Soft Computing Applications, Szeged-Arad, Romania, 29 July–1 August 2009; pp. 111–114.
4. Tache, F.L. Trust model for consumer protection (TMCP). In Proceedings of the 4th International Workshop on Soft Computing Applications, Arad, Romania, 15 July–17 July 2010; pp. 107–112.
5. Robinson, S.; Cattaneo, A.; El-Said, M. Updating and Estimating a Social Accounting Matrix Using Cross Entropy Methods. *Econ. Syst. Res.* **2001**, *13*, 47–64. [CrossRef]
6. Dervis, K.; de Melo, J.; Robinson, S. *General Equilibrium Models for Development Policy*; The World Bank: Washington, DC, USA, 1982.
7. Liang, Q.; Wei, Y. Distributional impacts of taxing carbon in China: Results from the CEEPA model. *Appl. Energy* **2012**, *92*, 545–551. [CrossRef]
8. Radu, R.I.; Mihai, I.; Isai, V. Considerations Regarding the Assessment Capacity and Recognition in Accounting of Human Capital. *Risk Contemp. Econ.* **2017**, 135–145. [CrossRef]
9. Shan, Y.; Liu, J.; Liu, Z.; Xu, X.; Shao, S.; Wang, P.; Guan, D. New provincial CO_2 emission inventories in China based on apparent energy consumption data and updated emission factors. *Appl. Energy* **2016**, *184*, 742–750. [CrossRef]
10. Meng, X.; Siriwardana, M.; McNeill, J. The Environmental and Economic Impact of the Carbon Tax in Australia. *Environ. Resour. Econ.* **2012**, *54*, 313–332. [CrossRef]
11. Wang, P.; Dai, H.; Ren, S.; Zhao, D.; Masui, T. Achieving Copenhagen target through carbon emission trading: Economic impacts assessment in Guangdong Province of China. *Energy* **2015**, *79*, 212–227. [CrossRef]
12. Qi, T.; Weng, Y. Economic impacts of an international carbon market in achieving the INDC targets. *Energy* **2016**, *109*, 886–893. [CrossRef]
13. Stua, M. Evidence of the clean development mechanism impact on the Chinese electric power system's low-carbon transition. *Energy Policy* **2013**, *62*, 1309–1319. [CrossRef]
14. Cardenete, M.A.; Roberto, L. How modes of transport perform differently in the economy of Andalusia. *Transp. Policy* **2018**, *66*, 9–16. [CrossRef]
15. Czamanski, S. Intergenerational Transfers in a Framework of Fused Regional Accounts. In *Regional Science Perspectives for the future*, 1st ed.; Chatterji, M., Ed.; Macmillan Press Ltd.: London, UK, 1997; pp. 108–126.

16. Dragomir, F.L.; Dumitriu, C.Ș.; Bărbulescu, A. Recommendation Systems—Modeling Abusive Clauses in E-commerce. In Proceedings of the 2021 International Conference on Electrical, Computer, Communications and Mechatronics Engineering (ICECCME), Mauritius, 7–8 October 2021; pp. 1–4. Available online: https://ieeexplore.ieee.org/document/9590828 (accessed on 27 November 2021).
17. Bărbulescu, A.; Dumitriu, C.S.; Dragomir, F.-L. Detecting Aberrant Values and Their Influence on the Time Series Forecast. In Proceedings of the 2021 International Conference on Electrical, Computer, Communications and Mechatronics Engineering (ICECCME), Mauritius, 7–8 October 2021; pp. 1–5. Available online: https://ieeexplore.ieee.org/document/9591085 (accessed on 27 November 2021).
18. Dumitriu, C.Ș.; Dragomir, F.-L. Modeling the Signals Collected in Cavitation Field by Stochastic and Artificial Intelligence Methods. In Proceedings of the 2021 13th International Conference on Electronics, Computers and Artificial Intelligence (ECAI), Pitesti, Romania, 1–3 July 2021; pp. 1–4.
19. Cai, W.; Cowan, T. SAM and regional rainfall in IPCC AR4 models: Can anthropogenic forcing account for southwest Western Australian winter rainfall reduction? *Geophys. Res. Lett.* **2006**, *33*. [CrossRef]
20. Cazcarro, I.; Pac, R.D.; Sánchez-Chóliz, J. Water Consumption Based on a Disaggregated Social Accounting Matrix of Huesca (Spain). *J. Ind. Ecol.* **2010**, *14*, 496–511. [CrossRef]
21. Rizwan, N.; Shikoh, S.; Davies, S.; Moeen, M.S.; Rana, A.; Haider, Z. Assessing the economic cost of depleting groundwater in Balochistan: A Social Accounting Matrix (SAM) multiplier approach. *IFPRI Discussion Paper* **2021**, 1–44. [CrossRef]
22. Harun, M.; Zakariah, A.; Azali, M. Constructing a Social Accounting Matrix Framework to Analyse the Impact of Public Expenditure on Income Distribution in Malaysia. *arXiv* **2020**, arXiv:2001.03488.
23. Banerjee, O.; Cicowiez, M.; Vargas, R.; Horridge, M. *Construction of an Extended Environmental and Economic Social Accounting Matrix from a Practitioner's Perspective*; Laborales y Sociales (CEDLAS), Centro de Estudios Distributivos, Universidad Nacional de La Plata: La Plata, Argentina, 2019.
24. Kotsopoulos, N.; Haitsma, G.; Connolly, M.P.; Standaert, B. Estimating the money flow in the economy attributed to rotavirus disease and vaccination in the Netherlands using a Social Accounting Matrix (SAM) framework. *Expert Rev. Pharm. Outcomes Res.* **2020**, *20*, 603–612. [CrossRef]
25. Llop, M. The role of saving and investment in a SAM price model. *Ann. Reg. Sci.* **2010**, *48*, 339–357. [CrossRef]
26. Fuentes-Saguar, P.D.; Mainar-Causapé, A.J.; Ferrari, E. The Role of Bioeconomy Sectors and Natural Resources in EU Economies: A Social Accounting Matrix-Based Analysis Approach. *Sustainability* **2017**, *9*, 2383. [CrossRef]
27. Skuras, D.; Psaltopoulos, D. Estimating Spatial Employment Impacts of the CAP through Social Accounting Analysis. In Proceedings of the European Association of Agricultural Economists, 160th Seminar, Warsaw, Poland, 1–2 December 2016. [CrossRef]
28. Angel, J.; García, D.; Maldonado, N. Revisión de metodologías para la construcción de Matrices de Contabilidad Social Regionales (MCSR). *Ensayos Econ.* **2017**, *27*, 125–149. [CrossRef]
29. Czamanski, D.; Broitman, D. Information and communication technology and the spatial evolution of mature cities. *Socio-Econ. Plan. Sci.* **2017**, *58*, 30–38. [CrossRef]
30. Gribincea, C. Improving Energy Management in the Food Industry Using the Motivational and Prediction Factors Evaluation and Energy Efficiency Measurement System. *Contemp. Econ. J.* **2016**, *1*, 84–92.
31. Mainar-Causapé, A.; Ferrari, E.; McDonald, S. *Social Accounting Matrices: Basic Aspects and Main Steps for Estimation*; EUR 29297 EN, JRC Technical Reports; Publications Office of the European Union: Luxembourg, 2018. [CrossRef]
32. Mitra-Kahn, B.H. WP 2008-1 Debunking the Myths of Computable General Equilibrium Models. Schwartz Center for Economic Policy Analysis and Department of Economics, The New School for Social Research, Working Paper Series, 2008, pp. 2–81. Available online: https://www.economicpolicyresearch.org/images/docs/research/economic_growth/SCEPA%20Working%20Paper%202008-1_Kahn.pdf (accessed on 27 November 2021).
33. Ionescu, R.-V. Regional Accounting and Regional Development. *J. Accunting Manag.* **2020**, *10*, 148–153.
34. Round, J.I. Social Accounting for Regional Economic Systems. In *Integrated Analysis of Regional Systems*; Batey, P., Madden, M., Eds.; Pion: London, UK, 1996; pp. 90–106.
35. Hewings, G.J.D.; Sonis, M.; Jensen, R.C. Fields of Influence of Technological Change in Input-Output Models. *Pap. Reg. Sci.* **1988**, *64*, 25–36. [CrossRef]

36. Landsburg, S.E.; Feinstone, L.J. *Macroeconomics*; McGraw-Hill College: New York, NY, USA, 1996.
37. Nordhaus, W.; Tobin, J. Is Growth Obsolete? In *Economic Research: Retrospect and Prospect, Volume 5, Economic Growth*; National Bureau of Economic Research, Inc.: Cambridge, MA, USA, 1972; pp. 1–80.

International Journal of
Environmental Research and Public Health

MDPI

Article

The Role of Corporate Social Responsibility and Corporate Image in Times of Crisis: The Mediating Role of Customer Trust

Chih-Cheng Chen [1], Asif Khan [1,*], Tanaporn Hongsuchon [2,*], Athapol Ruangkanjanases [2], Yen-Tzu Chen [3], Ornlatcha Sivarak [4] and Shih-Chih Chen [5]

1 Department of Marketing and Distribution Management, College of Management, National Kaohsiung University of Science and Technology, Kaohsiung 824005, Taiwan; volvic@nkust.edu.tw
2 Chulalongkorn Business School, Chulalongkorn University, Bangkok 10330, Thailand; athapol@cbs.chula.ac.th
3 Department of Information and Learning Technology, National University of Tainan, Tainan 70005, Taiwan; yentzu@gm2.nutn.edu.tw
4 Mahidol University International College, Mahidol University, Nakhon Pathom 73170, Thailand; ornlatcha.siv@mahidol.ac.th
5 Department of Information Management, National Kaohsiung University of Science and Technology, Kaohsiung 824005, Taiwan; scchen@nkust.edu.tw
* Correspondence: khan_asif04@yahoo.com (A.K.); tanaporn.h@chula.ac.th (T.H.)

Abstract: The purpose of this research is to empirically examine relationships between a multi-dimensional set of corporate social responsibility (CSR) initiatives, numerous dimensions of customer trust, and corporate image in an emerging economy. It also analyzes the mediating effect of customer trust on the relationship between CSR and corporate image. This study focuses on two of the most well-known hotel chains situated in Pakistan. Close-ended, self-administered questionnaires were circulated amongst a total of 300 hotel customers. The research data was analyzed using a partial least square-structural equation modeling (PLS-SEM) model. The results revealed that economic, legal, and ethical CSR significantly impacted corporate image, while philanthropic CSR did not affect the corporate image. However, economic, legal, and philanthropic CSRs were found to be in a significant relationship with customer trust, while ethical CSR was not in a significant relationship with customer trust. Finally, customer trust fully mediated the relationship between economic and legal CSR with corporate image, whereas it partially mediated the relationship between ethical and philanthropic CSR. This study is unique from earlier CSR research based on an assessment of the connection between CSR dimensions and corporate image to examine customers' trust in an emerging economy, especially in times of crisis.

Keywords: corporate social responsibility; multi-dimensional CSR; corporate image; customer trust; emerging economy; times of crisis; smart PLS; mediation

1. Introduction

Corporate Social Responsibility (CSR) describes how a company manages its industry and takes responsibility for its social impact. Corporate social responsibility encompasses various characteristics like economic dependence, legal conformity, ethical requirement, and societal influences [1]. CSR has been suggested to benefit the reciprocally advantageous long-term and reliable relations with its participants [2]. Customers are key participants of a corporation, hence, exploring corporate social responsibility from the perception of customers has progressively drawn the attention of investigators and experts, especially in the service industry [3]. Furthermore, times of crisis are described as the complex challenges faced by the companies. These challenges are mostly related to the strategic focus of the companies in times of economic downturns. According to public opinions, financial challenges and profit-making ability are deemed as the core aspects of a company in times of crisis. In contrast, other social challenges and responsibilities of the business are important but ignored in previous research, however, these challenges are supported by some of the previous research papers [4–6].

Consequently, corporations are expected to fulfill ethical and social responsibilities rather than utilizing them as a differentiating approach to achieve organizational authenticity [7]. The growing awareness and insight of CSR initiatives have driven CSR activities as a competitive strategy between firms.

Corporations consider the use of CSR strategies crucial in determining organizational objectives for enhancing corporate image (CI) and profitability by recognizing the need and significance of CSR activities [8]. Customers are extra positive to corporations that enthusiastically publicize their corporate social responsibility programs as compared to those corporations that would not promote their CSR activities [9]. Corporations' CSR methods have significantly influenced corporate image in a positive manner and caused the largest growth in market share [10]. Therefore, many corporations have utilized CSR activities as a distinctive management approach. A corporation's CSR execution can, as a result, have both a negative and a positive impact. As CSR becomes essential, both as a key academic course and a component of the corporate plan, customers are following up on corporations' commitment in CSR more enthusiastically than earlier. The corporate image that is achieved as a consequence from CSR procedures may possibly enhance customer social accountability conduct and the association among the company and customers [11].

Customers will participate actively like the firm's employee if he/she has an optimistic image of the corporation [12]. Corporate social responsibility additionally operates as a marketing instrument since it provides to set a constructive corporate image [1,13,14]. Numerous investigations have recognized the growing association concerning corporate image and corporate social responsibility initiatives. Corporate social responsibility is a crucial component in enhancing corporate image. Corresponding to a study performed in Korea confirmed that corporate achievements of financial and legal corporate social responsibility policies had an immediate and significant impact on the corporate image [15]. Moreover, a significant association between corporate social responsibility and the corporate image was exhibited to impact market share [16,17]. To be precise, companies' legal and ethical status concludes in a constructive corporate image of the company. Furthermore, companies are expected to engage in socially responsible endeavors by their customers, and the customers express their gratitude to the companies' behaviors by purchasing their products [18]. A few research scholars claimed that customers who believe admirably of companies are highly prone to engage in long-term relations with those companies [19].

Corporate social responsibility has a significant influence on business interactions with customers, and disreputable marketing conduct negatively affects the attitudes of customers, social conduct, and satisfaction. The business and its customers can be deemed corporate allies and their relationships are significantly influenced by their belief in mutual trust [20,21]. Furthermore, services industries have to handle several additional interactions with their customers in comparison to fast-moving consumer goods (FMCG) industries [21]. Therefore, in a service commerce's competitive framework, businesses can not merely introduce trust via truthful, and honest communication initiatives, but they also need to produce trust at each particular interaction phase, which forms a positive customer experience in the minds of customers, specifically when customers communicate with the frontline staff [22]. Hence, service industries have to build and represent their dedication to corporate social responsibility policies and programs thoroughly at all the various interaction points creating the customer experience [23]. In addition, the innovative digitalized and linked atmosphere additionally presents customers the likelihood of networking considerably more immediately with businesses [24,25]. Moreover, corporate social responsibility's relationship with customers and company's characteristics [26] causes mediation in the relationship between corporate social responsibility programs and company's assessments [27]. Customers' trust related to a corporation and its products is strengthened by the effective execution of CSR initiatives. [27]. Although customers' trust is an important factor to be examined, yet limited research has been conducted to explore the role of customers' trust within the framework of CSR. This research has utilized the rising multi-dimensional view of this construct.

To address the previous research inadequacies of CSR related to the measurement and conceptualization of CSR and customers' trust, this research study provides and empirically examines the research model that integrates the relationships between a multi-dimensional set of CSR initiatives namely legal, ethical, economic, and philanthropical CSR proposed by Carroll [28] and a numerous dimensions of customer trust containing integrity, experience, and benevolence, based on trust theory [29] and corporate image in an emerging economy. This research attempts to address at least four key research gaps related to CSR. First, we examine how CSR helps support corporate image. Second, we explore the relationship of CSR with customer trust. The third research gap covers the impact of customer trust on corporate image. This contributes to the fourth research gap, which is built on prior work by assessing the mediating role of trust on CSR to illustrate the influence of corporate social responsibility on corporate image.

2. Theoretical Background and Hypotheses Development

2.1. Corporate Social Responsibility (CSR) and Corporate Image (CI)

Carroll [28] conceptualized the CSR model by proposing to integrate four accountabilities: economic (delivering required products and services), ethical (implementation of the ethical conduct), legal (compliance to policies), and philanthropic (participating in volunteer activities). Furthermore, Carroll [28] stressed that the advantages gained by the company from CSR might also impact its stakeholders. A stakeholder can be described as "an entity or a group which might impact or is impacted by the fulfillment of the corporation's objectives" [30].

CI, achieved by the company's performance towards CSR initiatives, can be defined as the subjective view of customers related to the performance in terms of the stakeholders' societal concerns [8]. Corporate image is characterized as the reaction to the amount of trust, concepts, and thoughts the communities have in the direction of a corporation [31]. Furthermore, it is also related to the stakeholders' perception regarding the necessary measures taken by the company for the betterment of its stakeholders. Corporate image is an intangible asset that can improve customers' behavior intention including customers' need fulfillment, commitment, and repurchase intention to endorse [8]. Corporate Image is significant for achieving trade gains, hence the significance of social accountability in terms of establishing an optimistic image of a corporation is enhanced [32]. CSR integrates CI in the minds of customers and a positive corporate reputation is achieved. A corporation's reputation is a critical tactical source for achieving viable gain [33]. On the Contrary, not implementing corporate social responsibilities can eventually cause an adverse impact on the company. Previous research suggested that companies that honestly take measures for their social responsibilities and provided an optimistic image to their stakeholders were further expected to generate strong financial outcomes [34]. Effective CSR implementation can be achieved by the active simultaneous participation of external and internal stakeholders; hence it can enable a company to forecast and take benefit of rapidly changing social environments and beliefs. Service firms, like any other company, are required to be in harmony with sociocultural, socioeconomic, and environmental activities. Earlier studies confirm the relationships among corporate social responsibility and corporate image by verifying that a company's corporate social responsibility methods significantly impact the company's image, consumer attitudes and the company's ([8,11,35]. These initiatives additionally enhance relations among the customers and the company [10,36]. Park et al. (2014) have claimed that a company's realization of legal and economic corporate social responsibility activities had a significant impact on a company's reputation, however, both philanthropic and ethical corporate social responsibility activities had a significant impact. Plewa et al. [11] presented that acquaintance of customers with a company's Corporate Volunteering (CV) initiative is significantly associated with customer insights of the corporate image and customer acknowledgment of other placed motivations, furthermore, customers' perceptions of a company's corporate social responsibility reputation are significantly associated to the company's image. Consequently, it can be inferred that corporate social responsibility initiatives can improve a firm's corporate image for shareholders. In the research studies related to hospitality, Kim et al. [10] uncovered that each element of corporate social responsibility (ethical, economic, philanthropic, and legal) with the exception of legal accountability had a significant impact on the CI in the casino business. Ghaderi et al. [37] confirmed that each aspect of corporate social responsibility has direct and positive effect on the performance of the hotel.

Previous research on corporate social responsibility uncovered that corporate social responsibility has a significant association with corporate image, suggesting the utilization of corporate social responsibility as the instrument to improve corporate image. In additional words, when service suppliers operate well at corporate social responsibility, customers will create a constructive impression of them. This mutual association has been endorsed by current literature [38–41]. Popoli [42] also assert that corporate social responsibility has a significant impact on improving customers' views on a corporation's image. According to Hillenbrand, Money, and Pavelin [43], an improvement in the company's image might be a consequence of a company's philanthropic contributions, in that case, if the initiative and motivations related to the donation are perceived as optimistic. Additionally, for a company to achieve a responsible corporation reputation, the company is necessary to be viewed as a well-behaved corporation by its stakeholders (i.e., being professional in conducting company's interests, transparent, sustainable, and reduce adverse social effects) and with decent intentions (i.e., being reliable, honorable, and honestly care about the people).

B. Kim, Lee, & Kang [44] hypothesized that corporate social responsibility performances have a significant impact on company reputation in the framework of tourism. Lee, Kim, & Ham [45] uncovered that CSR affects brand trust and brand image. Thus, it is evident from the empirical and theoretical perspective that if the CSR initiatives are perceived optimistically by the stakeholders, they might be more favorable in leading towards the corporate image. Hence, established on Carroll's [28] four corporate social responsibility aspects and the previous study, we recommend the following hypotheses.

Hypotheses 1a (H1a). *Economic (CSR) positively influences corporate image (CI) in times of crisis.*

Hypotheses 1b (H1b). *Legal (CSR) positively influences corporate image (CI) in times of crisis.*

Hypotheses 1c (H1c). *Ethical (CSR) positively influences corporate image (CI) in times of crisis.*

Hypotheses 1d (H1d). *Philanthropical (CSR) positively influences corporate image (CI) in times of crisis.*

2.2. Corporate Social Responsibility and Customer Trust

Customer trust is the topic of significant efforts to describe it. For Barber (1983) trust is defined as a group of "socially realized and verified beliefs" that individuals have of other individuals or organizational bodies. Trust builds as a consequence of a company's belief that the trustee is trustworthy, sincere, and compassionate [46]. According to the customer's perspective trust can be defined as the customer's belief that a company will operate based on the expectations concerning its capability, goodwill, and integrity. Trust is perceived as a multidimensional concept [47], though most of the time it has been theorized and operationalized as a unidimensional global concept [27,48]. The customers and brand can be deemed corporate partners, whose relationships are impacted by their individual opinions of shared trust [20]. Consequently, trust can be described as the belief that every corporate partner should perform with reliability and trustworthiness throughout their collaborations. Conventionally, numerous researchers have recommended reliability and integrity as essential dimensions of trust. Moreover, corporate partners are prone to build trust by staying trustworthy, altruistic, and benevolent [21]. In this research study, the three-dimensional description of customer trust proposed by Mayer & Davis [47] is adopted, which comprises integrity, expertise, and social benevolence.

The viewpoint regarding the dearth of devious conduct between corporate partners is likewise vital for trust advancement, as is the viewpoint that the brand works reasonably, accountably, and conscientiously for its customers [20]. Various researchers have demonstrated that customer assessments that the business performs in a socially accountable way are significantly associated with customer trust in that business [49–51]. Analyzing customer experiences of corporate social responsibility, Vlachos et al. [52] recommended a framework linking customer opinions of the business's motivations for accepting corporate social responsibility measures to customer trust. Generally, socially accountable conduct is crucial, since a business, which is recognized as socially conscientious is further expected to be trustworthy by its customers [51]. Similarly, in the service industry, García de los Salmones et al. [53] discovered that the ethical conduct of a customer services business has a significant influence on customer trust. Furthermore, Choi and La [54] uncovered that corporate social responsibility has a significant effect on customer trust in several service industries including financial services, restaurants, and airlines. In the hotel business, Martínez and Rodríguez del Bosque [50] offered statistical proof of a significant impact of corporate social responsibility on customer trust.

A community's ethical view regarding the company is vital to construct a reliable connection, hence companies are more motivated to engage in socially responsible programs to express their dedication to the community [55]. According to Kim et. al [56], CSR is found to be one of the top approaches to stimulate trust in customers. Trust can be described as "the belief of ethically acceptable behavior" [57]. Firms, engaged in CSR initiatives, discovered CSR to deliver advantages like customer loyalty, customer satisfaction, good image, and high market value [48]. Performing company functions in an ethical fashion affects the complete image of the company's products or services and enhances customer trust [58]. An optimistic view of the company concerning CSR will impact consumer trust. Trust in a service industry is greatly linked to experiences of service provider's honesty, integrity, and morality [54]. Paine [59] asserts that devotion to moral norms offers the foundation for trust that improves to create repute, and strengthens the supply of value services. Similarly, ethical conduct by the staff of a business has a significant influence on customer trust.

These research studies provide evidence that CSR initiatives must place trust in the minds of customers' regarding the company's societal concern intent to engage in CSR initiatives to establish a positive impact on corporate image. In the model (Figure 1), the three types of trust are positioned as mediators of the effects that the four types of CSR initiatives have on corporate image.

Hypotheses 2a (H2a). *Economic (CSR) positively influences customer trust in times of crisis.*

Hypotheses 2b (H2b). *Legal (CSR) positively influences customer trust in times of crisis.*

Hypotheses 2c (H2c). *Ethical (CSR) positively influences customer trust in times of crisis.*

Hypotheses 2d (H2d). *Philanthropical (CSR) positively influences customer trust in times of crisis.*

2.3. Customer Trust and Corporate Image

The collaboration among employees and customers to produce an image must turn out to be an attractive study. According to a research finding, service companies like hotels were indicated as brands. Consequently, the values of a company are characterized by brands. Corporate image is an element of the argument regarding brands [60]. Based on this argument it can be underlined that whenever an employee presents a brand via collaborative initiatives with customers, the view regarding the company's image can be influenced. Service companies like hotels perform corporate image by agents of supervisors in conveying and delivering services to customers [61]. The managers and employees of the company deliver values to customers which in turn becomes optimistic impressions and beliefs [61,62].

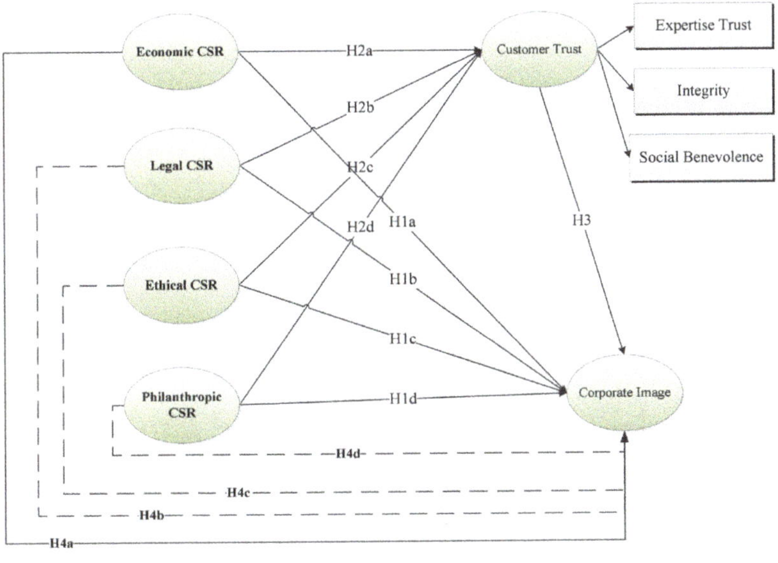

Figure 1. Theoretical Framework.

Trust is an essential concept in several academic disciplines, particularly in theories related to marketing and organizational management. In a provided exchange association, trust is described as the degree of trustworthiness ensured by the service provider to the customer, and it was demonstrated to be a vital aspect in retaining a constructive connection between the business and the customer in marketing. Customer trust is regarded as customers' trustworthiness about a business that is defined by a business's ability to genuinely fulfill the promises made to the customers. Since the corporate image is created by trustworthy initiatives of a company, hence, trust is deemed as a critical element in the success of a business. Providing agreed value is crucial to developing an optimistic repute. As trustworthiness is fragile, there is a great effort to recapture trustworthiness after it is lost [63]. Trust was additionally discovered to be the antecedent component of corporate image [15,63].

The hotel industry's psychological image can be described by several methods, comprising trust, favorability, status, and recognition. Corresponding to the opinion of the hotel managers the corporate image is exhibited by the customers' trust in the hotel [60]. It is also found that the hotel management finds trust to be a major factor for attracting visitors to the hotel. Hence, it implies that each hotel should be able to develop a psychological understanding of the attitudes of customers so that they can be motivated to experience the same brand one more time [64,65]. Privacy and safety are found to be vital factors in determining trust in a hotel. Hence, managers at a hotel are found to be paying close attention to ensuring the privacy and security of customers [60].

Based on the following discussions it can be proposed that:

Hypothesis 3 (H3). *Customer trust has a significant association with the corporate image in times of crisis.*

2.4. Mediating Role of Customer Trust

If a company is trusted by the customers, the customers would be more committed to facing risks, and therefore, this risk-taking conduct would have certain constructive consequences on the business [29]. A company's CSR initiatives are found to be an important factor in deciding the perception of customers' trust in the company. By participating in CSR programs, a business demonstrates to customers that it is concerned regarding the outcomes of its actions (benevolence) and supports some key values, such as reducing its adverse impacts on the community and the ecosystem (integrity) [66].

Consumer trust is influenced by the presence of principles that the customers and the company communicate. Concerning CSR programs, this conduct offers knowledge about business personality and principles, and it is valuable for boosting overall trust in the direction of the company [50]. As Hosmer [67] reveals, by introducing ethical and trustworthy values into businesses' tactical decision-making practices companies can improve the trust of all shareholders, as well as customers. The view that a business is moral and trustworthy promotes trust-based relations established in the principle that each exchange partners' activities will be plausible ahead of any legal or contractual limitations [51]. In an endorsement of this viewpoint, Pivato et al. [48] additionally recommended that "the establishment of the trust is one of the greatest direct outcomes of a business's societal functioning" or the direct or highly immediate consequence of CSR actions. Social relationships have been implemented primarily via customer trust in marketing relationship studies. Trust has been identified as the presence of a connection where one associate that is the customer in this study, trusts in the other associate that is the hotel in this study in terms of integrity and reliability [3,68]. Additionally, customer experiences of trust correlate to the business's thoughtfulness and reliability beyond its competence [69]. Therefore, it has been indicated that a business's real commitment to corporate social responsibility actions concerning its customers is useful for enhancing overall trust and decreasing distrust for the business [52]. Moreover, studies by Nicki [3], Swaen and Chumpitaz [51], and Garcı ́a de los Salmones et al. [53] discovered a significant correlation between a business's corporate social responsibility and customer trust in the service industry indicating that trust is the direct or most immediate result of a business's CSR initiatives.

According to the results of the study by Triatmanto et al [60] respondents approved that the psychological insight of the corporate image was certainly perceived as trust, awareness reputation, and favorability. Trust was found to be the most vital indicator from the four mentioned indicators, which was viewed optimistically by the respondents, indicating that in the hotel business, customers are more involved with hotels that are perceived to be trustworthy. Safety and privacy offered by a hotel can earn the trust of a hotel [70,71]. According to the model (Figure 1), the customers' trust is placed as a mediator of the impacts that the CSR programs have on corporate image:

Hypotheses 4a (H4a). *Customer trust mediates the association between economic CSR and corporate Image.*

Hypotheses 4b (H4b). *Customer trust mediates the association between legal CSR and corporate Image.*

Hypotheses 4c (H4c). *Customer trust mediates the association between ethical CSR and corporate Image.*

Hypotheses 4d (H4d). *Customer trust mediates the association between philanthropic CSR and corporate Image.*

3. Methodology

Sample and Procedure

This study focuses on two of the most well-known hotels situated in Pakistan. A total of 300 hotel customers staying in Peshawar and Islamabad cities were selected. Close-

ended self-administered questionnaires were circulated amongst the customers. Instead of requesting respondents merely whether they approve an opinion statement, the research paper used Likert scale items, in which the customers were requested how strongly they approve or disapprove with it, typically on a 7-point measure from 1 (=strongly disagree) to 7 (=strongly agree), with 4 demonstrating a neutral category.

A pretest will be conducted by a sample of 50 customers located in Peshawar city. Corporate social responsibility will be assessed by items recommended by [10] however, the items to measure Corporate image was applied from Chowdhury et al [72] and Kim et al [10] research study. Furthermore, McKnight et al [46] methodology was used to measure customer trust. The questionnaire is shared in the Appendix A. The hypothesis of this study will be tested using a structural equation model.

4. Data Analysis

Partial least squares (PLS) measurement was conducted using two measures. In the preliminary phase, the reliability and validity evaluation was conducted, whereas, in the next phase, the path coefficients and the structural model's explanatory power were analyzed and evaluated. The purpose of the two phases mentioned was to verify the construct's reliability and validity, including checking the relation among the constructs [73,74]. PLS has been applied and deemed as the finest tool for demonstrating the causal collaboration among constructs and consequently can handle model measurement items and construct variables simultaneously [75]. Moreover, because PLS uses simpler factors to measure the randomness and normality of the variables, it is found to be perfect for reviewing the association among constructs in the distribution of the irregular results. It also shares the advantages of assessing prediction models possessing dynamic qualities [76]. PLS was therefore considered to be more appropriate for this study as compared to other SEM analysis methodologies to assess the relations between construct variables, eradicate measurement errors, and prevent collinearity.

4.1. Convergent and Discriminant Validity

The associated external model measurements contained the internal consistency of every measurement item, the convergent validity, reliability, and differentiating validity of each layout. Employing an applicable loading of queries, the reliability of the results was analyzed. Factor loading's threshold value of individual reliability was considered to be 0.6 [77]. Individual reliabilities were based on this threshold value. All the observed variables in the study adhered to the criteria and went through the elimination process. Table 1 shows the composite reliability of each construct. The composite reliability (CR) values of all the variables were found to be higher than 0.7 [78] and suggested that the construct was adequate.

The factor loading, composite reliability, and the average variance extracted AVE factors for all construct variables were studied. A construct would be considered to possess an acceptable convergent validity if its related indicators were possessing values greater than 0.5 [79]. Table 1 reveals that the AVEs in this analysis is between 0.591 and 0.835 for hypothetical construct variables, suggesting that there is substantial convergence.

Discriminatory validity was utilized as a measurement to analyze the discrimination among different constructs and items. According to the results demonstrated in Table 2, the factor loading of each item exceeds the factor loading of other constructs, hence indicating possessing a fair discriminant validity [80].

The quality assessment of the model was done by measuring the Goodness of Fit (*GOF*), which was analyzed using Tenenhaus et al. [81] proposed model, calculated as follows:

$$GOF = \sqrt{\overline{AVE}} \times \sqrt{\overline{R^2}} = \sqrt{0.726 \times 0.697} = 0.711$$

Corresponding to the above-mentioned formula *AVE* is measuring the average variance, while *R* square is the coefficient of determination. According to the outcome, the *GOF* is 0.711, which achieves the 0.28 cut-off standards for a large impact size [82].

Table 1. Convergent validity.

Construct	Item Code	Factor Loading	Cronbach's Alpha	Composite Reliability	Average Variance Extracted (AVE)
Economic CSR	ECO1 ECO2 ECO3 ECO4	0.821 0.883 0.876 0.862	0.884	0.920	0.741
Legal CSR	LEG1 LEG2 LEG3	0.833 0.889 0.879	0.835	0.901	0.753
Ethical CSR	ETHI1 ETHI2 ETHI3	0.888 0.924 0.891	0.885	0.929	0.813
Philanthropical CSR	PHI1 PHI2 PHI3	0.803 0.790 0.675	0.870	0.920	0.793
Corporate image	CI1 CI2 CI3 CI4 CI5 CI6 CI7 CI8 CI9 CI10	0.735 0.756 0.809 0.786 0.830 0.832 0.745 0.705 0.719 0.759	0.923	0.935	0.591
Integrity	INT1 INT2 INT3 INT4	0.870 0.917 0.924 0.918	0.929	0.949	0.824
Expertise	EXP1 EXP2 EXP3	0.898 0.936 0.907	0.901	0.938	0.835
Benevolence	SOC1 SOC2 SOC3	0.911 0.909 0.851	0.870	0.920	0.794
Customer trust	Integrity Expertise Benevolence	0.926 0.907 0.866	0.944	0.952	0.666

Furthermore, standardized root mean square residual (SRMR) is characterized as the distinction between the studied relationship and the framework indicated relationship matrix. Hence, it lets evaluating the mean of the differences among studied and anticipated relationships as an indisputable scale of model fit standard. Consequently, if the model has an SRMR value of less than 0.08 it has a good model fit [83]. Henseler et al. [84] propose the standardized root mean square residual as a GOF gauge for PLS-SEM, which can be utilized to prevent model error. Additionally, Bentler-Bonett Normed Fit Index (NFI) is a phased gauge of GOF for a research model that is not influenced by the model's number of factors. The Normed Fit Index is the difference of 1 and Chi^2 divided by the model's Chi^2. Thus, the Normed Fit Index scores values between the range of 0 and 1. Normed Fit Index values exceeding 0.9 normally signify a satisfactory fit. According to the findings of smart PLS, the value of SRMR and NFI were 0.034 and 0.951, respectively. Given that SRMR < 0.08 and NFI > 0.90 the model is significant.

Table 2. Standardized factor loadings and cross-loadings of the outer model.

	Economic (CSR)	Ethical (CSR)	Legal (CSR)	Philanthropic (CSR)	Customer Trust	Corporate Image
ECO1	0.821	0.249	0.344	0.298	0.293	0.432
ECO2	0.883	0.247	0.403	0.320	0.326	0.502
ECO3	0.876	0.291	0.378	0.354	0.382	0.565
ECO4	0.862	0.321	0.433	0.374	0.405	0.595
ETHI1	0.298	0.888	0.477	0.622	0.540	0.508
ETHI2	0.263	0.924	0.507	0.643	0.546	0.535
ETHI3	0.317	0.891	0.596	0.696	0.567	0.594
LEG1	0.468	0.562	0.833	0.677	0.642	0.740
LEG2	0.391	0.505	0.889	0.665	0.599	0.669
LEG3	0.318	0.452	0.879	0.681	0.638	0.635
PHI1	0.342	0.696	0.714	0.905	0.652	0.629
PHI2	0.369	0.630	0.670	0.893	0.688	0.650
PHI3	0.342	0.619	0.696	0.874	0.726	0.663
EXP1	0.328	0.495	0.612	0.657	0.816	0.592
EXP2	0.311	0.499	0.598	0.633	0.838	0.579
EXP3	0.341	0.458	0.570	0.605	0.833	0.545
INT1	0.313	0.533	0.587	0.634	0.812	0.608
INT2	0.332	0.433	0.578	0.590	0.829	0.587
INT3	0.347	0.456	0.575	0.606	0.860	0.560
INT4	0.348	0.561	0.634	0.663	0.862	0.625
SOC1	0.375	0.510	0.538	0.624	0.735	0.574
SOC2	0.368	0.494	0.598	0.641	0.768	0.590
SOC3	0.316	0.552	0.608	0.666	0.804	0.604
CI1	0.490	0.521	0.650	0.567	0.537	0.735
CI2	0.590	0.462	0.663	0.598	0.590	0.809
CI3	0.584	0.456	0.568	0.542	0.563	0.786
CI4	0.567	0.462	0.638	0.572	0.581	0.830
CI5	0.519	0.446	0.597	0.568	0.559	0.832
CI6	0.456	0.522	0.613	0.610	0.554	0.745
CI7	0.363	0.418	0.495	0.453	0.493	0.705
CI8	0.325	0.406	0.533	0.476	0.458	0.719
CI9	0.343	0.435	0.646	0.551	0.518	0.759
CI10	0.441	0.519	0.633	0.624	0.645	0.756

Note 1: ECO CSR, Economic CSR; ETHI CSR, Ethical CSR; LEG CSR, Legal CSR; PHI CSR, Philanthropic CSR; EXP, Expertise trust; INT, Integrity trust; SOC, Social Benevolence; CI, Corporate Image.

4.2. Empirical Results

The hypothesis of this study was analyzed by using the internal PLS model. The path coefficients are the direction and power of the correlation among the constructs that signify cause and effect among the assessed latent and variables. Furthermore, the model's analytical capability can be demonstrated by the value of the R square. The degree of all the path coefficients was analyzed by using the bootstrapping approach. Re-sampling the data was used to improve the estimated limit value [85]. Consequently, this approach was adopted by the research study to examine the significance among variables. The findings of the study were divided into two models; model A of the study analyzed the relationship between CSR and corporate image without the mediating effect of customer trust, while model B integrated customer trust as a mediating variable.

According to the findings of model (A) highlighted in Table 3, and Figure 2, legal, ethical, and philanthropical responsibilities of CSR were all found to have a positive influence on the corporate image supporting H1b (β= 0.589, t-value= 7.805), H1c (β= 0.120, t-value= 2.191), and H1d (β= 0.159, t-value= 2.304), while not supporting H1a (β= 0.010, t-value=0.297), indicating that economic responsibility has no significant relationship with corporate image.

Table 3. Hypotheses results for model A.

Hypothesis	Path Coefficient	T Values	*p* Values	Results
H1a: Economic (CSR) -> Corporate image	0.010	0.297	0.766	Not Supported
H1b: Legal (CSR) -> Corporate image	0.589	7.805	0.000	Supported
H1c: Ethical (CSR) -> Corporate image	0.120	2.191	0.029	Supported
H1d: Philanthropic (CSR) -> Corporate image	0.159	2.304	0.042	Supported

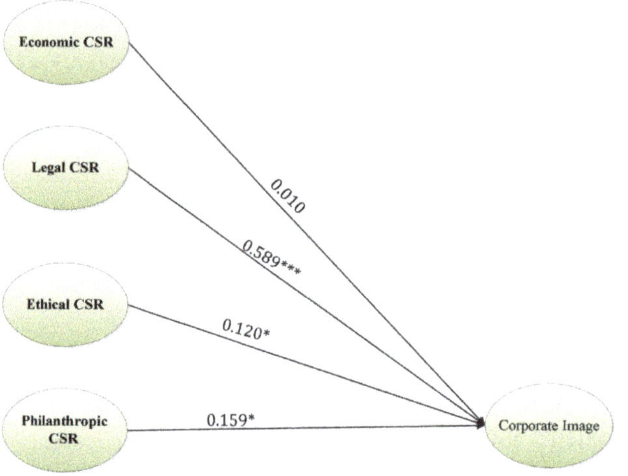

Figure 2. Results of the inner model A. Note: *** *p*-value < 0.001, * *p*-value < 0.05.

According to the findings of Model B highlighted in Table 4, and Figure 3, economic, legal, and philanthropical responsibilities of CSR were all found to have a positive influence on the corporate image supporting H1a (β= 0.293, t-value=6.80), H1b (β= 0.394, t-value=6.198), and H1c (β= 0.106, t-value=2.332), while not supporting H1d (β= 0.091, t-value=1.323), indicating that philanthropic responsibility has no significant relationship with corporate image. According to the statistical results, the relationship between CSR and corporate image has an incremental significance by including customer trust as a mediator.

Table 4. Hypotheses results for Model B.

Hypothesis	Path Coefficient	T Values	*p* Values	Results
H1a: Economic (CSR) -> Corporate image	0.293	6.080	0.000	Supported
H1b: Legal (CSR) -> Corporate image	0.394	6.198	0.000	Supported
H1c: Ethical (CSR) -> Corporate image	0.106	2.332	0.020	Supported
H1d: Philanthropic (CSR) -> Corporate image	0.091	1.323	0.186	Not Supported
H2a: Economic (CSR) -> Customer trust	0.076	1.936	0.053	Supported
H2b: Legal (CSR) -> Customer trust	0.272	3.627	0.000	Supported
H2c: Ethical (CSR) -> Customer trust	0.085	1.249	0.212	Not Supported
H2d: Philanthropic (CSR) -> Customer trust	0.471	5.761	0.000	Supported
H3: Customer trust -> Corporate image	0.178	3.504	0.000	Supported

The economic, legal, and philanthropic responsibilities of CSR influence customer trust, therefore H2a (β = 0.076, t-value = 1.936), H2b (β = 0.272, t-value = 3.627), and H2d (β = 0.471, t-value = 5.753) are supported. Ethical responsibility in CSR is not found to have an influence on corporate image (β = 0.085, t-value = 1.249); thus, H2d is not supported. Furthermore, customer trust was also found to have a significant impact on corporate image (β = 0.178, t-value = 3.504).

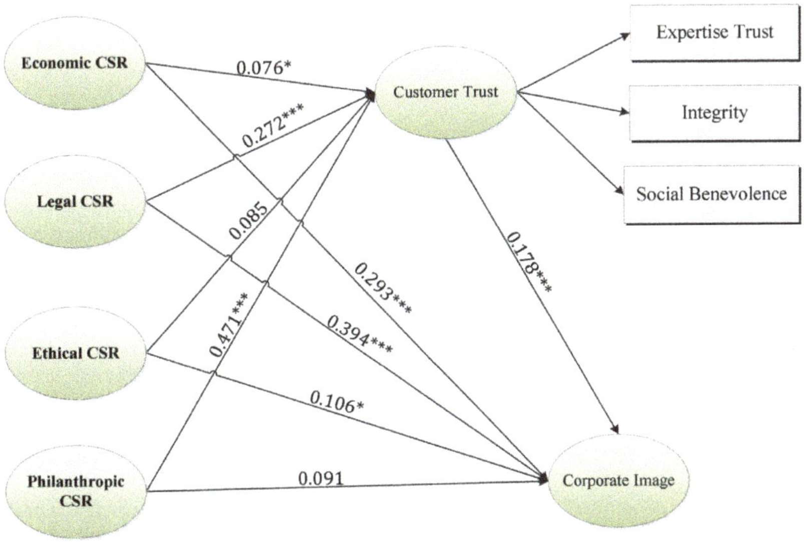

Figure 3. Results of the inner model B. Note: *** p-value < 0.001, * p-value < 0.05.

This study applied activity theory by Kofod-Petersen & Cassens [86] and the indirect effects as indicated in Table 5, generated by Smart pls to test the mediation results. According to the results shown in Table 5, customer trust fully mediates the relationship between economic and legal CSR with corporate image, while it partially mediates ethical and philanthropic CSRs' relationship with corporate image.

Table 5. Hypotheses and Mediating effects.

Hypothesis	Indirect Effects	Mediation
Economic (CSR) -> customer trust -> corporate image	0.014	Full
Legal (CSR) -> customer trust -> corporate image	0.048	Full
Ethical (CSR) -> customer trust -> corporate image	0.015	Partial
Philanthropic (CSR) -> customer trust -> corporate image	0.084	Partial

5. Discussion

This study is linked to the success of the hospitality marketing strategy; hence, it was imperative to perform an in-depth examination of the corporate image of the hotel. This study provides the framework to describe how the hotel's corporate image and customers' trust can be impacted by the four dimensions of corporate social responsibility. This framework will support other scholars in the hotel industry to comprehend customers' conduct built on their experiences of multidimensional CSR initiatives, corporate image, and customer trust.

With the growth of corporate social influence, CSR initiatives have been considered as a crucial component for a company's management. There is a requirement to recognize customers' opinions of CSR behaviors for potential corporate profitability. Consequently, this research examines the impact of multidimensional corporate social responsibility initiatives on corporate image. The findings revealed persuasive evidence stating customers' viewpoints regarding the CSR initiatives of a company could encourage their trust in the company. Each of the CSR constructs was found to have a significant impact on corporate image except, philanthropic CSR. The results of this study are somewhat similar to the study by Kim et al. [87]. According to their findings, ethical, economic, philanthropic, and legal responsibility, influenced corporate image and customer's citizenship behavior. The outcomes are also consistent with the generally recognized belief [15,88] that CSR significantly impacts the corporate image. However, in terms of the insignificant relationship of philanthropic CSR and CI, this study's results are somewhat similar to the research study by Park et al. [15]. According to their study, a company's ethical responsibilities did not have a significant impact on the CI of the company. This study delivers empirical inferences for businesses by validating the result of CSR initiatives as a principal factor in developing customers' trust as an organizational objective in the hotel business. It implies that the higher a company is understood to be involved in behaviors such as establishing a reasonable pricing strategy and generating jobs, the greater its corporate image is perceived by the customers. Additionally, companies' voluntary endeavors in favor of ecological sustainability and civil rights generate a positive attitude and a decent image. Furthermore, customers tend to have a constructive image of a business that conforms with rules and laws. Finally, a company requires to meet the expectation of the customers, perceiving the company to be a decent representative of society by partaking in or supporting social wellbeing. The outcomes indicate that to reinforce the corporate image, companies must give more consideration to the economic, legal, and ethical dimensions of corporate social responsibility.

According to the results, all CSR constructs had a significant impact on customer trust, except ethical responsibility. The research outcomes are consistent with the previous studies in the framework of customers' environmental activities [48] concerning the constructive influence of customers' corporate social responsibility experiences on their trust. When customers consider that a hotel worries about the outcomes of its functions on the environment and the community, they deem the hotel as a benevolent business, and they will trust it more. A study by Shafieizadeh & Tao [66] examined the impact of customers' views of a restaurant menu that comprises local food knowledge and its fundamental mechanism. The outcomes revealed that assessments of menu information influenced customers' views regarding the restaurant's openness and CSR initiatives significantly and additionally affected customers' trust significantly, but indirectly, via perceived corporate social responsibility actions. However, the insignificant relationship of ethical responsibility and trust was not found to be similar with other research studies. Previous researches found ethical responsibility to be in a significant relationship with customer trust [54,89].

Furthermore, the results of this study showed a positive and significant relationship between corporate image and customer trust. A study by Triatmanto et al. [60] revealed how the experiences and beliefs of hotel management in East Java enhance the corporate image as a marketing strategy of a hotel. Managers of the hospitality industry were selected as research respondents for this study. The findings demonstrated that the hotel management should comprehend the hotel's corporate image to maintain customers' trust in the hotel. Corresponding to the view of hotel management corporate image is exhibited by the trust presented by the hotel [90,91]. The managers in the hospitality industry also think that the hotel can acquire many guests if the customers trust the hotel. This implies that each hotel should be able to develop psychological recognition in the opinions of customers so that they can be driven to experience the same hotel again [64].

This research intended to build an enhanced understanding of the connection between corporate social responsibility and corporate image by contemplating a broader variety of CSR programs and the position of customer trust as a mediator between the relationship of corporate social responsibility and corporate image. Results showed that amongst the four types of CSR programs, the company's activities of economic and legal responsibility were fully mediated by customer trust, while ethical and philanthropic responsibility were partially mediated by customer trust. These outcomes are somewhat similar to the studies of Jongchul et al.'s [92] and Yoon et al.'s [88], according to results customers have a tendency to attach intentions to the company's philanthropic initiatives, and that a view of honesty and trustworthiness in the motivations results in a constructive company assessment.

6. Theoretical Implications

The research has the following theoretical implications. The first is that despite having theoretical assistance for the association of corporate social responsibility and corporate image in numerous service fields, little investigations have empirically examined the impacts of CSR's four dimensions on corporate image and customers' trust in association with the hotel service industry. This study is unique from earlier CSR research based on an assessment of the connection between CSR dimensions and corporate image to examine customers' trust in the company. Moreover, the dimensional composition of hotel corporate social responsibility was verified by examining the range of validity and reliability. Furthermore, the corporate social responsibility scale was demonstrated to be efficient in calculating the customers' attitude, trust, and perception regarding the service industry. Therefore, this scale might be utilized to describe additional variables, including customers' pro-social conduct, loyalty, and post-purchase conduct. Hence, the findings of this research can assist to build innovative information and expand to subsequent studies [1].

This research indicates that a company's corporate social responsibility initiatives affect the corporate image, which additionally affects the development of trust among customers and companies. Via the evaluation of the framework of CSR, customers' trust and corporate image were observed to be vital to a workable relationship. This study can hence be a beginning point in examining the association between corporate social responsibility and corporate image in customers' trust. It is assumed that customers recognize a company because its features are expressive, or parallel to their individual features or the features that they seek to possess. It is found that corporate social responsibility constantly plans a business's philanthropical and considerate principles that underline the uniqueness or character of the company, therefore it could be utilized as a powerful instrument by companies to create convincing images that appeal to customers' societal and emotional wants and encourage trust to a service company [3,93]. Certainly, the present research findings discovered that corporate social responsibility strengthens the customers' identification with a business in addition to their trust in that business. This conclusion develops the opinion that the blend of both viewpoints proposes an additional combined and complete method to understand the path from corporate social responsibility to the loyalty of customers, therefore offering managers with an added insight regarding the role and value of corporate social responsibility in developing trustworthy associations with customers.

Consequently, it was feasible to evaluate factors that impact corporate social responsibility and corporate image. By the formation and confirmation of subfactors of corporate social responsibility and corporate image, it facilitates to comprehend the four types of CSR and corporate image dimensions that impact customers' trust. A company's economic, legal and ethical CSR have a major effect on the corporate image of that company. Corporate image has an impact on making a suggestion, and that suggestion has an impact on the creation of customers' trust. This research improves the current information by demonstrating the mediation impact of customers' trust on the association between economic and legal CSR, and corporate image. Once customers consider that a hotel is striving to be understandable to them, by offering comprehensive information regarding the hotel's actions, they believe that it appreciates the expectations of its stakeholders, and hence the customers trust the hotel more.

7. Managerial Implications

The industrial and managerial implications of this research study are as follows. Hotels must try to enhance their corporate image, as the image is impacted by both the four dimensions of CSR and customers' trust. Corporate social responsibility was found to have an effect on corporate image, and economic, legal, and ethical corporate social responsibility initiatives were found to have a significant impact on corporate image whereas philanthropic responsibilities had no significant impact on corporate image. Based on this conclusion, operators can concentrate on economic CSR to boost the corporate image and promote customers' trust. Economic CSR initiatives produce profit via the delivery of attractive services. Customers wish for quality services at a satisfactory price. Firms can meet economic CSR initiatives by offering services much better than customers' beliefs. A company's economic initiatives mostly ignore the ecosystem or social responsibilities. Economic corporate social responsibility initiatives must hence be endorsed for profit-making purposes as a marketing strategy and an attractive answer to the social and ecological difficulties faced by a company. The hotel industry is engaged in organizing environmentally friendly marketing related to the ethical responsibilities to avoid pollution in the environment. Regarding legal responsibilities, the hotel industry must conform with sanitation and security procedures. Ethical and legal corporate social responsibility initiatives are considered to be vital, particularly in a competitive market. To satisfy philanthropic CSR, firms have maintained to organize charitable events or sponsor donations besides giving extra benefits to their employees. Businesses are now needed to engage with their society and give earnings back to society.

The results of this study can be utilized by employees to promote customers' trust, which can be useful to businesses. Maintaining constructive connections with customers can assist a business. Businesses want optimistic communications with customers to boost customers' trust. A business can build a community to accelerate the interaction between customers. Furthermore, if customers are paid with a souvenir or a coupon for their work and time, they may gain an emotional inclination to assist the business. As a consequence, customers will be extra loyal to the business.

Managers ought to be careful and tactical in using ethical and philanthropic responsibilities. Once a company performs philanthropic initiatives for a worthy reason, the company expects that customers consider a constructive acknowledgment regarding the company's motivations. Though businesses must contemplate the optimistic impacts of corporate social responsibility on their employees with discretion, as they might also possess some detrimental adverse outcomes like the staffs' inclination to engage in extra hard work and therefore result in labor dependence [94]. Accountable entrepreneurship is an enduring action and its initiation into the business delivers even greater advantages when there is an awareness for these initiatives [95,96].

This study made further practical contributions in offering hotels management understandings into the insight of corporate social responsibility dimensions and evaluating a hotel's corporate social responsibility operations. Consequently, hotel commerce must signify the necessity of smart customers and society, alongside worldwide developments regarding environmental safety. A hotel can comprehend its competition by frequently assessing and evaluating its corporate social responsibility endeavors with other hotels. Moreover, corporate social responsibility initiatives would additionally help enable internal organizational marketing by keeping decent relationships with personnel [1]. Service managers need to concentrate on corporate image protection and take into attention the significance of a corporation's image for their shareholders. More precisely, by skillfully controlling corporate image and corporate social responsibility as the prediction/interaction instrument of the company, they can encourage business relationships that may stimulate long-term relations and trust with customers [3,97].

8. Limitations and Future Research

This research has some shortcomings that have the possibility for potential research. The survey of this research was conducted in Pakistan; hence it has a shortage of representativeness and self-selection bias. To produce more generalized conclusions, the research survey can be done in numerous countries. Moreover, Pakistan is an emerging economy, future research can be conducted in developed economies and their results can be compared. Corporate image is an individual construct, therefore for a thorough investigation in the service perspective, several attitudinal and cognitive antecedents of corporate social responsibility should be considered for future potential research.

Furthermore, although Carroll's four CSR dimensions have been used recently in the service industry research [98,99]. Carroll's four corporate social responsibility dimension model has been extensively presented in the studies related to the hotel industry. Nevertheless, the hotel business varies from other businesses in conditions of stakeholders, customers, policies, organizational culture, and products due to its distinctive qualities that are indivisible, and intangible [100]. Additionally, the business neglects to indicate an expanding understanding of ecology, sustainability, renewable resource, and ecological safety [1,101–104]. Hence, future researchers can utilize the modified version of Carroll's CSR model while studying the service industry

Finally, since customers can act as effective agenda planners via various online platforms, they can become key influencers in times of crisis. Hence, future researchers can target the impact of customers communication on the periods of pre and post-crisis situations related to CSR.

9. Conclusions

The purpose of this is to analyze the connection between CSR dimensions and corporate image to examine customers' trust in an emerging economy, especially in times of crisis. This research empirically examines the relationships between a multi-dimensional set of corporate social responsibility (CSR) initiatives, numerous dimensions of customer trust, and corporate image in an emerging economy. It also analyzes the mediating effect of customer trust on the relationship between CSR and corporate image. The results revealed that economic, legal, and ethical CSR significantly impacted corporate image, while philanthropic CSR did not affect the corporate image. However, economic, legal, and philanthropic CSRs were found to be in a significant relationship with customer trust, while ethical CSR was not in a significant relationship with customer trust. Finally, customer trust fully mediated the relationship between economic and legal CSR with corporate image, whereas it partially mediated the relationship between ethical and philanthropic CSR.

Author Contributions: Conceptualization, C.-C.C.; Formal analysis, A.K., T.H., A.R. and Y.-T.C.; Investigation, A.K.; Methodology, C.-C.C., A.K., A.R. and Y.-T.C.; Supervision, T.H., S.-C.C. and O.S.; Validation, A.R. and Y.-T.C.; Writing—original draft, A.K., C.-C.C., S.-C.C., O.S., A.R., T.H. and Y.-T.C.; Writing—review & editing, A.K., C.-C.C., S.-C.C., A.R., O.S., T.H. and Y.-T.C. All authors have read and agreed to the published version of the manuscript.

Funding: This research received no external funding.

Informed Consent Statement: Informed consent was obtained from all subjects involved in the study.

Conflicts of Interest: The authors declare no conflict of interest.

Appendix A

Scales

Corporate Social Responsibility

- The hotel improves the tourism industry.
- The hotel generates employment through its operations.
- The hotel strives to activate the local economy.
- The hotel strives to achieve sustainable growth.
- The hotel properly implements health and safety rules and regulations.
- The hotel has established appropriate regulations for customers to abide by.
- The hotel strives to abide by regulations related to its customers' well-being.
- The hotel has established ethical guidelines for business activities.
- The hotel tries to become an ethically trustworthy company.
- The hotel makes efforts to fairly treat customers.
- The hotel participates in a variety of volunteer activities by starting the company's volunteer group.
- The hotel supports social welfare projects for the underprivileged.
- The hotel supports education programs.

Corporate Image (CI)

- I think the hotel emphasizes the rights of customers.
- I have good impressions of the hotel.
- In my opinion, the hotel has a good image in the minds of consumers.
- I think the service value provided by the hotel is high.
- I think the employees are very friendly.
- The appearance of the hotel is appealing.
- The area around the hotel is clean.
- The hotel is located in a nice area.
- The prices at the hotel are fair.
- I obtain value for my money at the hotel.

Consumer Trust

- The hotel performs its role of providing hoteling services very well.
- Overall, the hotel is a capable and proficient hoteling services provider.
- In general, the hotel is deeply knowledgeable about customer care.
- The hotel is truthful in its dealings with me.
- I would characterize the hotel as honest.
- The hotel would keep its commitments.
- The hotel is sincere and genuine.
- I believe that the hotel would act in my best interest.
- If I required help, the hotel would do its best to help me.
- The hotel is interested in my well-being, not just its own.

References

1. Wong, A.K.F.; Kim, S.S. Development and validation of standard hotel corporate social responsibility (CSR) scale from the employee perspective. *Int. J. Hosp. Manag.* **2020**, *87*, 102507. [CrossRef]
2. Fatma, M.; Khan, I.; Rahman, Z. The effect of CSR on consumer behavioral responses after service failure and recovery. *Eur. Bus. Rev.* **2016**, *28*, 583–599. [CrossRef]
3. Glaveli, N. Corporate social responsibility toward stakeholders and customer loyalty: Investigating the roles of trust and customer identification with the company. *Soc. Responsib. J.* **2021**, *17*, 367–383. [CrossRef]
4. Bansal, P.; Jiang, G.F.; Jung, J.C. Managing responsibly in tough economic times: Strategic and tactical CSR during the 2008–2009 global recession. *Long Range Plan.* **2015**, *48*, 69–79. [CrossRef]
5. Karaibrahimoglu, Y.Z. Corporate social responsibility in times of financial crisis. *Afr. J. Bus. Manag.* **2010**, *4*, 382.
6. Fehre, K.; Weber, F. Challenging corporate commitment to CSR: Do CEOs keep talking about corporate social responsibility (CSR) issues in times of the global financial crisis? *Manag. Res. Rev.* **2016**, *39*, 1410–1430. [CrossRef]
7. Lee, S.; Seo, K.; Sharma, A. Corporate social responsibility and firm performance in the airline industry: The moderating role of oil prices. *Tour. Manag.* **2013**, *38*, 20–30. [CrossRef]
8. Pérez, A.; Del Bosque, I.R. Corporate social responsibility and customer loyalty: Exploring the role of identification, satisfaction and type of company. *J. Serv. Mark.* **2015**, *29*, 15–25. [CrossRef]
9. Tian, Z.; Wang, R.; Yang, W. Consumer Responses to Corporate Social Responsibility (CSR) in China. *J. Bus. Ethics* **2011**, *101*, 197–212. [CrossRef]
10. Kim, H.L.; Rhou, Y.; Uysal, M.; Kwon, N. An examination of the links between corporate social responsibility (CSR) and its internal consequences. *Int. J. Hosp. Manag.* **2017**, *61*, 26–34. [CrossRef]
11. Plewa, C.; Conduit, J.; Quester, P.G.; Johnson, C. The Impact of Corporate Volunteering on CSR Image: A Consumer Perspective. *J. Bus. Ethics* **2015**, *127*, 643–659. [CrossRef]
12. Yi, Y.; Gong, T. Customer value co-creation behavior: Scale development and validation. *J. Bus. Res.* **2013**, *66*, 1279–1284. [CrossRef]
13. Blombäck, A.; Scandelius, C. Corporate heritage in CSR communication: A means to responsible brand image? *Corp. Commun. Int. J.* **2013**, *18*, 362–382. [CrossRef]
14. Martínez, P.; Pérez, A.; Del Bosque, I.R. CSR influence on hotel brand image and loyalty. *Acad. Rev. Latinoam. Adm.* **2014**, *27*, 267–283. [CrossRef]
15. Park, J.; Lee, H.; Kim, C. Corporate social responsibilities, consumer trust and corporate reputation: South Korean consumers' perspectives. *J. Bus. Res.* **2014**, *67*, 295–302. [CrossRef]
16. Famiyeh, S.; Kwarteng, A.; Dadzie, S.A. Corporate social responsibility and reputation: Some empirical perspectives. *J. Glob. Responsib.* **2016**, *7*, 258–274. [CrossRef]
17. Khuong, M.N.; An, N.K.T.; Hang, T.T.T. Stakeholders and Corporate Social Responsibility (CSR) programme as key sustainable development strategies to promote corporate reputation—evidence from vietnam. *Cogent Bus. Manag.* **2021**, *8*, 1917333. [CrossRef]
18. Becker-Olsen, K.L.; Cudmore, B.A.; Hill, R.P. The impact of perceived corporate social responsibility on consumer behavior. *J. Bus. Res.* **2006**, *59*, 46–53. [CrossRef]
19. Barry, J.M.; Dion, P.; Johnson, W. A cross-cultural examination of relationship strength in B2B services. *J. Serv. Mark.* **2008**, *22*, 114–135. [CrossRef]
20. Singh, J.J.; Iglesias, O.; Batista-Foguet, J.M. Does Having an Ethical Brand Matter? The Influence of Consumer Perceived Ethicality on Trust, Affect and Loyalty. *J. Bus. Ethics* **2012**, *111*, 541–549. [CrossRef]
21. Iglesias, O.; Markovic, S.; Bagherzadeh, M.; Singh, J.J. Co-creation: A Key Link Between Corporate Social Responsibility, Customer Trust, and Customer Loyalty. *J. Bus. Ethics* **2018**, *163*, 151–166. [CrossRef]
22. Markovic, S.; Iglesias, O.; Singh, J.J.; Sierra, V. How does the Perceived Ethicality of Corporate Services Brands Influence Loyalty and Positive Word-of-Mouth? Analyzing the Roles of Empathy, Affective Commitment, and Perceived Quality. *J. Bus. Ethics* **2015**, *148*, 721–740. [CrossRef]
23. Sierra, V.; Iglesias, O.; Markovic, S.; Singh, J.J. Does Ethical Image Build Equity in Corporate Services Brands? The Influence of Customer Perceived Ethicality on Affect, Perceived Quality, and Equity. *J. Bus. Ethics* **2017**, *144*, 661–676. [CrossRef]
24. Ramaswamy, V.; Ozcan, K. Brand value co-creation in a digitalized world: An integrative framework and research implications. *Int. J. Res. Mark.* **2016**, *33*, 93–106. [CrossRef]
25. Ind, N.; Iglesias, O.; Markovic, S. The co-creation continuum: From tactical market research tool to strategic collaborative innovation method. *J. Brand Manag.* **2017**, *24*, 310–321. [CrossRef]
26. Sen, S.; Bhattacharya, C. Does Doing Good Always Lead to Doing Better? Consumer Reactions to Corporate Social Responsibility. *J. Mark. Res.* **2001**, *38*, 225–243. [CrossRef]
27. Castaldo, S.; Perrini, F.; Misani, N.; Tencati, A. The Missing Link Between Corporate Social Responsibility and Consumer Trust: The Case of Fair Trade Products. *J. Bus. Ethics* **2009**, *84*, 1–15. [CrossRef]
28. Carroll, A.B. The pyramid of corporate social responsibility: Toward the moral management of organizational stakeholders. *Bus. Horiz.* **1991**, *34*, 39–48. [CrossRef]
29. Mayer, R.C.; Davis, J.H.; Schoorman, F.D. An Integrative Model of Organizational Trust. *Acad. Manag. Rev.* **1995**, *20*, 709–734. [CrossRef]

30. Hannan, M.T.; Freeman, J. Structural Inertia and Organizational Change. *Am. Sociol. Rev.* **1984**, *49*, 149–164. [CrossRef]
31. Adeniji, A.A.; Osibanjo, A.O.; Abiodun, J.; Oni-Ojo, E.E. Corporate Image: A Strategy for Enhancing Customer Loyalty and Profitability. *J. South Afr. Bus. Res.* **2015**, *2015*, 1–12. [CrossRef]
32. Martínez, P.; del Bosque, I.R. Sustainability dimensions: A source to enhance corporate reputation. *Corp. Reput. Rev.* **2014**, *17*, 239–253. [CrossRef]
33. Keh, H.T.; Xie, Y. Corporate reputation and customer behavioral intentions: The roles of trust, identification and commitment. *Ind. Mark. Manag.* **2009**, *38*, 732–742. [CrossRef]
34. Mohr, L.A.; Webb, D.J. The effects of corporate social responsibility and price on consumer responses. *J. Consum. Aff.* **2005**, *39*, 121–147. [CrossRef]
35. Lombart, C.; Louis, D. A study of the impact of Corporate Social Responsibility and price image on retailer personality and consumers' reactions (satisfaction, trust and loyalty to the retailer). *J. Retail. Consum. Serv.* **2014**, *21*, 630–642. [CrossRef]
36. Russo, A.; Perrini, F. Investigating Stakeholder Theory and Social Capital: CSR in Large Firms and SMEs. *J. Bus. Ethics* **2010**, *91*, 207–221. [CrossRef]
37. Ghaderi, Z.; Mirzapour, M.; Henderson, J.C.; Richardson, S. Corporate social responsibility and hotel performance: A view from Tehran, Iran. *Tour. Manag. Perspect.* **2019**, *29*, 41–47. [CrossRef]
38. Ozdora-Aksak, E.; Ferguson, M.A.; Duman, S.A. Corporate social responsibility and CSR fit as predictors of corporate reputation: A global perspective. *Public Relat. Rev.* **2016**, *42*, 79–81. [CrossRef]
39. Bianchi, E.C.; Bruno, J.M.; Sarabia-Sanchez, F.J. The impact of perceived CSR on corporate reputation and purchase intention. *Eur. J. Manag. Bus. Econ.* **2019**, *28*, 206–221. [CrossRef]
40. Alvarado-Herrera, A.; Bigne, E.; Aldas-Manzano, J.; Curras-Perez, R. A Scale for Measuring Consumer Perceptions of Corporate Social Responsibility Following the Sustainable Development Paradigm. *J. Bus. Ethics* **2017**, *140*, 243–262. [CrossRef]
41. Rivera, J.; Bigne, E.; Curras-Perez, R. Effects of Corporate Social Responsibility perception on consumer satisfaction with the brand. *Span. J. Mark. ESIC* **2016**, *20*, 104–114. [CrossRef]
42. Popoli, P. Linking CSR strategy and brand image: Different approaches in local and global markets. *Mark. Theory.* **2011**, *11*, 419–433. [CrossRef]
43. Hillenbrand, C.; Money, K.; Pavelin, S. Stakeholder-Defined Corporate Responsibility for a Pre-Credit-Crunch Financial Service Company: Lessons for How Good Reputations are Won and Lost. *J. Bus. Ethics* **2011**, *105*, 337–356. [CrossRef]
44. Kim, B.; Lee, S.; Kang, K.H. The moderating role of CEO narcissism on the relationship between uncertainty avoidance and CSR. *Tour. Manag.* **2018**, *67*, 203–213. [CrossRef]
45. Lee, S.; Kim, B.; Ham, S. Strategic CSR for airlines: Does materiality matter? *Int. J. Contemp. Hosp. Manag.* **2018**, *30*, 3592–3608. [CrossRef]
46. McKnight, D.H.; Choudhury, V.; Kacmar, C. Developing and Validating Trust Measures for e-Commerce: An Integrative Typology. *Inf. Syst. Res.* **2002**, *13*, 334–359. [CrossRef]
47. Mayer, R.C.; Davis, J.H. The effect of the performance appraisal system on trust for management: A field quasi-experiment. *J. Appl. Psychol.* **1999**, *84*, 123–136. [CrossRef]
48. Pivato, S.; Misani, N.; Tencati, A. The impact of corporate social responsibility on consumer trust: The case of organic food. *Bus. Ethics A Eur. Rev.* **2007**, *17*, 3–12. [CrossRef]
49. Lin, J.; Lu, Y.; Wang, B.; Wei, K.K. The role of inter-channel trust transfer in establishing mobile commerce trust. *Electron. Commer. Res. Appl.* **2011**, *10*, 615–625. [CrossRef]
50. Martínez, P.; del Bosque, I.R. CSR and customer loyalty: The roles of trust, customer identification with the company and satisfaction. *Int. J. Hosp. Manag.* **2013**, *35*, 89–99. [CrossRef]
51. Swaen, V.; Chumpitaz, R.C. Impact of Corporate Social Responsibility on Consumer Trust. *Rech. Appl. Mark.* **2008**, *23*, 7–34. [CrossRef]
52. Vlachos, P.A.; Tsamakos, A.; Vrechopoulos, A.P.; Avramidis, P.K. Corporate social responsibility: Attributions, loyalty, and the mediating role of trust. *J. Acad. Mark. Sci.* **2009**, *37*, 170–180. [CrossRef]
53. Crespo, Á.H.; Del Bosque, I.R.; Sánchez, M.M.G.D.L.S. The influence of perceived risk on Internet shopping behavior: A multidimensional perspective. *J. Risk Res.* **2009**, *12*, 259–277. [CrossRef]
54. Choi, B.; La, S. The impact of corporate social responsibility (CSR) and customer trust on the restoration of loyalty after service failure and recovery. *J. Serv. Mark.* **2013**, *27*, 223–233. [CrossRef]
55. Islam, T.; Islam, R.; Pitafi, A.H.; Xiaobei, L.; Rehmani, M.; Irfan, M.; Mubarak, M.S. The impact of corporate social responsibility on customer loyalty: The mediating role of corporate reputation, customer satisfaction, and trust. *Sustain. Prod. Consum.* **2021**, *25*, 123–135. [CrossRef]
56. Kim, J.; Cho, K.; Park, C.K. Does CSR Assurance Affect the Relationship between CSR Performance and Financial Performance? *Sustainability* **2019**, *11*, 5682. [CrossRef]
57. Hosmer, L.T. Trust: The Connecting Link between Organizational Theory and Philosophical Ethics. *Acad. Manag. Rev.* **1995**, *20*, 379–403. [CrossRef]
58. DeConinck, J.B. The effect of organizational justice, perceived organizational support, and perceived supervisor support on marketing employees' level of trust. *J. Bus. Res.* **2010**, *63*, 1349–1355. [CrossRef]

59. Paine, J.B.; Organ, D.W. The cultural matrix of organizational citizenship behavior: Some preliminary conceptual and empirical observations. *Hum. Resour. Manag. Rev.* **2000**, *10*, 45–59.
60. Triatmanto, B.; Respati, H.; Wahyuni, N. Towards an understanding of corporate image in the hospitality industry East Java, Indonesia. *Heliyon* **2021**, *7*, e06404. [CrossRef]
61. Wallace, E.; De Chernatony, L. Service Employee Performance: Its Components and Antecedents. *J. Relatsh. Mark.* **2009**, *8*, 82–102. [CrossRef]
62. Dominguez, A.A. The impact of human resource disclosure on corporate image. *J. Hum. Resour. Costing Account.* **2011**, *15*, 279–298. [CrossRef]
63. Song, H.; Ruan, W.; Park, Y. Effects of Service Quality, Corporate Image, and Customer Trust on the Corporate Reputation of Airlines. *Sustainability* **2019**, *11*, 3302. [CrossRef]
64. Sarkar, S.; Singh, P. Strategising CSR in addressing sustainable development goals using a scorecard approach. *World Rev. Sci. Technol. Sustain. Dev.* **2019**, *15*, 313–329. [CrossRef]
65. Xhema, J.; Metin, H.; Groumpos, P. Switching-Costs, Corporate Image and Product Quality effect on Customer Loyalty: Kosovo Retail Market. *IFAC-PapersOnLine* **2018**, *51*, 287–292. [CrossRef]
66. Shafieizadeh, K.; Tao, C.-W.W. How does a menu's information about local food affect restaurant selection? The roles of corporate social responsibility, transparency, and trust. *J. Hosp. Tour. Manag.* **2020**, *43*, 232–240. [CrossRef]
67. Hosmer, L.T. Strategic planning as if ethics mattered. *Strat. Manag. J.* **2007**, *15*, 17–34. [CrossRef]
68. Bozic, B. Consumer trust repair: A critical literature review. *Eur. Manag. J.* **2017**, *35*, 538–547. [CrossRef]
69. Colquitt, J.A.; Rodell, J.B. Justice, Trust, and Trustworthiness: A Longitudinal Analysis Integrating Three Theoretical Perspectives. *Acad. Manag. J.* **2011**, *54*, 1183–1206. [CrossRef]
70. Ariffin, S.; Yusof, J.M.; Putit, L.; Shah, M.I.A. Factors Influencing Perceived Quality and Repurchase Intention Towards Green Products. *Procedia Econ. Financ.* **2016**, *37*, 391–396. [CrossRef]
71. Giovanis, A.N.; Zondiros, D.; Tomaras, P. The Antecedents of Customer Loyalty for Broadband Services: The Role of Service Quality, Emotional Satisfaction and Corporate Image. *Procedia-Soc. Behav. Sci.* **2014**, *148*, 236–244. [CrossRef]
72. Chowdhury, J.; Reardon, J.; Srivastava, R. Alternative Modes of Measuring Store Image: An Empirical Assessment of Structured versus Unstructured Measures. *J. Mark. Theory Pract.* **1998**, *6*, 72–86. [CrossRef]
73. Anderson, J.C.; Gerbing, D.W. Structural equation modeling in practice: A review and recommended two-step approach. *Psychol. Bull.* **1988**, *103*, 411. [CrossRef]
74. Hulland, J. Use of partial least squares (PLS) in strategic management research: A review of four recent studies. *Strateg. Manag. J.* **1999**, *20*, 195–204. [CrossRef]
75. Petter, S.; Straub, D.; Rai, A. Specifying Formative Constructs in Information Systems Research. *MIS Q.* **2007**, *31*, 623–656. [CrossRef]
76. Chin, W.W.; Newsted, P.R. Structural equation modeling analysis with small samples using partial least squares. *Stat. Strateg. Small Sample Res.* **1999**, *1*, 307–341.
77. Hair, J.F., Jr.; Babin, B.J.; Anderson, R.E. *A Global P-Erspect-Ivie*; Kennesaw State University: Kennesaw, GA, USA, 2010.
78. Chin, W.W. The partial least squares approach to structural equation modeling. *Mod. Methods Bus. Res.* **1998**, *295*, 295–336.
79. Fornell, C.; Larcker, D.F. *Structural Equation Models with Unobservable Variables and Measurement Error: Algebra and Statistics*; Sage Publications: Los Angeles, CA, USA, 1981.
80. Hair, J.F., Jr.; Hult, G.T.M.; Ringle, C.; Sarstedt, M. *A Primer on Partial Least Squares Structural Equation Modeling (PLS-SEM)*; Sage Publications: Los Angeles, CA, USA, 2016.
81. Tenenhaus, M.; Vinzi, V.E.; Chatelin, Y.-M.; Lauro, C. PLS path modeling. *Comput. Stat. Data Anal.* **2005**, *48*, 159–205. [CrossRef]
82. Wetzels, M.; Odekerken-Schröder, G.; Van Oppen, C. Using PLS Path Modeling for Assessing Hierarchical Construct Models: Guidelines and Empirical Illustration. *MIS Q.* **2009**, *33*, 177–195. [CrossRef]
83. Hu, L.T.; Bentler, P.M. Cutoff criteria for fit indexes in covariance structure analysis: Conventional criteria versus new alternatives. *Struct. Equ. Model. Multidiscip. J.* **1999**, *6*, 1–55. [CrossRef]
84. Henseler, J.; Dijkstra, T.K.; Sarstedt, M.; Ringle, C.M.; Diamantopoulos, A.; Straub, D.W.; Calantone, R.J. Common beliefs and reality about PLS: Comments on Rönkkö and Evermann. *Organ. Res. Methods* **2014**, *17*, 182–209. [CrossRef]
85. Purvis, R.L.; Sambamurthy, V.; Zmud, R.W. The Assimilation of Knowledge Platforms in Organizations: An Empirical Investigation. *Organ. Sci.* **2001**, *12*, 117–135. [CrossRef]
86. Kofod-Petersen, A.; Cassens, J. Using activity theory to model context awareness. In *International Workshop on Modeling and Retrieval of Context*; Springer: Berlin, Germany, 2015; pp. 1–17.
87. Kim, M.; Yin, X.; Lee, G. The effect of CSR on corporate image, customer citizenship behaviors, and customers' long-term relationship orientation. *Int. J. Hosp. Manag.* **2020**, *88*, 102520. [CrossRef]
88. Yoon, Y.; Gurhan-Canli, Z.; Schwarz, N. The Effect of Corporate Social Responsibility (CSR) Activities on Companies with Bad Reputations. *J. Consum. Psychol.* **2006**, *16*, 377–390. [CrossRef]
89. Coulter, K.S.; Coulter, R.A. The effects of industry knowledge on the development of trust in service relationships. *Int. J. Res. Mark.* **2003**, *20*, 31–43. [CrossRef]
90. Balmer, J.; Greyser, S. *Revealing the Corporation: Perspectives on Identity, Image, Reputation, Corporate Branding and Corporate Level Marketing*; Routledge: Oxfordshire, UK, 2003.

91. Boulding, K.E. General systems theory—The skeleton of science. *Manag. Sci.* **1956**, *2*, 197–208. [CrossRef]
92. Seongkon, L.; Gento, M.; Matsushima, J.; Jongchul, H. Competitiveness analysis of international journal paper and patent on carbon capture and storage technology: In the case of government supported research institutes and major universities. *AFORE* **2013**, 293.
93. Chung, K.-H.; Yu, J.-E.; Choi, M.-G.; Shin, J.-I. The Effects of CSR on Customer Satisfaction and Loyalty in China: The Moderating Role of Corporate Image. *J. Econ. Bus. Manag.* **2015**, *3*, 542–547. [CrossRef]
94. Brieger, S.A.; Anderer, S.; Fröhlich, A.; Bäro, A.; Meynhardt, T. Too Much of a Good Thing? On the Relationship Between CSR and Employee Work Addiction. *J. Bus. Ethics* **2019**, *166*, 311–329. [CrossRef]
95. Kotowska, B.; Martyniuk, T. Reporting of Corporate Social Responsibility in Smes Sector in Poland. 2015. Available online: https://ideas.repec.org/a/scn/000ven/50136.html (accessed on 14 June 2021).
96. Rózsa, Z.; Belás, J.; Khan, K.A.; Zvaríková, K. Corporate social responsibility and essential factors of personnel risk management in SMEs. *Pol. J. Manag. Stud.* **2021**, *23*, 449–463.
97. Jeffrey, S.; Rosenberg, S.; McCabe, B. Corporate social responsibility behaviors and corporate reputation. *Soc. Responsib. J.* **2019**, *15*, 395–408. [CrossRef]
98. Lee, S.; Han, H.; Radic, A.; Tariq, B. Corporate social responsibility (CSR) as a customer satisfaction and retention strategy in the chain restaurant sector. *J. Hosp. Tour. Manag.* **2020**, *45*, 348–358. [CrossRef]
99. Kim, Y.; Lee, S.S.; Roh, T. Taking Another Look at Airline CSR: How Required CSR and Desired CSR Affect Customer Loyalty in the Airline Industry. *Sustainability* **2020**, *12*, 4281. [CrossRef]
100. Lovelock, C.; Gummesson, E. Whither services marketing? In search of a new paradigm and fresh perspectives. *J. Serv. Res.* **2004**, *7*, 20–41. [CrossRef]
101. Ettinger, A.; Grabner-Kräuter, S.; Terlutter, R. Online CSR communication in the hotel industry: Evidence from small hotels. *Int. J. Hosp. Manag.* **2018**, *68*, 94–104. [CrossRef]
102. Supanti, D.; Butcher, K.; Fredline, L. Enhancing the employer-employee relationship through corporate social responsibility (CSR) engagement. *Int. J. Contemp. Hosp. Manag.* **2015**, *27*, 1479–1498. [CrossRef]
103. Tamajón, L.G.; Font, X. Corporate social responsibility in tourism small and medium enterprises evidence from Europe and Latin America. *Tour. Manag. Perspect.* **2013**, *7*, 38–46. [CrossRef]
104. Zientara, P.; Zamojska, A.; Nikodemska-Wołowik, A.M. CSR, age management and altruism: The role of future time perspective and personal altruistic convictions. *Przedsiębiorczość i Zarządzanie* **2018**, *19*, 439–454.

International Journal of
Environmental Research and Public Health

MDPI

Article

Corporate Social Responsibility Disclosure: Responding to Investors' Criticism on Social Media

Yuming Zhang and Fan Yang *

School of Management, Shandong University, Jinan 250100, China; zhangym@sdu.edu.cn
* Correspondence: fanyang@mail.sdu.edu.cn; Tel.: +86-183-6611-1863

Abstract: Companies use corporate social responsibility (CSR) disclosures to communicate their social and environmental policies, practices, and performance to stakeholders. Although the determinants and outcomes of CSR activities are well understood, we know little about how companies use CSR communication to manage a crisis. The few relevant CSR studies have focused on the pressure on corporations exerted by governments, customers, the media, or the public. Although investors have a significant influence on firm value, this stakeholder group has been neglected in research on CSR disclosure. Grounded in legitimacy theory and agency theory, this study uses a sample of Chinese public companies listed on the Shanghai Stock Exchange to investigate CSR disclosure in response to social media criticism posted by investors. The empirical findings show that investors' social media criticism not only motivates companies to disclose their CSR activities but also increases the substantiveness of their CSR reports, demonstrating that companies' CSR communication in response to a crisis is substantive rather than merely symbolic. We also find that the impact of social media criticism on CSR disclosure is heterogeneous. Non-state-owned enterprises, companies in regions with high levels of environmental regulations, and companies in regions with local government concern about social issues are most likely to disclose CSR information and report substantive CSR activities. We provide an in-depth analysis of corporate CSR strategies for crisis management and show that crises initiated by investors on social media provide opportunities for corporations to improve their CSR engagement.

Keywords: corporate social responsibility disclosure; social media criticism; investors; crisis management; SOEs; NSOEs; regulatory pressure

1. Introduction

The disclosure of corporate social responsibility (CSR) has increased significantly in recent years, receiving growing attention from both academics and practitioners [1,2]. CSR disclosure reflects a company's attitudes toward the interests of various stakeholders and its commitment to sustainable development [3]. Communicating CSR has significant benefits, such as improving customer loyalty and brand recognition, reducing the risk of government sanctions, lowering the cost of equity capital, and increasing competitive advantage and long-run value [4–7]. Studies have identified the specific antecedents and consequences of CSR disclosure decisions [1,4]. However, few attempts have been made to investigate companies' CSR disclosure strategies in response to crises, especially those instigated by investors.

Crises are situations that can have devastating consequences for an organization. As a typical crisis, investors' criticism on social media can seriously damage a company's reputation and increase its business risks [8]. The literature has largely explored companies' CSR disclosure decisions in response to pressure from governments, customers, the media, or the public [9]. Although investors are essential stakeholders in capital markets, investor-initiated pressure has been neglected in the research on CSR disclosure. Today, social media platforms (e.g., Facebook and Twitter) allow investors, especially small investors, to publicly voice their concerns. This may have serious consequences for firms in the firing line, as negative feedback on organizations spreads rapidly on social media [10]. Social media criticism posted by investors therefore poses a considerable threat to companies' image and legitimacy. To minimize the associated risks, companies are likely to conduct CSR communication campaigns to manage stakeholder perceptions [11]. Focusing on crises generated by investors' social media criticism, this study investigates whether companies respond to crises by disclosing CSR activities.

However, companies' CSR disclosures may not fully reflect their CSR behaviors. An important issue, which remains under-explored in the literature, is the extent to which CSR disclosures are symbolic or substantive. Although many companies issue CSR reports on their social and environmental policies, practices, and performance, these disclosures may be little more than a strategic response to resolve crises rather than demonstrating substantive effort [12]. A frequently cited example is the "Beyond Petroleum" campaign by British Petroleum (BP), which makes frequent claims about its plans to invest in renewable energy to reduce global warming. However, the firm was criticized for its negative environmental impact at the Johannesburg Earth Summit [12]. Nevertheless, most studies have focused on the likelihood of companies' disclosing CSR activities and paid little attention to the quality of the CSR communication [1,13]. To help fill this research gap, we provide in-depth insights into whether companies take substantive CSR actions or merely act symbolically in response to investors' social media criticism.

We are also interested in assessing whether companies' responses to social media criticism vary depending on the need for CSR communication. Social media criticism posted by investors may create varying degrees of difficulty for companies with diverse attributes, leading to heterogeneous CSR strategies. For example, Chinese state-owned enterprises (SOEs) controlled by central or local governments have considerable access to political support, even when they are heavily criticized by stakeholders [14]. As non-state-owned enterprises (NSOEs) lack government endorsement, they may be more vulnerable to criticism [13]. Therefore, the need to use communication strategies to manage societal perceptions in times of crisis is expected to be greater among NSOEs. We thus verify whether the influence of social media criticism on CSR disclosure varies between SOEs and NSOEs. In addition, regulatory pressure is a key determinant of CSR implementation [15]. When local governments place greater emphasis on environmental and social issues, CSR disclosure is considered more important. As a result, the intensity of government environmental regulation and social concern may influence companies' decisions on CSR disclosure in response to a crisis. Therefore, we also investigate whether the effect of social media criticism on CSR disclosure differs across regions with higher and lower levels of regulatory pressure.

While CSR disclosure strategies have been widely discussed in the context of Western economies [1,4,5], relatively few studies have focused on this issue in emerging markets such as China. It is crucial to address CSR disclosure strategies in China, an increasingly important global player in CSR, for the following three reasons. First, China's economic and manufacturing growth in the last few decades has brought significant environmental and social problems. Second, although CSR is an increasingly important item on corporate agendas in China, the quality of Chinese companies' CSR disclosures has been questioned [14]. Third, while investors are the main participants in Chinese markets, formal legal protection for this group is weak. Social media provide a new channel for investors to influence corporate decision making [16]. Based on legitimacy theory and agency theory, we find that Chinese listed companies are more likely to disclose CSR activities when facing more criticism on social media from investors. In addition, companies facing more criticism are more likely to elaborate on the specific CSR actions taken, indicating that their responses are not merely symbolic. Furthermore, our analysis suggests that these responses are heterogeneous. The effects of social media criticism on CSR disclosure choice and substantiveness are more pronounced among NSOEs than

SOEs. In addition, such criticism only has a significant effect on CSR disclosure in regions with high levels of environmental and social concern.

We contribute to the literature in several ways. First, we extend the CSR disclosure research from the perspective of crisis management. Studies have systematically explored the motivations for and outcomes of CSR activities and their disclosure [17,18]. However, CSR disclosure and its symbolic strategies in times of crisis have been underexplored. We attempt to fill this research gap by assessing both the probability and substantiveness of CSR disclosure in response to crises. Second, although investors are a powerful group with the ability to influence a company's direction [19], studies have mainly focused on the demands of other stakeholders (e.g., governments and customers) [9,20]. We thus focus on the pressure exerted by investors through criticism on social media platforms. We use machine learning to identify such criticism and are able to correlate corporate responses with the intensity of social media criticism. Third, our findings suggest that CSR disclosure strategies in response to crises vary depending on company ownership and government intervention, providing in-depth insights into companies' CSR communication behavior in times of crisis. Furthermore, we offer guidance for regulators on promoting CSR engagement and disclosure.

The rest of this paper is organized as follows. Section 2 introduces the institutional background. Section 3 presents the theoretical background, discusses the literature, and develops our hypotheses. Section 4 details the methodology. In Section 5, we present our empirical findings. Section 6 details further analyses of the heterogeneous impact of social media criticism. Section 7 concludes the study by describing its implications and limitations.

2. Institutional Background

2.1. CSR Disclosure in China

China is the world's largest emerging economy. Although the country differs from the developed countries in which CSR originated [13], China is rapidly becoming a critical player in CSR. In the 1990s, when CSR initiatives were already a core business strategy in Western countries, Chinese enterprises rarely engaged in CSR [21]. To some extent, the growth of the Chinese economy at that time came at the expense of environmental considerations. Unsurprisingly, given the critical influence of the government on business and the economy in China [22], the growing emphasis on social and environmental responsibility is mainly guided by government policy. The Chinese government has begun to realize the need to balance the pursuit of economic growth with environmental protection and social development [23]. In 2003, the Scientific Outlook on Development was introduced in the Third Plenary Session of the 16th Central Committee, seeking to direct the economy toward comprehensive, coordinated, and sustainable development. Subsequently, the goal of building a harmonious society was introduced in the central government's 11th Five-Year Plan. As a component of both China's Scientific Outlook on Development and its plan to build a harmonious society, CSR is clearly on the national strategic agenda.

In terms of CSR disclosure, it was not until 2006 that CSR was explicitly recognized in company law in China [2]. In September 2006, the Shenzhen Stock Exchange (SZSE) issued its "Guidelines for Corporate Social Responsibility of Listed Companies." Companies listed on the SZSE are expected to behave in a socially responsible manner and make voluntary disclosures on their performance. In 2008, the Shanghai Stock Exchange (SSE) released two sets of guidelines regarding listed companies' social responsibility and environmental information disclosure. In the same year, the State-owned Assets Supervision and Administration Commission of the State Council (SASAC) released a document on CSR for central-government-controlled SOEs, encouraging these companies to demonstrate social and environmental responsibility and voluntarily disclose their CSR. At present, companies included in the SZSE 100 index are required to publish reports on their social responsibility. In the SSE, three types of listed companies have been required to publish CSR reports since 2008, namely, companies listed in the Corporate Governance Index, companies that list shares overseas, and companies in the financial sector [13]. Other companies listed on both stock exchanges are encouraged to make CSR disclosures on a voluntary basis. In the short history of CSR disclosure in China, government promotion has rendered CSR disclosure an increasingly important component of business, attracting the attention of various stakeholders.

Figure 1 presents the number of Chinese A-share listed companies that disclose CSR information, according to data from the China Security Markets and Accounting Research (CSMAR) database. Due to severe data limitations before 2010, we analyze only data from 2010. As shown, Chinese listed companies gradually increased their CSR disclosure practices from 2010 to 2019. In 2017, the number of voluntary CSR disclosures exceeded the number of mandatory disclosures for the first time. From that year onward, a stable increase in the proportion of voluntary CSR disclosure can be observed. In the latest available year (2019), 597 of the 1018 CSR disclosures issued were voluntary, three times greater than in the starting year, 2010. These numbers indicate that Chinese listed companies are gradually recognizing the value of voluntary disclosure. However, there is still a significant gap between China and Western countries in terms of the level of CSR disclosure. To supplement the research on emerging markets, it is crucial to assess Chinese firms' social responsibility initiatives and disclosure strategies.

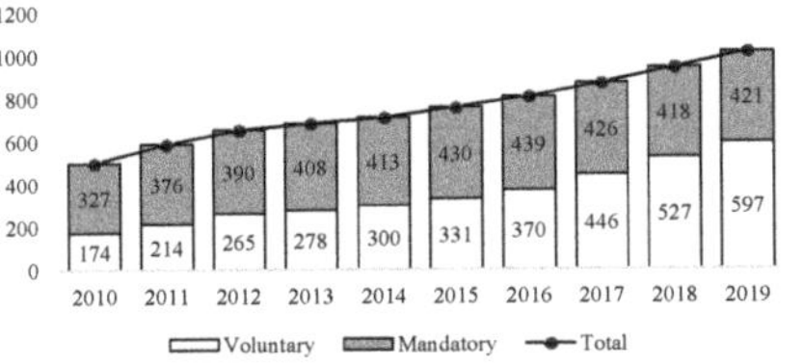

Figure 1. The number of CSR disclosure reports issued by Chinese listed firms from 2010 to 2019.

2.2. *The Use of Social Media in Capital Markets and Potential Crises*

We focus on small investors as company stakeholders. Whereas developed capital markets are dominated by institutional investors, small investors are the main participants in emerging markets. In China, small investors account for 99.77% of stock market participants (according to Chinese statistics, the number of investors at the end of January 2021 was 179,869,200, of which natural persons numbered 179,448,300 (data source: China Securities Depository and Clearing Corporation Limited, CSDC)) and thus play an important role in corporate governance. How best to respond to the demands and manage the perceptions of this group is a vital question for companies in emerging markets. In the last two decades, the managers of listed companies have sought to interact with large institutional stakeholders through road shows, conference calls, and site visits [10]. However, they have neglected small investors, as the formal legal protections for such investors are relatively weak in emerging economies [16]. Therefore, this group has had to seek alternative channels, such as new forms of media [24,25], to influence company decisions [26].

Along with the growing use of information technology in capital markets, social media platforms have become an increasingly important tool for firm–investor communication [10]. In 2013, the U.S. Securities and Exchange Commission (SEC) issued guidelines that explicitly approved companies' use of social media platforms to announce information (see https://www.sec.gov/news/press-release/2013-2013-51htm#.VM9R3u8rfc, accessed on 10 July 2021)). In the same year, the SSE built a formal social media platform known as E-interactive (see http://sns.sseinfo.com, accessed on 10 July 2021)), aiming to encourage two-way interaction between listed companies and investors. Since then, Chinese market participants, especially small investors, have had a direct line with which to communicate with managers. Given their interactive nature, social media have changed not only the process of companies' information dissemination but also corporate governance [27]. Social media provide investors with the opportunity to process and disseminate information, potentially challenging top managers in a public forum. However, social media are a double-edged sword, as they can trigger a crisis by broadcasting damaging news to a wider audience, thereby accelerating the spread of negative sentiments. Due to the unpredictability of the fallout from social media criticism, firms have lost a certain amount of control over their information environments [28]. As a result, if an investor publicly denounces a company's actions on social media, the company will treat the event as a crisis, irrespective of whether the accusation is true. Social media criticism sometimes goes viral, with devastating consequences for corporate reputation. It is therefore vital for companies to respond adequately to social media criticism.

3. Theoretical Background and Hypothesis Development

3.1. Theoretical Background

Although many CSR studies have been conducted, no single theory frames the issue of CSR in response to social media criticism by investors. While some studies have discussed the mechanisms of companies' CSR engagement and disclosure using either institutional theory, legitimacy theory, stakeholder theory, or agency theory [29,30], our study has a multi-theoretical framework: we use legitimacy theory and agency theory to analyze CSR communication strategies in response to crises.

Legitimacy theory, widely used in CSR studies [31], stipulates that in a social system, there is a social contract between corporations and society. A company needs to seek and maintain legitimacy by complying with social values and must operate conforming to societal expectations [32]. Legitimacy is critical capital that provides organizations with access to resources allocated by stakeholders, brings competitive advantages, and enhances their long-run value [4,7]. Failing to respond to public expectations regarding legitimate conduct usually results in sanctions against the offending business. In this study, we focus on criticism posted on social media by investors that posed a threat to organizational legitimacy and plunges companies into crisis. According to legitimacy theory, an organization can rebuild its reputation by communicating its commitment to society rather than appearing to take actions that are motivated by self-interest [33]. As a result, legitimacy theory provides an appropriate framework to explain companies' CSR disclosure behavior in times of crisis.

Agency theory has also been widely used in the literature on CSR disclosure, as it links various corporate governance mechanisms to CSR decision making in corporations [18,29]. According to agency theory, effective mechanisms have an impact on managerial CSR decisions [34]. For example, Majeed et al. [18] found that institutional investors, independent directors, foreign nationals, and female directors were most likely to support CSR-related activities, and that there were significant associations between these identity markers and the extent of CSR reporting [35]. As a significant source of crisis for a company, investor-driven social media pressure also plays a governance role: investors' posts serve to monitor decisions in a corporation by airing public opinion, as indicated by Ang et al. [16]. Therefore, this theory provides insights into agency issues regarding CSR disclosure and how the fallout from crisis, including crises caused by social media criticism, can be overcome through effective governance mechanisms.

3.2. Literature Review

Corporate disclosures are a prerequisite for the efficient allocation of resources in capital markets and for building stakeholder confidence [36]. Corporations recognize that disclosing CSR activities is a key way of cultivating legitimacy, as it enables them to demonstrate their efforts to become more socially responsible and accountable [31]. Furthermore, CSR is an important mechanism for building corporate reputation and prestige [3,37]. Studies have posited that CSR disclosure helps companies to attract institutional investors [38,39], enhances companies' relationships with stakeholders and the government [11], reduces the cost of equity capital [5,17], enhances companies' reputation, gives companies a competitive advantage over their rivals [40], and enhances companies' long-term performance and value [7]. With widespread recognition of the importance of CSR disclosure in business, a large and growing body of literature has examined the determinants that drive CSR disclosure. From the perspective of legitimacy, CSR reporting serves as a communication strategy and legitimizing tool to influence public perceptions of companies [31]. Given the public's tremendous influence on businesses, companies have an incentive to provide CSR disclosures when they face pressure from investors, governments, customers, media representatives, and mimetic stakeholders [9,41]. Furthermore, strategic decisions such as CSR disclosure is a function of corporate governance mechanisms [29]. A number of studies have documented a significant relationship between CSR disclosure and firm ownership, board structure, internal control, and top management team composition [1,18,29]. Amid the extensive research on CSR disclosures and various crises, there has been much exploration of how companies conduct CSR activities to manage crises in the face of pressure from customers, governments, the media and the public. However, there is minimal empirical evidence of strategic CSR activities in response to crises instigated by investors, particularly investors' criticism on social networks.

As an important form of non-financial disclosure, CSR disclosures are expected to contain comprehensive and in-depth information regarding companies' policies, practices, and performance in the social and environmental domains [42]. Unlike financial disclosure, which is mandatory and verifiable, CSR disclosure is unregulated in China; it is mainly published on a voluntary basis and lacks a widely enforced reporting framework. As a result, CSR disclosure lacks external audit and regulatory oversight [42]. Whereas financial reports frequently use quantifiable data to illustrate a company's financial performance, CSR disclosure primarily provides qualitative textual information related to a company's sustainable development practices in areas such as production safety, environmental protection, and community welfare [17]. Due to the descriptive and unverifiable nature of CSR disclosure, disclosure quality plays a prominent role in determining the effectiveness of CSR communication and in managing stakeholders' perceptions of companies' CSR activities [1]. Du and Yu [42] argued that CSR reports released by companies should convey useful information to market participants and improve information transparency. Lee et al. [13] posited that state subsidies influence Chinese firms' decisions on whether to disclose extensive CSR information, citing political cost considerations. Nevertheless, a few studies have documented that companies often comply with stakeholder demands by strategically supplying CSR disclosures, although of low quality and containing limited information. For example, Lyon and Maxwell [12] criticized companies for using a "greenwashing" (greenwashing refers to the organizational practice of strategically disclosing environmental information but failing to fully demonstrate the organization's environmental impact to deflect attention from its environmentally unfriendly or less savory activities) communication strategy to publicize environmental actions that they have not actually taken and to mask their actual environmental practices, thereby misleading the public. Taking an institutional perspective, Marquis and Qian [14] also showed that companies in emerging markets often respond only symbolically to government requests for CSR reporting. Therefore, there is so far limited and inconclusive evidence on whether companies provide CSR disclosure in a substantive way when under pressure or facing threats.

3.3. Hypothesis Development

3.3.1. CSR Disclosure Decision in Response to Social Media Criticism

CSR decisions in corporations are made under social pressure in social environments. Based on legitimacy theory, companies face increasing pressure and criticism from stakeholders and are thus increasingly expected to offer voluntary CSR disclosure to address increased threats to their organizational legitimacy [31]. In contrast to traditional, often one-way communication methods such as press releases and conference calls, social media create richer channels for the dissemination of valuable information among market participants [43]. Although social media platforms provide some advantages for companies, they can also create challenges to the management of the flow of information; due to the platforms' interactive qualities, companies have little control over what users post. As a result, companies have become vulnerable to threats to their organizational prestige [10]. When investors use social media to publicly criticize a company, their negative comments are widely disseminated to other users and impact perceptions of the company. Social media criticism posted by investors negatively affects companies' reputation and thus their performance and stock prices. Such posts also increase the probability of companies' being investigated by regulators, which may expose their illegal or unethical activities, further impairing organizational legitimacy [32]. Furthermore, the loss of legitimacy may lead to regulatory penalties, damage business networks, and limit companies' access to necessary resources. To minimize these adverse effects, companies strive to present themselves as good corporate citizens to stakeholders [3]. The most efficient way for companies to improve their reputation is to implement legitimization strategies, such as voluntary CSR disclosure to declare their CSR initiatives, to strengthen the trust of investors and other stakeholders. According to Deegan [44] and Cho and Patten [31], companies seeking to create reputational capital can use communication strategies such as social and environmental disclosures. Similarly, by portraying companies in a positive light and influencing societal perceptions accordingly, the disclosure of CSR activities can serve as a crisis management tool to foster legitimacy in response to crises brought by social media criticism.

From the perspective of corporate governance, we posit that social media criticism predicts the decision to disclose CSR information given its monitoring role. Although numerous CSR studies carried out in Western contexts have emphasized the managerial over investment tendency in CSR, there is a comparative lack of enthusiasm for CSR engagement among companies in emerging countries. Due to the separation of ownership and control in corporations [45], those in managerial positions are often the owner's agents. These agents do not bear all the consequences of CSR for a firm's long-term value [34]. Instead, managerial CSR decisions become myopic because substantial financial resources are needed to support these activities, which often give rise to short-run performance volatility [46]. According to agency theory, effective governance mechanisms can play a monitoring role in mitigating agency issues affecting managerial decisions [47]. For example, a variety of factors, such as institutional ownership, board independence and media coverage, can have positive impacts on CSR decisions [29,35]. Zhou et al. [16] found that attention garnered through investors' social media posts encouraged companies to take timely corrective action to redress violations, confirming that public criticism on social media is an effective mechanism of corporate governance. Based on the aforementioned argument, we believe that social media criticism posted by investors can play an important role in motivating managers to make value-added decisions by behaving more ethically, thereby resulting in voluntary CSR disclosure.

CSR disclosure serves as a legitimizing tool used by companies to communicate with stakeholders, as it helps mitigate the effects of potential losses due to increasing criticism. Moreover, social media criticism exposes companies' decisions to greater monitoring, which encourages CSR involvement and disclosure. As such, we propose the following hypothesis to guide our empirical investigation:

Hypothesis 1 (H1). *Companies subject to high levels of social media criticism by investors are more likely to disclose voluntary CSR information.*

3.3.2. CSR Disclosure Substantiveness in Response to Social Media Criticism

Arguing that a company's disclosure strategies are not usually scrutinized by stakeholders, some research has failed to consider the substantiveness of information disclosure [48]. However, with increasing attention devoted to CSR practices, CSR reports that contain inaccurate or overly positive descriptions carry significant risks for companies, especially those subject to pressure from critical stakeholders. Research on CSR disclosure strategy has also suggested that deliberately failing to provide substantive CSR disclosures has adverse consequences for companies, as stakeholders (e.g., the public, media, government) might expose the companies' lies and punish them accordingly [14]. The Chinese newspaper *Southern Weekly* releases an annual "greenwashing list" detailing unethical behavior by Chinese corporations, particularly greenwashing. In 2017, *Southern Weekly*'s greenwashing list included FAW Group, a company that publicized its "green factory and green industrial chain" program in one of its CSR reports. Although seemingly an environmentally responsible program, the report ignored FAW Group's questionable practices, including poor pollutant treatment and excessive emissions of harmful waste gas. The public reacted angrily to the company's dishonesty. As a result, FAW Group was criticized and fined by the government. The FAW Group incident demonstrates the ways in which corporate CSR actions are monitored by stakeholders: symbolic (non-substantive) CSR gestures not only increase the risk of disrepute but also have negative economic outcomes. Investors' social media criticism places companies under the watchful eye of sophisticated stakeholders such as analysts, auditors, the government, and the media. Therefore, in times of crisis, failing to provide substantive CSR disclosures is likely to exacerbate the spread of negative publicity via social media, increasing the threat to organizational legitimacy. To rebuild the confidence of stakeholders and reduce business risk, companies are likely to cultivate a positive image by engaging in substantive CSR disclosure in response to social media criticism.

In addition, when companies publicize ethical actions that they have not actually taken in CSR reports, they engage in opportunistic behavior, which arises from agency problems. Given the monitoring role of social media [16,27], we expect social media criticism posted by investors to be closely associated with the substantiveness of CSR disclosures. Through substantive CSR actions, companies are able to make substantive progress, including the adoption of clean production methods, advancement of technological innovation, and increased research and development for green products. Such activities are conducive to reducing production costs, improving customer satisfaction, and increasing competitive advantage. On the contrary, responding merely symbolically to stakeholders' demands is not beneficial to a company's long-term value and may have devastating consequences if deception is discovered. Social media criticism posted by investors has an important influence on the ways in which a company operates. The negative publicity brought by stakeholders' criticism has a deterrent effect, encouraging companies to act in socially and environmentally responsible ways. This is in line with the argument of Campbell [30], and Marquis and Qian [14] that companies' reporting of symbolic or substantive CSR activities depends on the extent of external scrutiny or monitoring. It can be assumed that in crisis situations, in which companies are likely to be monitored and criticized by investors, companies are more likely to provide substantive CSR disclosures. We therefore hypothesize as follows:

Hypothesis 2 (H2). *Companies facing more social media criticism from investors are likely to engage in more substantive CSR disclosure.*

4. Methodology

4.1. Sample and Data

Our data come from several credible sources. Specifically, our CSR disclosure choice data come from the CSMAR database and our CSR disclosure substantiveness data come from an independent CSR ratings agency, Rankins CSR Ratings (RKS). The CSMAR database provides information on Chinese companies' CSR activities as disclosed in their CSR reports or annual reports. RKS provides highly credible information on the substantiveness of CSR reporting, in line with the Global Reporting Initiative (3.0). Studies have also shown it to be a credible source of data on the substantiveness of CSR reporting [13]. To collect data on social media criticism, we use Python to crawl all comments posted by investors on each listed company on the E-interactive platform, which is discussed in Section 2. This platform is especially useful for investigating our hypotheses for two reasons. First, as it was created by a stock exchange, the E-interactive platform differs significantly from other online channels (e.g., Facebook, Twitter, Weibo): it serves participants in the stock market, especially investors and companies, and thus to a great extent avoids interference from other agents, such as consumers. Using this platform can help researchers observe investors' comments on a company, providing a useful method of measuring the extent of a crisis. Second, the platform features a specialized Q&A section and communication on the E-interactive platform is initiated by investors rather than companies. According to the rules of the SSE, if companies receive questions or criticism from investors, they must reply or take relevant actions in a timely manner. Therefore, investors' concerns on this platform are expected to have a more significant influence on corporate decision making than posts on other social media. The information on institutional ownership information comes from the Wind Financial Database (Wind). All other relevant data are obtained from the CSMAR database.

To investigate CSR disclosure choice, we base our sample selection on all Chinese companies listed on the SSE from 2013 to 2019. We use 2013 as the start date because the SSE developed the E-interactive platform in that year. Prior to this year, there was no formal social media platform for small investors to publicly interact with the management of the firms listed on the SSE. We restrict our sample to non-financial companies. Table 1 illustrates the details of our sample. Panel A presents our sample selection process for testing reporting choice. Of the 8703 observations for 2013 to 2019, we eliminate 2253 observations that feature mandatory CSR reports, as we consider only voluntary CSR reporting choice. We then eliminate 451 observations with missing values for the variables used in the subsequent empirical tests. This selection process results in a final sample of 5999 firm-year observations. Panel B provides the yearly distribution of the observations and demonstrates that the percentage of Chinese firms that voluntarily disclosed CSR information increased gradually across the sample years. For example, the years with the smallest and largest proportions of firms that voluntarily disclosed CSR information are 2013 and 2019, at 14.216% and 23.931%, respectively.

Table 1. Sample selection and distribution.

Panel A: Sample Selection Process for CSR Disclosure Choice					**No. of Observations**		
Initial firm-year sample from 2013 to 2019					8703		
Less: Observations that are mandated to disclose CSR information					(2253)		
Observations with missing values for variables					(451)		
Final sample for testing disclosure choice					5999		
Panel B: Sample Distribution for CSR Disclosure Choice by Fiscal Year							
	2013	2014	2015	2016	2017	2018	2019
# of firm-years	612	622	679	776	1000	1094	1216
% of voluntary CSR disclosures	14.216	14.791	16.348	16.237	17.700	21.298	23.931
Panel C: Sample Selection Process for CSR Disclosure Substantiveness					**No. of Observations**		
Initial firm-year sample from 2013 to 2017					2249		
Less: Observations with missing values for variables					(150)		
Final sample for testing disclosure substantiveness					2099		
Panel D: Sample Distribution for CSR Disclosure Substantiveness by Fiscal Year							
		2013	2014	2015	2016	2017	
# of firm-years		384	393	412	438	472	
Average RKS score		41.261	43.312	42.761	43.507	43.023	

Note: This table presents our sample selection process for CSR disclosure choice (Panel A) and yearly distribution (Panel B), and the sample selection process for CSR disclosure substantiveness (Panel C) and yearly distribution (Panel D).

To investigate the substantiveness of firms' CSR reporting, we use data for the period 2013 to 2017, as the most recent open dataset on firms' CSR reporting is only available from RKS up to 2017. Following Lee et al. [13], we incorporate companies that are required to issue CSR reports into our sample to provide comprehensive evidence of the substance of CSR disclosure and maximize the sample size. Panel C summarizes the sample selection process. The sample is limited to companies with CSR reports rated by RKS. Due to missing values for CSR reporting rating scores and other variables, the final sample for the test is reduced to 2099 firm-year observations, slightly less than the initial sample of 2249. Panel D provides the yearly distribution of the sample. The average rating score over the whole sample period does not exceed 50 out of 100, indicating that the substantiveness of Chinese listed companies' CSR disclosure is poor.

4.2. Variable Definitions

4.2.1. CSR Disclosure

We focus not only on CSR disclosure choice but also on the substance of CSR activities reported. Thus, we consider two dependent variables. First, we use an indicator variable, CSR, to designate a company's CSR disclosure choice. We assign CSR a value of 1 if a company voluntarily issued a standalone CSR report or disclosed CSR-related information in its annual report in a given year; otherwise, we assign CSR a value of 0.

Second, we assess the extent to which CSR disclosure reflects substantive CSR activities. Following Marquis and Qian [14], we use the extent to which CSR disclosure is substantive (RKS) as another dependent variable, which is measured as an overall rating score of CSR reporting from an entirely independent CSR rating agency, RKS, which has been widely used by researchers [14,18]. Specifically, on the basis of data gathered from CSR reports as well as other communications such as websites and press releases, each firm's CSR reporting is evaluated in four dimensions. The first is an overall evaluation based on a firm's CSR strategy, the extent of stakeholders' participation in CSR activities, the comparability of CSR disclosure across time, the innovativeness of CSR activities, and the extent of external auditing. The second is a content evaluation based on the extent of the leadership and organizational system in place for implementing CSR activities. The third is a technical evaluation based on the transparency, regularity, and availability of CSR information. The fourth is an industrial evaluation that focuses on CSR activities associated with industry-specific factors. The overall rating score for CSR disclosure substantiveness ranges from 0 to 100. As such, we take the natural logarithm of the rating score as the dependent variable.

4.2.2. Social Media Criticism Posted by Investors

We focus on how companies strategically manage specific crises brought by social media criticism through CSR communication. Unlike past studies [9], we focus exclusively on companies criticized by investors on social media platforms to understand the unique characteristics of this type of criticism and its effects on organizations. We identify the magnitude of a crisis according to the volume of criticism posted over time.

Moreover, we identify the criticisms themselves. On the E-interactive platform, individual investors can publish positive as well as negative comments on a company. A growing body of capital market and information disclosure research has conducted textual analyses to examine the tone and sentiment of corporate annual reports, press releases, conference calls, and media reports [49–51]. In this study, we also distinguish between positive and negative posts based on investors' tone, using textual analysis methods. There are two feasible approaches to conducting textual analysis: the dictionary-based approach and the machine learning method. The former approach uses an algorithm in which a computer program reads the text and classifies words (or phrases) into different categories (i.e., positive versus negative) based on a dictionary (word list). For instance, a general-purpose dictionary such as the Harvard General Inquirer is often used to perform textual analysis. Loughran and McDonald [52] developed a financial emotion word list (LM list) that captures positive and negative words in the accounting and finance contexts, which has been widely used in capital market research [42,49].

The alternative method, machine learning, can automatically infer the content of a text and classify documents with subjective opinions based on big data and deep learning techniques. In this study, we use machine learning instead of the dictionary-based method for several reasons. First, very few word lists are appropriate for use in research on Chinese capital markets. Li [53] argued that dictionary-based approaches are not ideal for finance research, even though this method has been used extensively in the fields of Western languages and culture. In the Chinese context, researchers have usually translated the English words in the LM dictionary into Chinese and measured tone by calculating negative/positive word frequencies based on the translated word lists [54]. However, this process introduces considerable bias and renders the method inapplicable to the Chinese context, as there are significant differences in linguistic elements such as word meanings, expressions, sentence structure, and cultural elements between the Chinese and English languages. Second, dictionary-based approaches do not take sentence context into consideration. For instance, if an investor is talking about revenue, "increase" should be treated as a positive word; however, the word is likely to have a negative meaning in the context of cost [53]. Fortunately, the machine learning approach can address these problems.

We use Senta, an open-source sentiment classification system established by Baidu that uses the Bidirectional Long Short-Term Memory (Bi-LSTM) model, to perform our sentiment analysis. The LSTM model is a type of recurrent neural network model that overcomes the vanishing gradient problem. The model learns to store only relevant content based on training [55]. The Bi-LSTM model has been pre-trained with large corpora and is intended for widespread use in various domains, such as e-commerce, tourism, media, finance, and law. The model accepts the input of a given sentence and automatically gives a positive sentiment score (ranging from 0 to 1) and a negative sentiment score (ranging from 0 to 1) for specific texts. The effectiveness of the Bi-LSTM model is high; a recent study found that the model's accuracy with a test set exceeded 85% [56]. According to the metrics of sentiment analysis, comments on the E-interactive platform that receive scores higher than 0.5 are identified as negative and therefore defined as "criticism". We calculate the natural logarithm of 1 plus the total number of criticisms posted by investors about a company on the E-interactive platform in a given year to proxy for social media criticism (CRITICISM).

4.3. Model Specification

To test H1, we estimate the probability of a company's disclosing CSR information. As a dummy variable is used as the dependent variable, a probit regression model is applied as follows:

$$\begin{aligned}\Pr(\mathrm{CSR}_{i,t}) &= \alpha_0 + \alpha_1\mathrm{CRITICISM}_{i,t} + \alpha_2\mathrm{SIZE}_{i,t} + \alpha_3\mathrm{LEV}_{i,t} + \alpha_4\mathrm{ROA}_{i,t} + \alpha_5\mathrm{TOBINQ}_{i,t} \\ &+\alpha_6\mathrm{INSH}_{i,t} + \alpha_7\mathrm{FSH}_{i,t} + \alpha_8\mathrm{OUTDIR}_{i,t} + \alpha_9\mathrm{BOARD}_{i,t} + \alpha_{10}\mathrm{SOE}_{i,t} \\ &+\mathrm{Industry} + \mathrm{Year} + \varepsilon_{i,t}\end{aligned} \quad (1)$$

To test H2, we use ordinary least squares (OLS) regression to examine the relationship between criticism and the substance of CSR disclosure as follows:

$$\begin{aligned}\mathrm{RKS}_{i,t} &= \beta_0 + \beta_1\mathrm{CRITICISM}_{i,t} + \beta_2\mathrm{SIZE}_{i,t} + \beta_3\mathrm{LEV}_{i,t} + \beta_4\mathrm{ROA}_{i,t} + \beta_5\mathrm{TOBINQ}_{i,t} \\ &+\beta_6\mathrm{INSH}_{i,t} + \beta_7\mathrm{FSH}_{i,t} + \beta_8\mathrm{OUTDIR}_{i,t} + \beta_9\mathrm{BOARD}_{i,t} + \beta_{10}\mathrm{SOE}_{i,t} \\ &+\mathrm{Industry} + \mathrm{Year} + \mu_{i,t}\end{aligned} \quad (2)$$

where i indexes firm and t indexes time. The dependent variable of CSR disclosure choice, CSR, is a dummy variable that equals 1 if firm i voluntarily issues a standalone CSR report or discloses CSR information in its annual report in year t, and 0 otherwise. RKS is the natural logarithm of the overall rating score of CSR disclosure substantiveness for a firm in year t, obtained from RKS. The independent variable, CRITICISM, is the natural logarithm of 1 plus the volume of criticism (negative posts) posted by investors on firm i via the E-interactive platform in year t. We estimate Equations (1) and (2) with a focus on α_1 and β_1, the coefficients for CRITICISM, which are expected to be significantly positive if companies tend to disclose CSR information and issue substantive CSR disclosures in a severe crisis arising from social media criticism.

To eliminate potential confounding effects, we introduce a series of control variables that may impact CSR disclosure choice or quality to the regression model. Following Lee et al. [13], we expect larger firms to face more public pressure, to have more financial resources to engage in CSR activities, and therefore to provide more substantive disclosures. As a result, we include SIZE, which is computed as the natural logarithm of the book value of assets at the end of year t. Firm leverage increases business risk, which in turn requires companies to make CSR disclosures [57]. We measure leverage (LEV) using the ratio of total debt divided by total assets at the end of year t. Following the argument of Li et al. [46] that well-performing companies may have greater incentives to disclose their CSR activities to stakeholders, return on assets (ROA) (the ratio of net income divided by total assets in year t) should be controlled. Higher-growth firms may either have greater resource constraints that inhibit their ability to issue good CSR reports [13] or have more motivation to voluntarily initiate non-financial disclosure to reduce the cost of capital [17]. Therefore, there is no way to predict with certainty a company's growth opportunity and CSR disclosure. We therefore measure growth opportunity by Tobin's Q (TOBINQ), which is computed as the ratio of the market value to the book value of assets in year t. Majeed et al. [18] documented a variety of elements related to corporate governance that have significant effects on companies' CSR engagement and disclosure decisions. To capture these effects, we include several governance-related control variables: institutional ownership (INSH), the percentage of stock holdings by institutional investors at the end of year t; ownership concentration (FSH), the percentage of stock holdings by the first largest shareholder at the end of year t; independent directors (OUTDIR), the proportion of independent directors on the board in year t; and board size (BOARD), proxied by the natural logarithm of the number of directors on the board in year t. In the Chinese context, SOEs are encouraged by the state to be model corporate citizens, and are therefore more likely than NSOEs to engage in CSR activities and demonstrate their CSR initiatives through substantive disclosure [41]. We therefore include SOE in the regression model to specify whether a firm is an SOE. Finally, dummy variables representing China Securities Regulatory Commission (CSRC) two-digit industry membership and year fixed effects are included in all of the regressions. The specifications of the variables used in our empirical analyses are presented in Table 2.

Table 2. Variable definitions.

Variables	Definition
Dependent variables	
CSR	Dummy variable that equals 1 if a firm voluntarily either issues a standalone CSR report or discloses CSR information in its annual report in year *t*, and otherwise 0
RKS	The natural logarithm of the overall rating score of CSR reporting substantiveness for a firm in year *t*, obtained from RKS
Independent variable	
CRITICISM	The natural logarithm of 1 plus the volume of criticism of a firm that investors post on the E-interactive platform in year *t*
Control variables	
SIZE	The natural logarithm of the book value of assets at the end of year *t*
LEV	The ratio of total debt divided by total assets at the end of year *t*
ROA	Return on assets ratio, defined as net income divided by total assets in year *t*
TOBINQ	The ratio of the market value to the book value of assets in year *t*

Table 2. *Cont.*

Variables	Definition
INSH	The sum of the percentage of stock holdings by institutional investors at the end of year *t*
FSH	The percentage of stock holdings by the first largest shareholder at the end of year *t*
OUTDIR	The proportion of independent directors on the board in year *t*
BOARD	The natural logarithm of the number of directors on the board in year *t*
SOE	Indicator variable that equals 1 if a firm's ultimate shareholder is the state in year *t*, and otherwise 0
Industry	Dummy variable that represents industry (CSRC two-digit industry code)
Year	Dummy variable representing the year

5. Empirical Findings

5.1. Descriptive Statistics

Table 3 presents descriptive statistics for the variables used in our analyses. To mitigate the influence of outliers, all of the continuous variables are winsorized at the 1st and 99th percentiles. The mean value of CSR is 0.186, with a standard deviation of 0.389, which indicates that Chinese companies that voluntarily disclosure CSR information account for only 18.6% of the observations in our sample. The average CSR disclosure substantiveness is 3.711 and the corresponding original value is 40.895, with minimum and maximum values of 21.200 and 82.517, respectively. This means that, on average, Chinese companies' CSR reports contain only limited information on specific CSR activities, although there are big differences between companies in the sample. Our results show that CRITICISM has an average value of 2.816 and an original value of 15.710. The standard deviation for CRITICISM is 1.175 and the minimum and maximum values for CRITICISM are 0.000 and 5.298, respectively. These results imply that, on average, a firm in our sample was criticized by investors 16 times on the E-interactive platform each year, with significant variation in the extent of crisis across companies. In particular, the most heavily criticized firm received approximately 199 negative posts in the focal period, while a few firms did not receive any criticism on the platform. The average value of institutional ownership (INSH) is 0.386, suggesting that the average ratio of institutional ownership of our sample is 38.6%. Regarding the other control variables, the average firm has a SIZE value of 22.185, leverage of 0.454, return on assets of 0.033, Tobin's Q of 2.295, largest shareholder ownership of 0.365, and board size of 2.134. On average, independent directors make up 37.3% of a firm's board members. SOEs account for 42.9% of the observations. Overall, the statistical distributions of the above variables are consistent with previous studies [13].

Table 3. Sample descriptive statistics.

Variables	Obs.	Mean	Median	SD	Min	Max
CSR	5999	0.186	0.000	0.389	0.000	1.000
RKS	2099	3.711	3.670	0.297	3.054	4.413
CRITICISM	5999	2.816	2.890	1.175	0.000	5.298
SIZE	5999	22.185	22.089	1.254	19.452	27.955
LEV	5999	0.454	0.436	0.219	0.070	0.966
ROA	5999	0.033	0.034	0.066	−0.280	0.192
TOBINQ	5999	2.295	1.677	1.880	0.876	12.401
INSH	5999	0.386	0.398	0.235	0.000	0.921
FSH	5999	0.365	0.343	0.154	0.080	0.768
OUTDIR	5999	0.373	0.333	0.050	0.333	0.571
BOARD	5999	2.134	2.197	0.193	1.609	2.708
SOE	5999	0.429	0.000	0.495	0.000	1.000

Note: This table presents descriptive statistics for the main variables. The variables are defined in Table 2. All of the variables except the dummy variables are winsorized at the 1% and 99% levels.

5.2. Pearson Correlation Analysis

Table 4 shows the Pearson correlation matrix for the main variables. The correlation between CSR and CRITICISM is 0.062, significant at the 1% level. The preliminary correlation results indicate a positive relationship between social media criticism and the possibility of CSR disclosure, which lends initial support for H1. The correlation between RKS and CRITICISM is 0.025, but it is not statistically significant. The two dependent variables have positive significant correlations with SIZE, LEV, INSH, FSH, and BOARD. The correlations between CSR, RKS, and SOE are also significantly positive, in line with our expectation that state-owned enterprises are more likely to disclose CSR activities and issue high-quality CSR reports. Moreover, the two CSR variables have positive relationships with TOBINQ. Finally, as the maximum pairwise correlation between OUTDIR and BOARD is −0.560, below the maximum threshold of 0.7 suggested by Lind et al. [58], multicollinearity is not a serious concern in this study. Although most of the results are consistent with our expectations, Pearson correlation analysis does not simultaneously control for other variables. We examine the relationships more rigorously in subsequent analyses.

Table 4. Pearson correlation matrices.

Variables	1	2	3	4	5	6	7	8	9	10	11	12
1-CSR	1											
2-RKS	−0.044	1										
3-CRITICISM	0.062 ***	0.025	1									
4-SIZE	0.258 ***	0.541 ***	0.151 ***	1								
5-LEV	0.074 ***	0.229 ***	−0.053 ***	0.413 ***	1							
6-ROA	−0.016	0.009	0.060 ***	0.010	−0.435 ***	1						
7-TOBINQ	−0.096 ***	−0.197 ***	−0.034 ***	−0.473 ***	−0.067 ***	−0.067 ***	1					
8-INSH	0.168 ***	0.340 ***	−0.042 ***	0.412 ***	0.184 ***	−0.013	0.003	1				
9-FSH	0.058 ***	0.191 ***	−0.083 ***	0.219 ***	−0.033 **	0.184 ***	−0.198 ***	0.279 ***	1			
10-OUTDIR	−0.004	0.064 ***	0.051 ***	−0.032 **	0.012	−0.029 **	0.076 ***	−0.060 ***	0.004	1		
11-BOARD	0.089 ***	0.240 ***	−0.072 ***	0.247 ***	0.127 ***	−0.028**	−0.125 ***	0.171 ***	0.037 ***	−0.560 ***	1	
12-SOE	0.140 ***	0.219 ***	−0.119 ***	0.254 ***	0.247 ***	−0.156 ***	−0.075 ***	0.377 ***	0.164 ***	−0.083 ***	0.246 ***	1

Note: This table presents Pearson correlation matrices of main variables. The variables are defined in Table 2. All variables except dummy variables are winsorized at the 1% and 99% levels. ** and *** indicate significance at the 5% and 1% levels, respectively.

5.3. Test of H1: CSR Disclosure Choice

Table 5 presents probit regression estimates of the probability of a company's disclosing CSR information. Column (1) introduces CSR as the dependent variable and controls for other determinants of CSR disclosure identified by previous studies as well as industry and year fixed effects. It shows that the coefficient of CRITICISM is positive, as predicted, and significant at the 1% level (coefficient = 0.066, z-stat = 3.788). The empirical results suggest that being criticized more severely by investors on social media platforms results in companies' making voluntary CSR disclosures, supporting H1. Based on the marginal effect reported in Column (2), a 1% increase in CRITICISM increases the likelihood of companies' issuing CSR disclosure by 0.016%. Our findings indicate that in response to an increasing crisis brought by social media criticism posted by investors, listed companies are more likely to disclose their CSR activities voluntarily. The findings are in line with our argument that listed companies anticipate the negative consequences of a crisis when faced with increasing investor criticism on social media platforms. To mitigate the negative effects of this criticism, companies are expected to conduct crisis management and rebuild legitimacy using CSR disclosure to communicate their social and environmental initiatives to stakeholders. In addition, as Zhou et al. [16] and Ang et al. [27] documented using the principal–agent framework, social media criticism by investors serves as an effective mechanism of corporate governance, as it forces managers to make value-added decisions, including voluntary CSR disclosure [18].

Table 5. Test of H1: Social media criticism posted by investors and the probability of CSR disclosure.

Variables	Expected Sign	Dep. Var. = Prob (CSR)	
		(1)	(2)
		Coefficient	Marginal Effect
CRITICISM	+	0.066 *** (3.788)	0.016
SIZE	+	0.202 *** (10.585)	0.050
LEV	+	−0.423 *** (−3.542)	−0.104
ROA	+	−1.057 *** (−2.939)	−0.261
TOBINQ	?	−0.028 * (−1.943)	−0.007
INSH	+	0.560 *** (5.652)	0.138
FSH	?	−0.225 (−1.624)	−0.056
OUTDIR	+	0.852 * (1.837)	0.210
BOARD	+	0.290 ** (2.324)	0.072
SOE	+	0.239 *** (5.414)	0.059
Intercept	?	−6.376 *** (−12.680)	
Year effect		Yes	
Industry effect		Yes	
Obs.		5999	
Pseudo R^2		0.077	

Note: This table presents probit regression estimates for social media criticism and voluntary CSR disclosure choice. The variables are defined in Table 2. All of the variables except the dummy variables are winsorized at the 1% and 99% levels. The z-statistics are reported in brackets. *, **, and *** indicate significance at the 10%, 5%, and 1% levels, respectively.

The signs of the coefficients on most of the control variables are as expected, apart from LEV and ROA. For example, the coefficient of SIZE is significantly positive in the regression, as expected, suggesting that large firms have greater incentives to voluntarily disclose their CSR actions. INSH also has a positive coefficient, consistent with the argument that institutional investors place a high value on social achievements and reputation when investing in firms, and companies with higher institutional ownership are more likely to voluntarily issue CSR reporting [18]. The variable BOARD is positively related to CSR disclosure choice, implying that board size has a positive influence on companies' voluntary CSR disclosure. Moreover, the coefficients on SOE are significantly positive as expected, indicating that Chinese SOEs engage more actively in CSR activities than non-SOEs and have greater incentives to make CSR disclosure decisions. Firm leverage (LEV) and return on assets (ROA) also have significant coefficients, but their relationships with the probability of CSR disclosure are negative in this case, indicating that poor-performing and low-leverage Chinese firms are more likely to issue CSR reports or disclose CSR information in their annual reports. The results are consistent with the findings of other relevant studies in the Chinese context [1,13].

5.4. Test of H2: CSR Disclosure Substantiveness

Above, we establish that companies tend to disclose CSR information to manage stakeholders' perceptions. To test H2, we investigate the substance of the CSR disclosures released by conducting further analyses. Table 6 reports the results of the OLS regression model of CSR reporting substantiveness in response to social media criticism, controlling for other factors that are also related to the dependent variables. We note that the coefficient of CRITICISM is positive and statistically significant at the 5% level (coefficient = 0.011, t-stat = 2.389), lending support for our second hypothesis, H2. Therefore, we can conclude that increasing social media criticism posted by investors pushes companies to issue CSR reports with more substantive details that reflect what they have actually done to address the issues raised in the criticism. Conversely, if companies only strategically issue symbolic reports that are uninformative, investors and stakeholders are likely to become increasingly angry and resentful, especially in times of crisis. Companies recognize that providing substantive details in CSR reports is a useful way of managing stakeholders' perceptions and regaining legitimacy: effective communication regarding company initiatives through CSR actions provide a transparent means of pacifying investors and other stakeholders in times of crisis. As a result, companies are more likely to publish greater substantive CSR reports to enhance their reputation and legitimacy in response to social media criticism posted by investors.

Table 6. Test of H2: Social media criticism posted by investors and CSR disclosure substantiveness.

Variables	Expected Sign	Dep. Var. = RKS
		Coefficient
CRITICISM	+	0.011 ** (2.389)
SIZE	+	0.081 *** (16.061)
LEV	+	−0.067 (−1.632)
ROA	+	−0.046 (−0.331)
TOBINQ	?	0.015 *** (2.651)
INSH	+	0.172 *** (5.874)
FSH	?	0.073 * (1.830)
OUTDIR	+	0.047 (0.428)
BOARD	+	0.143 *** (4.872)
SOE	+	0.040 *** (2.967)
Intercept	?	1.271 *** (9.736)
Year effect		Yes
Industry effect		Yes
Obs.		2099
Adj R^2		0.366

Note: This table presents OLS regression results for social media criticism and the substantiveness of CSR disclosure. The variables are defined in Table 2. All of the variables except the dummy variables are winsorized at the 1% and 99% levels. The t-statistics are reported in brackets. *, **, and *** indicate significance at the 10%, 5%, and 1% levels, respectively.

Regarding the control variables, most of the results are as expected. Specifically, the significantly positive coefficients of SIZE and BOARD support the findings of Cabeza-García et al. [1] that firm size and board size have positive effects on the substance of CSR reporting. The growth opportunity (TOBINQ) of firms is positively related to CSR disclosure substantiveness, probably because Chinese firms with greater growth opportunities are motivated to initiate detailed CSR disclosure to acquire financial resources for growth from stakeholders. Consistent with Majeed et al. [18], we still find institutional ownership (INSH) to be positively related to the substantiveness of CSR reporting. SOE has a significant coefficient of determination, which is consistent with the assumption stated in the previous section that Chinese SOEs are encouraged to conduct activities that are beneficial to society and the environment, and thus are more likely to engage in more substantial CSR disclosures than NSOEs. Moreover, while the variable FSH is positively correlated with CSR disclosure substantiveness, this is not statistically significant, and there is also no evidence pointing to a relationship between LEV, ROA, OUTDIR, and the dependent variable.

5.5. Robustness Checks

5.5.1. Alternative Proxy for CSR Disclosure Substantiveness

To ensure the reliability of our findings, we perform a robustness test by replicating the main tests with an alternative measure of CSR disclosure substantiveness. In addition to the ratings score used in our main tests, which is a continuous variable, RKS ranks companies each year according to their overall score for CSR reporting substantiveness on 17 levels, ranging from CC to AA+. AA+ is reserved for the highest-quality CSR reports, which include the greatest amount of substantive detail, and CC is reserved for the lowest-quality CSR reports, which are symbolic and/or uninformative. Following Lee et al. [13], we conduct robustness tests with this alternative dependent variable (RKS_rank), which ranges from 1 to 17. A Poisson regression model is therefore employed, as the variable RKS_rank is count based. When RKS_rank is taken as the dependent variable, the results reported in Table 7 still show a positive and significant relation between social media criticism posted by investors and CSR disclosure substantiveness at the 5% level (coefficient = 0.017, z-stat = 2.368). Thereafter, most of the control variables have signs in line with our expectations. These findings suggest that the main hypothesis is still valid, even after employing alternative methods to measure the degree of substantiveness of CSR activities.

Table 7. Robustness check: Alternative proxy for CSR disclosure substantiveness.

Variables	Dep. Var. = RSK_Rank
	Coefficient
CRITICISM	0.017 ** (2.368)
SIZE	0.121 *** (15.533)
LEV	−0.103 (−1.538)
ROA	0.061 (0.262)
TOBINQ	0.018 * (1.888)
INSH	0.279 *** (5.931)
FSH	0.071 (1.131)
OUTDIR	0.002 (0.009)
BOARD	0.204 *** (4.481)

Table 7. *Cont.*

Variables	Dep. Var. = RSK_Rank
	Coefficient
SOE	0.049 **
	(2.183)
Intercept	−1.729 ***
	(−8.042)
Year effect	Yes
Industry effect	Yes
Obs.	2099
Pseudo R^2	0.110

Note: This table reports the results of using an alternative measure of CSR disclosure substantiveness. The variables are defined in Table 2. All of the variables except the dummy variables are winsorized at the 1% and 99% levels. The z-statistics are reported in brackets. *, **, and *** indicate significance at the 10%, 5%, and 1% levels, respectively.

5.5.2. Condensed Sample

Our sample contains a small number of companies not subject to any social media criticism posted by individual investors. In the primary analysis above, the variable CRITICISM takes a value of 0, as these observations were not actually threatened by a specific crisis in our sample period. To further enhance the robustness of our evidence, we eliminate these observations, ensuring that the observations in the condensed sample are all subject to social media criticism. We thus use 5820 and 2014 observations to test CSR disclosure choice and substantiveness, respectively. We estimate Equations (1) and (2) and present the results in Table 8. Column (1) shows that in the probit regression where CSR is taken as the independent variable, CRITICISM still has a positive and significant coefficient (coefficient = 0.081, z-stat = 4.175). When RKS is added as the dependent variable, the results in Column (2) also show a positive and significant relationship, albeit slightly weaker, between social media criticism and the substantiveness of CSR disclosure. Most of the control variables are in line with our expectations. Overall, the robustness checks validate our main findings after changing the sample.

Table 8. Robustness check: Using condensed sample.

Variables	Dep. Var. = Prob (CSR)	Dep. Var. = RKS
	(1)	(2)
	Coefficient	Coefficient
CRITICISM	0.081 ***	0.009 *
	(4.175)	(1.701)
SIZE	0.201 ***	0.083 ***
	(10.346)	(16.031)
LEV	−0.396 ***	−0.087 **
	(−3.266)	(−2.081)
ROA	−1.045 ***	−0.099
	(−2.877)	(−0.698)
TOBINQ	−0.026 *	0.014 **
	(−1.793)	(2.493)
INSH	0.553 ***	0.177 ***
	(5.482)	(5.822)
FSH	−0.228	0.062
	(−1.621)	(1.496)

Table 8. *Cont.*

Variables	Dep. Var. = Prob (CSR)	Dep. Var. = RKS
	(1)	(2)
	Coefficient	Coefficient
OUTDIR	0.856 *	0.023
	(1.818)	(0.205)
BOARD	0.265 **	0.148 ***
	(2.090)	(4.933)
SOE	0.239 ***	0.035 **
	(5.328)	(2.480)
Intercept	−6.358 ***	1.251 ***
	(−12.432)	(9.363)
Year effect	Yes	Yes
Industry effect	Yes	Yes
Obs.	5820	2014
Pseudo R^2/Adj R^2	0.076	0.370

Note: This table presents the regression results for the condensed sample. The variables are defined in Table 2. All of the variables except the dummy variables are winsorized at the 1% and 99% levels. The z-statistics/t-statistics are reported in brackets. *, **, and *** indicate significance at the 10%, 5%, and 1% levels, respectively.

6. Further Analysis

As the need for CSR communication is different for companies with different attributes, CSR disclosure strategies in response to crises are expected to be heterogeneous. Property rights structure and government regulation lead to different legitimacy positions and corporate decision making on strategic CSR disclosure [41,59]. Therefore, the heterogeneous responses to social media criticism are influenced by company ownership and regulatory pressure. In this section, we analyze the heterogeneous effects of social media criticism posted by investors on the probability and substantiveness of CSR disclosure across SOEs and NSOEs and across regions with different levels of local government concern about environmental and social issues.

6.1. Effects on SOEs and NSOEs

Our empirical results indicate that SOEs are more likely than NSOEs to disclose CSR information and provide better CSR communication in reports. SOEs pay more attention to social responsibility because they are encouraged by the state to behave in socially and environmentally responsible ways [29,41]. This sub-section discusses the results of our investigation into whether SOEs and NSOEs behave differently with regard to CSR disclosure in response to social media criticism posted by investors.

To examine this issue, we partition the sample into SOEs and NSOEs and look at the effects of social media criticism on these two groups. As reported in Columns (1) and (2) of Table 9, the coefficient of CRITICISM is positive but statistically insignificant for the SOE group. However, CRITICISM has a significantly positive coefficient for the NSOEs group, and the difference between the coefficients for these groups is statistically significant. These observations suggest that a positive relationship between social media criticism and the probability of CSR disclosure only exists for NSOEs. Columns (3) and (4) report the estimation with RKS as the dependent variable. It also shows an insignificant relationship between CRITICISM and RKS for SOEs. The coefficient of CRITICISM is significantly positive and larger in the NSOE group than in the SOE group, confirming that NSOEs are more likely to issue substantive CSR reports in response to social media criticism.

These findings, although interesting, are not surprising. In emerging markets, political connections are an important form of capital, as business practices are heavily influenced by the government. Compared with SOEs, who enjoy innate legitimacy, Chinese NSOEs have less access to key resources due to their lack of government support, particularly during times of crisis. Social media criticism is therefore more likely to have negative effects on the organizational legitimacy and reputation capital of NSOEs, as SOEs operate with the endorsement of the government even if their reputation is partially damaged. To mitigate the adverse effects of social media criticism by investors, NSOEs are more likely to disclose their CSR activities and provide more substantive details on these actions to enhance their legitimacy. Our findings support the argument of Marquis and Qian [14] that compared with NSOEs, SOEs have greater legitimacy due to their inherent political ties and thus fewer incentives to engage in activities such as CSR reporting to seek access to resources.

Table 9. Differential effects on SOEs versus NSOEs.

Variables	Dep. Var. = Prob (CSR)		Dep. Var. = RKS	
	(1)	(2)	(3)	(4)
	SOEs	NSOEs	SOEs	NSOEs
CRITICISM	0.025 (0.998)	0.103 *** (4.052) [p-value = 0.031]	0.000 (0.014)	0.024 *** (2.946) [p-value = 0.007]
SIZE	0.227 *** (6.851)	0.220 *** (7.915)	0.088 *** (13.793)	0.115 *** (10.401)
LEV	−0.805 *** (−4.658)	−0.143 (−0.831)	−0.048 (−1.038)	−0.231 *** (−2.809)
ROA	−1.959 *** (−3.582)	−0.243 (−0.502)	0.110 (0.685)	−0.716 *** (−2.665)
TOBINQ	−0.036 (−1.440)	−0.016 (−0.861)	0.015 ** (2.155)	0.032 *** (3.438)
INSH	0.565 *** (3.542)	0.441 *** (3.365)	0.202 *** (5.839)	0.028 (0.518)
FSH	0.168 (0.834)	−0.680 *** (−3.420)	0.016 (0.334)	0.209 *** (2.692)
OUTDIR	0.931 (1.478)	0.215 (0.299)	0.067 (0.532)	−0.207 (−0.860)
BOARD	0.429 ** (2.487)	−0.004 (−0.020)	0.106 *** (3.210)	0.255 *** (4.036)
Intercept	−6.994 *** (−9.264)	−5.993 *** (−7.793)	1.435 *** (7.943)	0.353 (1.324)
Year effect	Yes	Yes	Yes	Yes
Industry effect	Yes	Yes	Yes	Yes
Obs.	2574	3425	1557	542
Pseudo R^2/Adj R^2	0.060	0.072	0.355	0.390

Note: This table reports heterogeneous effects for SOEs and non-SOEs. The variables are defined in Table 2. All of the variables except the dummy variables are winsorized at the 1% and 99% levels. The z-statistics/t-statistics are reported in brackets. The p-values for the differences between SOEs and NSOEs in the coefficients on CRITICISM are reported in square brackets. **, and *** indicate significance at the 5%, and 1% levels, respectively.

6.2. Effects of Regulatory Pressure: Environmental Regulation and Social Concerns

In their CSR activities, Chinese companies pay the most attention to environmental protection. (According to Hurun China Social Entrepreneurship 2020, 36% of Chinese CSR activities focus on environmental protection, ahead of poverty alleviation, employee labor protection, community welfare and so on.) The reason for this is that, for a long time, China's economic development has mainly taken place at the expense of its ecological environment, which has directly affected the health and well-being of its people. Other countries in the world have recognized and even condemned China's serious environmental problems. Thus, the Chinese government regards environmental issues as the most important aspect of CSR and has launched a series of relevant actions to deal with them, such as revising "environmental law" and restricting lending to highly polluting enterprises or even closing them down. Guided by government, enterprises therefore devote much effort to environmental protection. Compared with the most prominent environmental issues, social issues such as human rights and employment conditions receive relatively little attention.) As documented in the literature [11], government pressure is one of the most salient factors affecting a company's CSR behavior. We examine whether the effect of social media criticism posted by investors on strategic CSR disclosure is greater or smaller in regions with strict environmental regulations in place. We use local government spending on environmental protection scaled by budget expenditure each year to proxy for the intensity of local environmental regulation (REG). Our full sample is divided into two subgroups along the median of REG: companies in regions with high levels of environmental regulation (high-REG) and those based in regions with low levels of environmental regulation (low-REG). We then rerun the above models to account for these new subgroups. We observe in Columns (1) and (2) of Table 10 that the coefficient of CRITICISM is positive and statistically significant for the high-REG group and positive but insignificant for the low-REG subgroup. A test of the equality of the coefficients between the two groups implies that companies operating in regions where local governments place more emphasis on environmental protection are more likely to disclose CSR information in response to social media criticism. As indicated in Columns (3) and (4), the coefficient of CRITICISM is significantly positive only for the high-REG group, not for the low-REG group; however, the difference between the two groups is not statistically significant.

Table 10. Differential effects across regions with high and low levels of environmental regulation.

Variables	Dep. Var. = Prob (CSR)		Dep. Var. = RKS	
	(1)	(2)	(3)	(4)
	High-REG	Low-REG	High-REG	Low-REG
CRITICISM	0.097 ***	0.025	0.015 **	0.005
	(3.768)	(1.012)	(2.342)	(0.792)
		[p-value = 0.045]		[p-value = 0.281]
SIZE	0.225 ***	0.285 ***	0.085 ***	0.085 ***
	(8.523)	(8.353)	(12.403)	(9.925)
LEV	−0.522 ***	−0.572 ***	−0.044	−0.078
	(−3.065)	(−3.299)	(−0.763)	(−1.330)
ROA	−1.417 ***	−0.709	−0.102	0.214
	(−2.898)	(−1.331)	(−0.535)	(1.055)
TOBINQ	−0.019	−0.016	0.027 ***	0.003
	(−0.948)	(−0.768)	(3.364)	(0.417)
INSH	0.615 ***	0.285 *	0.126 ***	0.210 ***
	(4.471)	(1.914)	(3.222)	(4.666)
FSH	−0.258	−0.112	0.034	0.147 **
	(−1.339)	(−0.556)	(0.615)	(2.444)
OUTDIR	−0.261	1.855 ***	0.096	−0.031
	(−0.407)	(2.686)	(0.615)	(−0.195)
BOARD	0.246	0.211	0.086 **	0.219 ***
	(1.434)	(1.140)	(2.125)	(5.078)
SOE	0.243 ***	0.252 ***	0.047 **	0.044 **
	(3.985)	(3.843)	(2.310)	(2.332)
Intercept	−6.458 ***	−8.336 ***	1.242 ***	1.011 ***
	(−9.432)	(−9.989)	(7.161)	(4.597)
Year effect	Yes	Yes	Yes	Yes
Industry effect	Yes	Yes	Yes	Yes
Obs.	3069	2930	1059	1040
Pseudo R^2 / Adj R^2	0.090	0.078	0.417	0.327

Note: This table presents the subgroup analysis for regions with different levels of environmental regulation. The variables are defined in Table 2. All of the variables (except the dummy variables) are winsorized at the 1% and 99% levels. The z-statistics/t-statistics are reported in brackets. The p-values for the differences between the high-REG and low-REG sub-samples in the coefficients on CRITICISM are reported in square brackets. *, **, and *** indicate significance at the 10%, 5%, and 1% levels, respectively.

Although Chinese companies get most involved with environmental issues among the CSR activities, we cannot leave social issues unanalyzed, as they are important for improving people's well-being and promoting social harmony and stability [21]. Therefore, we add social issues to the study and test whether the impact of investors' social media criticism on CSR disclosure is greater or smaller in regions where local government is heavily concerned with social problems. We use the legal and institutional index (LI index) to proxy the level of local government concern for social issues. The LI index is one of five secondary indexes of the Marketization Index, which has been widely used in previous studies in the Chinese context [60–62]. The LI index evaluates the legal institutional environment in China's regions from several angles, including the protection of social rights, effectively capturing the extent of government emphasis on social issues. We partition our sample into two subgroups based on the median of the LI index: companies in regions with high government concern for social issues (high-LI) and those in regions with low government concern for social issues (low-LI). We then rerun the above models. In Columns (1) and (2) of Table 11, we find that the coefficient of CRITICISM is positive and significant for the high-LI subgroup but negative and insignificant for the low-LI subgroup. As shown in Columns (3) and (4), the coefficient of CRITICISM is also significantly positive only in the high-LI group.

Table 11. Differential effects across regions with high and low levels of social concern.

Variables	Dep. Var. = Prob (CSR)		Dep. Var. = RKS	
	(1)	(2)	(3)	(4)
	High-LI	Low-LI	High-LI	Low-LI
CRITICISM	0.119 *** (4.577)	−0.019 (−0.757) [p-value = 0.000]	0.012 * (1.714)	0.004 (0.782) [p-value = 0.137]
SIZE	0.283 *** (8.571)	0.310 *** (9.117)	0.082 *** (10.385)	0.066 *** (8.615)
LEV	−0.225 (−1.264)	−0.936 *** (−5.472)	0.090 (1.318)	−0.123 ** (−2.506)
ROA	−0.500 (−0.940)	−1.480 *** (−3.045)	0.165 (0.729)	0.075 (0.456)
TOBINQ	−0.027 (−1.211)	0.016 (0.789)	0.015 * (1.680)	0.008 (1.083)
INSH	0.306 ** (2.247)	0.466 *** (2.903)	0.168 *** (3.914)	0.157 *** (4.045)
FSH	−0.317 * (−1.651)	−0.218 (−1.048)	0.071 (1.120)	0.073 (1.442)
OUTDIR	0.449 (0.647)	0.160 (0.244)	0.126 (0.726)	−0.062 (−0.448)
BOARD	−0.416 ** (−2.126)	0.787 *** (4.626)	0.130 *** (2.767)	0.174 *** (4.731)
SOE	0.407 *** (6.436)	0.088 (1.384)	0.041 * (1.865)	0.053 *** (3.194)
Intercept	−6.826 *** (−8.431)	−9.301 *** (−11.584)	1.309 *** (6.897)	1.575 *** (8.440)
Year effect	Yes	Yes	Yes	Yes
Industry effect	Yes	Yes	Yes	Yes
Obs.	3081	2918	1061	1038
Pseudo R^2/Adj R^2	0.107	0.089	0.427	0.273

Note: This table presents the subgroup analysis for regions with different levels of social concern. The variables are defined in Table 2. All of the variables (except the dummy variables) are winsorized at the 1% and 99% levels. The z-statistics/t-statistics are reported in brackets. The p-values for the differences between the high-LI and low-LI sub-samples in the coefficients on CRITICISM are reported in square brackets. *, **, and *** indicate significance at the 10%, 5%, and 1% levels, respectively.

Overall, our results indicate that social media criticism has more obvious effects on CSR disclosure in regions where local governments attach greater importance to environmental and social issues. Given that enterprises in China are often dictated to by local governments, maintaining a good relationship with regulators gives companies better access to resources and support, which is critical to acquiring or maintaining a competitive advantage. Owing to the larger concern of increasing regulatory costs or sacrificing ties with local governments, listed companies in regions with higher levels of environmental regulation and social concerns tend to disclose CSR-related information and engage in more substantive CSR disclosures to showcase their commitment to social and environmental responsibility, as demanded by governments. Our findings also indicate that social media criticism from investors and regulatory pressure are effective in motivating companies to engage in CSR disclosure and substantive CSR behavior. These two external pressures—from investors and governments—work in tandem to achieve the same result.

7. Discussion

7.1. Practical Implications

First, this study has implications for the external stakeholders of listed companies in China. External stakeholders generally lack channels through which to voice their opinions on company operations, preventing them from playing a role in corporate governance. Studies have increasingly focused on the ways (e.g., conference calls, site visits) in which capital market participants can directly interact with companies or their managers [10,63]. However, this research has generally considered groups recognized as professional participants, such as institutional investors, analysts, and media representatives. Although non-professional groups (e.g., small shareholders, consumers, the public) are significant participants in the shaping of CSR actions, they have received little attention. We show that in the emerging market context, investor criticism posted on social media platforms can serve as a governance mechanism by prompting companies to release high-quality CSR disclosures. The widespread use of social media enables external stakeholders to play an effective role in corporate governance, publicly voicing their concerns to exert pressure on companies to reduce unethical and opportunistic behaviors.

Second, our findings have implications for policy makers in China. As corporations play a critical role in sustainable social and economic development, it is vital for policy makers to understand the factors that influence CSR. Our findings demonstrate that formal mechanisms such as environmental laws and regulations play a decisive role in CSR disclosure. Despite the growing popularity of CSR disclosure in China, many Chinese listed companies still provide only limited information on their CSR activities. Some companies even engage in "greenwashing" as a symbolic act. Our findings suggest that the growing number of crises linked to social media criticism increases the probability of a company engaging in voluntary CSR disclosure as well as substantive CSR reporting. In other words, social media criticism posted by investors can be an effective informal tool to influence the extent to which a company engages in CSR activities. Therefore, the Chinese government should strengthen its social responsibility governance. Regulators (e.g., the China Securities Regulatory Commission and stock exchanges) should advance the use of modern information technology in capital markets and provide direct channels for stakeholders to interact with managers to promote the sustainable development of listed companies. We find that the effects of social media criticism on CSR disclosure are more pronounced for NSOEs than for SOEs and for companies operating in regions with higher levels of environmental regulation and social concern. Therefore, multiple stakeholders should come together to guide CSR disclosure decisions.

7.2. Limitations

This study has several limitations that suggest directions for further investigation. First, we focus exclusively on companies' CSR responses to criticism by investors on social media. While our findings fill an important gap in the literature, we acknowledge that different crises have diverse consequences for organizations, requiring a variety of crisis management strategies. We do not consider the effects of internal or external crises initiated by other stakeholders. For example, if a company is fined by regulators for financial fraud, how can it use CSR to mitigate potential risk? Second, as our main purpose is to investigate companies' CSR decisions in response to crises, we do not empirically assess the outcomes of CSR disclosure. For example, do CSR disclosure choice and substantiveness minimize the corresponding adverse effects of social media criticism on organizational legitimacy? Third, we restrict our sample to public listed companies in China. We do not include unlisted private firms as they are not required to publicly disclose their CSR data and other financial data. Nevertheless, consideration of the CSR disclosure strategies of private firms is highly relevant to the line of research. Finally, we ask only whether the impact of social media criticism varies depending on ownership and regulatory pressure. We thus offer limited insights into heterogeneous CSR disclosure in response to crises. Do CSR disclosure decisions in times of crisis show different patterns across heavily polluted areas and other industrial sectors, or across companies with different political connections or board characteristics? Researchers should conduct comprehensive cross-sectional analyses to better understand the various attributes or situations that might affect a company's CSR practices.

8. Conclusions

In this study, we investigate the ways in which Chinese companies respond to a crisis using CSR disclosure strategies. Differing from studies that have examined a series of factors that render a company more or less likely to disclose CSR activities, such as political pressure, we focus on how firms strategically use CSR communication in response to crises brought on by social media criticism by investors. Based on legitimacy theory and agency theory and using panel data on Chinese public companies listed on the SSE, we arrive at the following conclusions.

First, we find that companies tend to disclose CSR activities to gain legitimacy when they receive a large volume of social media criticism from investors. Although some studies have confirmed the importance of CSR and demonstrated that CSR engagement can build reputational capital for companies [33], few have discussed the ways in which companies use CSR communication as a tool for risk management in response to crises, especially those due to investors' criticism. We focus on specific crises arising from negative comments by investors, a stakeholder group whose influence on CSR communication has not been adequately addressed in the literature [64]. Using the machine learning method, we identify criticism posted by investors via social media platforms and empirically test whether companies are more likely to voluntarily disclose CSR information when they are subjected to serious criticism on social media. Given that companies generally regard CSR disclosure as a legitimizing tool to communicate with investors and other participants, this practice can mitigate potential reputation damage resulting from social media criticism. Our results are consistent with those of Zhou et al. [16] and Ang et al. [27], confirming that investors play an effective monitoring role in corporate governance via their social media posts. This underscores the importance of investor criticism in forcing companies to avoid unethical behavior and engage in CSR disclosure.

Second, in addition to testing the propensity of companies to engage in CSR disclosure, which can be seen as a primarily symbolic act, we examine the extent to which CSR reporting reflects substantive CSR activities. CSR reporting in emerging economies has been criticized for its low quality and limited information content. However, these limitations have been neglected in studies of CSR disclosure in emerging markets. Using RKS rating data to evaluate the substantiveness of Chinese companies' CSR reports, we find that criticism posted on social media by investors exerts pressure on companies to provide more substantive and detailed CSR reports. As stakeholders tend to criticize reports that do not provide substantial details of the ways in which companies intend to respond to investor criticism, listed companies are likely to engage actively in CSR rather than merely expressing a symbolic commitment to CSR. Communicating substantive details in CSR reports can help companies maintain their legitimacy by giving stakeholders insights into CSR initiatives in times of crisis. We expand research on CSR disclosure and show that crises can provide opportunities for companies to enhance their corporate image through disclosure.

Finally, our further analyses demonstrate that the effects of criticism on CSR disclosure are heterogeneous. Compared with SOEs, NSOEs are more likely to voluntarily disclose CSR activities in times of crisis. For SOEs, social media criticism does not significantly predict the probability of either CSR disclosure or substantive reporting. As NSOEs lack political connections, crises pose a considerable threat to their reputational capital and organizational legitimacy. NSOEs are thus more likely than SOEs to engage in crisis management through CSR disclosure. Furthermore, social media criticism only affects CSR actions in regions where the local government attaches importance to environmental and social issues. In other words, companies that operate in regions with stricter environmental regulations and high concern for social problems are more likely to engage in CSR activities and, crucially, to provide more substantive CSR reports in response to crises. Our findings reveal the heterogeneous nature of CSR responses to social media criticism and show how regulatory pressure from the government affects companies' responses to investor criticism in terms of CSR disclosure and substantive engagement in CSR.

Author Contributions: Conceptualization, Y.Z. and F.Y.; methodology, F.Y.; software, F.Y.; validation, Y.Z. and F.Y.; formal analysis, F.Y.; investigation, Y.Z.; resources, Y.Z.; data curation, F.Y.; writing—original draft preparation, Y.Z. and F.Y.; writing—review and editing, Y.Z. and F.Y.; visualization, F.Y.; supervision, Y.Z.; project administration, Y.Z.; funding acquisition, Y.Z. All authors have read and agreed to the published version of the manuscript.

Funding: This research was funded by National Social Science Foundation of China's program, grant number 18BJY108.

Institutional Review Board Statement: Not applicable.

Informed Consent Statement: Not applicable.

Data Availability Statement: The data presented in this study are available on request from the corresponding author.

Acknowledgments: The authors would like to thank Tao Pan for his help with the machine learning method.

Conflicts of Interest: The authors declare no conflict of interest.

References

1. Cabeza-García, L.; Fernández-Gago, R.; Nieto, M. Do Board Gender Diversity and Director Typology Impact CSR Reporting? *Eur. Manag. Rev.* **2018**, *15*, 559–575. [CrossRef]
2. Hu, Y.Y.; Zhu, Y.; Tucker, J.; Hu, Y. Ownership influence and CSR disclosure in China. *Account. Res. J.* **2018**, *31*, 8–21. [CrossRef]
3. Birkey, R.N.; Michelon, G.; Patten, D.M.; Sankara, J. Does assurance on CSR reporting enhance environmental reputation? An examination in the U.S. context. *Account. Forum* **2019**, *40*, 143–152. [CrossRef]
4. Porter, M.E.; Kramer, M.R. The link between competitive advantage and corporate social responsibility. *Harv. Bus. Rev.* **2006**, *84*, 78–92.
5. Richardson, A.J.; Welker, M. Social disclosure, financial disclosure and the cost of equity capital. *Account. Organ. Soc.* **2001**, *26*, 597–616. [CrossRef]
6. Jo, H.; Harjoto, M.A. Corporate Governance and Firm Value: The Impact of Corporate Social Responsibility. *J. Bus. Ethics* **2011**, *103*, 351–383. [CrossRef]
7. Servaes, H.; Tamayo, A. The Impact of Corporate Social Responsibility on Firm Value: The Role of Customer Awareness. *Manag. Sci.* **2013**, *59*, 1045–1061. [CrossRef]
8. van der Meer, T.G.L.A.; Verhoeven, P.; Beentjes, H.W.J.; Vliegenthart, R. Communication in times of crisis: The stakeholder relationship under pressure. *Public Relat. Rev.* **2017**, *43*, 426–440. [CrossRef]
9. Fernandez-Feijoo, B.; Romero, S.; Ruiz, S. Effect of Stakeholders' Pressure on Transparency of Sustainability Reports within the GRI Framework. *J. Bus. Ethics* **2013**, *122*, 53–63. [CrossRef]
10. Miller, G.S.; Skinner, D.J. The Evolving Disclosure Landscape: How Changes in Technology, the Media, and Capital Markets Are Affecting Disclosure. *J. Account. Res.* **2015**, *53*, 221–239. [CrossRef]
11. Zhao, M. CSR-Based Political Legitimacy Strategy: Managing the State by Doing Good in China and Russia. *J. Bus. Ethics* **2012**, *111*, 439–460. [CrossRef]
12. Lyon, T.P.; Maxwell, J.W. Greenwash: Corporate environmental disclosure under threat of audit. *J. Econ. Manag. Strategy* **2011**, *20*, 3–41. [CrossRef]
13. Lee, E.; Walker, M.; Zeng, C. Do Chinese state subsidies affect voluntary corporate social responsibility disclosure? *J. Account. Public Policy* **2017**, *36*, 179–200. [CrossRef]
14. Marquis, C.; Qian, C. Corporate Social Responsibility Reporting in China: Symbol or Substance? *Organ. Sci.* **2014**, *25*, 127–148. [CrossRef]
15. See, G. Harmonious Society and Corporate Social Responsibility: Shaping the Factors That Drive Environment-Related CSR. *J. Int. Bus. Ethics* **2014**, *7*, 41.
16. Zhou, J.; Ye, S.; Lan, W.; Jiang, Y. The effect of social media on corporate violations: Evidence from Weibo posts in China. *Int. Rev. Financ.* **2020**. [CrossRef]
17. Dhaliwal, D.; Li, O.Z.; Tsang, A.; Yang, Y.G. Corporate social responsibility disclosure and the cost of equity capital: The roles of stakeholder orientation and financial transparency. *J. Account. Public Policy* **2014**, *33*, 328–355. [CrossRef]
18. Majeed, S.; Aziz, T.; Saleem, S. The Effect of Corporate Governance Elements on Corporate Social Responsibility (CSR) Disclosure: An Empirical Evidence from Listed Companies at KSE Pakistan. *Int. J. Financ. Stud.* **2015**, *3*, 530–556. [CrossRef]
19. Cheong, C.W.H.; Sinnakkannu, J.; Ramasamy, S. Reactive or proactive? Investor sentiment as a driver of corporate social responsibility. *Res. Int. Bus. Financ.* **2017**, *42*, 572–582. [CrossRef]
20. Zyglidopoulos, S.C.; Georgiadis, A.P.; Carroll, C.E.; Siegel, D.S. Does media attention drive corporate social responsibility? *J. Bus. Res.* **2012**, *65*, 1622–1627. [CrossRef]
21. Wang, L.; Juslin, H. The Impact of Chinese Culture on Corporate Social Responsibility: The Harmony Approach. *J. Bus. Ethics* **2009**, *88*, 433–451. [CrossRef]
22. Allen, F.; Qian, J.; Qian, M. Law, finance, and economic growth in China. *J. Financ. Econ.* **2005**, *77*, 57–116. [CrossRef]
23. See, G. Harmonious society and Chinese CSR: Is there really a link? *J. Bus. Ethics* **2009**, *89*, 1–22. [CrossRef]
24. Dai, L.; Parwada, J.T.; Zhang, B. The Governance Effect of the Media's News Dissemination Role: Evidence from Insider Trading. *J. Account. Res.* **2015**, *53*, 331–366. [CrossRef]

25. Miller, G.S. The press as a watchdog for accounting fraud. *J. Account. Res.* **2006**, *44*, 1001–1033. [CrossRef]
26. Dyck, A.; Volchkova, N.; Zingales, L. The corporate governance role of the media: Evidence from Russia. *J. Financ.* **2008**, *63*, 1093–1135. [CrossRef]
27. Ang, J.S.; Hsu, C.; Tang, D.; Wu, C. The role of social media in corporate governance. *Account. Rev.* **2021**, *96*, 1–32. [CrossRef]
28. Cade, N.L. Corporate social media: How two-way disclosure channels influence investors. *Account. Organ. Soc.* **2018**, *68–69*, 63–79. [CrossRef]
29. Lau, C.; Lu, Y.; Liang, Q. Corporate Social Responsibility in China: A Corporate Governance Approach. *J. Bus. Ethics* **2014**, *136*, 73–87. [CrossRef]
30. Campbell, J.L. Why would corporations behave in socially responsible ways? An institutional theory of corporate social responsibility. *Acad. Manag. Rev.* **2007**, *32*, 946–967. [CrossRef]
31. Cho, C.H.; Patten, D.M. The role of environmental disclosures as tools of legitimacy: A research note. *Account. Organ. Soc.* **2007**, *32*, 639–647. [CrossRef]
32. Dowling, J.; Pfeffer, J. Organizational legitimacy: Social values and organizational behavior. *Pac. Sociol. Rev.* **1975**, *18*, 122–136. [CrossRef]
33. Williams, R.J.; Barrett, J.D. Corporate philanthropy, criminal activity, and firm reputation: Is there a link? *J. Bus. Ethics* **2000**, *26*, 341–350. [CrossRef]
34. Jensen, M.C.; Meckling, W.H. Theory of the firm: Managerial behavior, agency costs and ownership structure. *J. Financ. Econ.* **1976**, *3*, 305–360. [CrossRef]
35. Oh, W.Y.; Chang, Y.K.; Martynov, A. The Effect of Ownership Structure on Corporate Social Responsibility: Empirical Evidence from Korea. *J. Bus. Ethics* **2011**, *104*, 283–297. [CrossRef]
36. Roberts, R.W. Determinants of corporate social responsibility disclosure: An application of stakeholder theory. *Account. Organ. Soc.* **1992**, *17*, 595–612. [CrossRef]
37. Odriozola, M.D.; Baraibar-Diez, E. Is Corporate Reputation Associated with Quality of CSR Reporting? Evidence from Spain. *Corp. Soc. Responsib. Environ. Manag.* **2017**, *24*, 121–132. [CrossRef]
38. Hoq, M.Z.; Saleh, M.; Zubayer, M.; Mahmud, K.T. The effect of CSR disclosure on institutional ownership. *Pak. J. Commer. Soc. Sci. PJCSS* **2010**, *4*, 22–39.
39. Yu, W.; Zheng, Y. Does CSR reporting matter to foreign institutional investors in China? *J. Int. Account. Audit. Tax.* **2020**, *40*. [CrossRef]
40. Saeidi, S.P.; Sofian, S.; Saeidi, P.; Saeidi, S.P.; Saaeidi, S.A. How does corporate social responsibility contribute to firm financial performance? The mediating role of competitive advantage, reputation, and customer satisfaction. *J. Bus. Res.* **2015**, *68*, 341–350. [CrossRef]
41. Zeng, S.X.; Xu, X.D.; Yin, H.T.; Tam, C.M. Factors that Drive Chinese Listed Companies in Voluntary Disclosure of Environmental Information. *J. Bus. Ethics* **2011**, *109*, 309–321. [CrossRef]
42. Du, S.; Yu, K. Do Corporate Social Responsibility Reports Convey Value Relevant Information? Evidence from Report Readability and Tone. *J. Bus. Ethics* **2020**. [CrossRef]
43. Elliott, W.B.; Grant, S.M.; Hobson, J.L.; Asay, S. Trader Participation in Disclosure: Implications of Interactions with Management. *Contemp. Account. Res.* **2020**, *37*, 68–100. [CrossRef]
44. Deegan, C. Introduction: The legitimising effect of social and environmental disclosures–a theoretical foundation. *Account. Audit. Account. J.* **2002**, *15*, 282–311. [CrossRef]
45. Fama, E.F.; Jensen, M.C. Separation of ownership and control. *J. Law Econ.* **1983**, *26*, 301–325. [CrossRef]
46. Li, Q.; Luo, W.; Wang, Y.; Wu, L. Firm performance, corporate ownership, and corporate social responsibility disclosure in China. *Bus. Ethics A Eur. Rev.* **2013**, *22*, 159–173. [CrossRef]
47. Jo, H.; Harjoto, M.A. The Causal Effect of Corporate Governance on Corporate Social Responsibility. *J. Bus. Ethics* **2011**, *106*, 53–72. [CrossRef]
48. Zajac, E.J.; Westphal, J.D. The social construction of market value: Institutionalization and learning perspectives on stock market reactions. *Am. Sociol. Rev.* **2004**, *69*, 433–457. [CrossRef]
49. Ertugrul, M.; Lei, J.; Qiu, J.; Wan, C. Annual Report Readability, Tone Ambiguity, and the Cost of Borrowing. *J. Financ. Quant. Anal.* **2017**, *52*, 811–836. [CrossRef]
50. Davis, A.K.; Ge, W.; Matsumoto, D.; Zhang, J.L. The effect of manager-specific optimism on the tone of earnings conference calls. *Rev. Account. Stud.* **2015**, *20*, 639–673. [CrossRef]
51. Davis, A.K.; Piger, J.M.; Sedor, L.M. Beyond the numbers: Measuring the information content of earnings press release language. *Contemp. Account. Res.* **2012**, *29*, 845–868. [CrossRef]
52. Loughran, T.; McDonald, B. When is a liability not a liability? Textual analysis, dictionaries, and 10-Ks. *J. Financ.* **2011**, *66*, 35–65. [CrossRef]
53. Li, F. The information content of forward-looking statements in corporate filings—A naïve Bayesian machine learning approach. *J. Account. Res.* **2010**, *48*, 1049–1102. [CrossRef]
54. Zhou, B.; Zhang, C.; Zeng, Q. Does the rhetoric always hide bad intention: Annual report's tone and stock crash risk. *China J. Account. Stud.* **2018**, *6*, 178–205. [CrossRef]

55. Chen, X.; Yan, H.; Yan, Q.; Zhang, X. *Machine Learning for Cyber Security: Third International Conference, ML4CS 2020, Guangzhou, China, October 8-10, 2020, Proceedings, Part II*; Springer Nature: Basingstoke, UK, 2020; Volume 12487.
56. Hameed, Z.; Garcia-Zapirain, B. Sentiment classification using a single-layered BiLSTM model. *Ieee Access* **2020**, *8*, 73992–74001. [CrossRef]
57. Ye, K.; Zhang, R. Do lenders value corporate social responsibility? Evidence from China. *J. Bus. Ethics* **2011**, *104*, 197–206. [CrossRef]
58. Lind, D.A.; Marchal, W.G.; Wathen, S.A. *Statistical Techniques in Business & Economics*; McGraw-Hill Education: New York, NY, USA, 2017.
59. Albareda, L.; Lozano, J.M.; Ysa, T. Public policies on corporate social responsibility: The role of governments in Europe. *J. Bus. Ethics* **2007**, *74*, 391–407. [CrossRef]
60. Xin, Z.; Xin, S. Marketization process predicts trust decline in China. *J. Econ. Psychol.* **2017**, *62*, 120–129. [CrossRef]
61. Wang, Y.; Chen, C.R.; Huang, Y.S. Economic policy uncertainty and corporate investment: Evidence from China. *Pac. Basin Financ. J.* **2014**, *26*, 227–243. [CrossRef]
62. Lucey, B.; Xiaoxue, W.; Yanfang, W.; Ying, X. Can financial marketization mitigate the negative effect of exchange rate fluctuations on exports? Evidence from Chinese regions. *Financ. Res. Lett.* **2020**, *34*. [CrossRef]
63. Jiang, X.; Yuan, Q. Institutional investors' corporate site visits and corporate innovation. *J. Corp. Financ.* **2018**, *48*, 148–168. [CrossRef]
64. Michelon, G.; Rodrigue, M. Demand for CSR: Insights from Shareholder Proposals. *Soc. Environ. Account. J.* **2015**, *35*, 157–175. [CrossRef]

International Journal of
Environmental Research and Public Health

MDPI

Article

The Mediating Role of Responsible Innovation in the Relationship between Stakeholder Pressure and Corporate Sustainability Performance in Times of Crisis: Evidence from Selected Regions in China

Hong Tian and Jiahui Tian *

Business School, Jilin University, Changchun 130012, China; tianhong2919@163.com
* Correspondence: tianjh19@mails.jlu.edu.cn; Tel.: +86-151-4307-9213

Abstract: Responsible innovation, as a new management paradigm that balances the need for profit growth and the appeal of social value, plays an important role in taking into account corporate economic, social and environmental performance. It provides new ideas for driving enterprises to become more risk-resistant and sustainable in times of crisis. However, existing research on responsible innovation has mostly focused on content issues, and there is a lack of sufficient research and empirical studies on its effectiveness in business organizations. Based on the stakeholder theory and the research logic of "pressure–behavior-performance", this study investigates the formation mechanism of responsible innovation and its impact on corporate performance. Through empirical research on 306 Chinese sample data, the results show that stakeholder pressure has a positive impact on corporate sustainability performance and responsible innovation plays a partially mediating role in this relationship. Flexible routine replication positively moderates the relationship between stakeholder pressure and responsible innovation, while positively moderating the mediating role that responsible innovation plays between stakeholder pressure and corporate sustainability performance. This study contributes to helping enterprises recognize the importance of responsible innovation in responding to stakeholder pressure and promoting corporate sustainability performance in times of crisis.

Keywords: responsible innovation; stakeholder pressure; corporate sustainability performance; flexible routine replication; corporate social responsibility

1. Introduction

The spread of COVID-19 has caused dramatic dynamic environmental changes, changeable market demand and systematic economic stagnation, which have brought great challenges to the survival and development of science and technology enterprises. In times of crisis, how to enhance the ability of enterprises to resist risks while maintaining sustainable production and development has become one of the focuses of research. Innovation is an effective way for enterprises to cope with uncertainty, enabling enterprises to remain dynamic and sustainable [1]. However, the reality is that innovative products such as big data not only bring huge market space and broad development prospects, but also come with a scientific and ethical crisis that challenges the legal and moral bottom line, such as information security and privacy leakage. With the increasing importance of stakeholders to corporate social responsibility and the continuous emergence of ethical dilemmas, academic and business scholars begin to pay attention to the "distinction between justice and benefit" in the new market environment, and to rethink the fundamental issue of "interest and morality". How can we avoid the "Collingridge's dilemma" [2] while enjoying the dividends of innovation? How to effectively address the reasonable balance between current innovative development and visionary planning, so as to enhance the ability of enterprises to resist risks? How to take into account the harmonious coexistence of economic, social and environmental benefits, so as to achieve sustainable development? These issues have become important topics that need to be addressed urgently.

The European Commission's Horizon 2020 Framework Plan proposes the concept of "Responsible Innovation" (RI), which suggests that there should be cooperation and matching between society and science and technology [3,4]. Responsible innovation emphasizes meeting future needs through collective management, and the process and result of innovation should be morally acceptable, sustainable and socially desirable [5]. Given the "balance" thought contained in responsible innovation, this concept has been introduced in business management research as a new management paradigm [6,7]. Responsible innovation will mitigate or even reverse the negative externalities of corporate activities and will create both economic benefits and business opportunities for enterprises [8,9]. However, much of the research on responsible innovation is currently focused on science and technology innovation [10] rather than business-driven innovation [11]. Enterprises are an important source of innovation [8], but for enterprises that pay attention to efficiency and cost, whether and why they are willing to adopt responsible innovation activities is an issue to be discussed. In addition, researchers have focused on the evaluation criteria and content issues of responsible innovation [12,13], but pay little attention to its implementation path and mechanism, that is, there is a lack of research on the motivation and impact of responsible innovation in the business field.

Stakeholder theory provides a theoretical basis for integrating business and social domain research [14]. Stakeholders provide resources and support for the long-term sustainability of enterprises and at the same time require enterprises to actively respond to the value proposition of the stakeholders [15]. Given that stakeholder rewards and penalties for sustainable performance will threaten the survival and growth of enterprises, enterprises are increasingly focusing on sustainability activities and devoting more resources to developing strategies, policies and practices that are consistent with sustainability and social responsibility goals in response to stakeholder pressure [16,17]. As a deliberative innovation mode in which stakeholders are included in innovation activities, responsible innovation can meet both economic benefits and sustainable development goals [7], and its innovation process and results will be affected by the value demands of stakeholders. It can be seen that there is an obvious logical relationship between stakeholder pressure and responsible innovation. Therefore, this study considers the role of stakeholder pressure on responsible innovation from a stakeholder perspective and then explores the impact of adopting this innovation model on the sustainable performance of enterprises. Furthermore, the ability of enterprises to effectively organize, search and reconstruct knowledge to match and meet the needs of responsible innovation also have a significant impact on corporate innovation effectiveness and sustainability performance [18]. Flexible routine replication, which relies on exploration capability, emphasizes more on the dynamic capability of enterprises, and can help enterprises break the old knowledge coupling, generate new knowledge combinations and create value [19]. Therefore, flexible routine replication is a new means for enterprises to create and solve problems [20], which is helpful for enterprises to acquire diversified knowledge to solve the problem of value co-creation between stakeholders and enterprises. This study also explores the moderating role of flexible routine replication in these influence paths.

In conclusion, based on the stakeholder theory, this study introduces responsible innovation into the research field of corporate strategic management, focuses on the promoting effect of stakeholder pressure on responsible innovation and the impact of responsible innovation on the sustainable performance of enterprises, and discusses the influencing mechanism under the contingency effect of flexible routine replication. This study can make contributions in the following aspects: First, it provides a new perspective on the "righteousness and profit debate", which is helpful for enterprises to solve the problem of harmonious coexistence of interests and morality. Second, it expands the cross research between stakeholder theory and corporate innovation management, which helps to promote the multi-subject co-governance of corporate innovation. Third, the knowledge and capability factors are extended to the research framework of responsible innovation, and the importance of knowledge management is revealed. In addition, this study provides a practical insight for balancing innovation independence and social responsibility, and promotes corporate sustainable development in times of crisis.

2. Theory and Hypotheses

2.1. Responsible Innovation

The concept of responsible innovation, proposed by Stilgoe et al. [5], has been widely accepted by academics to refer to the collective management of current science and innovation to meet future needs, and is more broadly defined as "innovation with society and innovation for society". Responsible innovation is a new concept based on governance approaches and innovation assessment, democratizing innovation through deliberative forms of governance such as stakeholder and public participation, specifically aiming to incorporate ethical and social concerns at the outset of innovation in order to avoid negative impacts of innovation [21,22]. Lubberink et al. [7] further propose a framework for responsible innovation in a business context and provide practices conducive to the implementation of responsible innovation. In the business context, responsible innovation covers the whole process of enterprise innovation, including stakeholder participation and prediction at the beginning of innovation, reflection and introspection in the innovation process, and the conformity of innovation results with moral and social expectations [9,12,23].

Unlike previous "risk management frameworks" that focused only on avoiding harm [24], or "social innovation" and "shared value" studies that focused only on doing good [25], the governance and responsibility logic contained in responsible innovation can simultaneously promote the dual results of avoiding harm and doing good [7,8,26]. Compared with the traditional innovation model, the characteristics of responsible innovation are mainly reflected in four aspects: anticipation, reflexivity, inclusion and responsiveness [5]. Anticipation refers to the systematic thinking of any possible impact of innovation in order to predict potential problems of innovation and evaluate available alternatives, aiming to form "proactive governance" [7]. Reflexivity implies that enterprises confront their activities, commitments and assumptions and become aware of the limitations of their knowledge. In addition, enterprises should examine how their value systems and beliefs influence the development of corporate innovation, not only by fulfilling their role tasks but also by taking on broader ethical responsibilities [5,21]. Inclusion implies that enterprises should leverage multi-stakeholder relationships to include lay members in responsible innovation activities, seeking to diversify inputs and delivery to governance [10]. Responsiveness refers to the fact that responsible innovation requires the ability to change shape or direction in response to stakeholder and public values and changing circumstances [27].

Studies have focused on the theoretical framework of responsible innovation [7], the innovation process [10], governance mechanisms, and from institutional scenarios, resource capacity [6,23] and corporate social responsibility [28] perspectives to explore the formation mechanism of corporate responsible innovation [29]. Based on the stakeholder theory, this study presents responsible innovation as a way for enterprises to respond to stakeholder demands and to balance the needs of corporate development with social value expectations to achieve strategic goals for sustainable development.

2.2. Stakeholder Pressure and Corporate Sustainability Performance

Corporate sustainability focuses on the integration of economic prosperity, environmental protection and social progress [17,30], which is considered as a corporate strategy for enterprises to seek the best business practices to meet and balance the needs of current and future stakeholders [31–33]. Corporate sustainability performance measures the extent to which enterprises include economic, environmental, social and governance factors in their operations [34,35], as well as the final impact these factors have on the enterprises and society, including economic performance, social performance and environmental performance [32,36,37]. Horisch et al. [38] have shown that the central themes of stakeholder theory and corporate sustainability research are similar in terms of creating long-term environmental, social and economic value for stakeholders and enterprises. Stakeholders are institutions, organizations, communities and individuals that may influence or be affected by specific organizations. Stakeholder pressure can prompt enterprises to adopt strategies and practices in line with the goal of social responsibility, to reduce agency problems while safeguarding their interests [15,39].

Currently, corporate responses to sustainability issues are influenced by the sustainability concerns of a growing number of stakeholders, and responsible behavior has been recognized as essential for corporate success and survival [9,40,41]. Enterprises must clarify their important stakeholder relationships, systematically evaluate the impact of corporate actions on stakeholders, and then actively adjust their responsible behaviors to maintain a mutually beneficial strategic partnership with stakeholders or reconcile differences [12,42]. On the one hand, the action of enterprises responding to the demands of stakeholders helps enterprises mobilize and share the capital, knowledge and technology of stakeholders [43], which helps enterprises form strategic partnerships with stakeholders [10,14] while promoting the formation of specific environmental and social capabilities [10,14]. In this way, enterprises can reduce the cost of solving sustainable development problems and improve their sustainable performance [8]. Moreover, enterprises focusing on growth and development integrate stakeholder pressure with enterprises' value chain by implementing social responsibility activities related to their main business [44], that is, creating shared value through strategic corporate social responsibility [25,45–47]. This multi-objective strategic model cannot only focus on and respond to the changing social and environmental concerns of stakeholders, but also provide opportunities and benefits for the core business of enterprises [48]. On the other hand, stakeholder pressure helps enterprises understand the preferences of stakeholders such as governments and consumers in terms of sustainability [49]. To enhance the effectiveness of corporate sustainability strategies and respond to stakeholders' sustainability needs, threats and opportunities to corporate sustainability strategies must be identified, as well as reducing and avoiding corporate risks and uncertainties [18,41]. Furthermore, enterprises' initiatives that incorporate social responsibility and stakeholder pressure into strategic corporate thinking can be seen as doing the right thing, thus helping to protect corporate reputation, improve corporate image and ensure the long-term sustainability of the company's objectives [9,23]. In summary, stakeholder pressure motivates enterprises to respond and fulfill their social and environmental responsibilities while focusing on economic efficiency, which helps enterprises improve corporate sustainability performance. Therefore, this paper proposes the following hypothesis:

Hypothesis 1 (H1). *Stakeholder pressure is positively related to corporate sustainability performance.*

2.3. The Mediating Effect of Responsible Innovation in an Association between Stakeholder Pressure and Corporate Sustainability Performance

According to the stakeholder theory, organizations establish relationships with several stakeholder groups and stakeholders can influence organizations' decisions [15]. On the one hand, as a form of governance in which enterprises include stakeholders and the public in a deliberative innovation model, responsible innovation can respond to the demands of stakeholders by discussing with stakeholders the underlying norms and values that can guide innovation in the desired direction [7]. Enterprises integrate the sustainability goals of different stakeholders, thus prompting corporate innovation processes and outcomes that are consistent with stakeholders' expectations of social and environmental responsibility [6,50,51]. On the other hand, responsible innovation facilitates the exchange of resources and capabilities between enterprises and stakeholders.

Enterprises reflect on potential problems in the existing innovation model, while assessing the feasibility of alternative solutions, thus achieving the goal of improving the efficiency and effectiveness of corporate innovation. In addition, responsible innovation can enhance investors' understanding and recognition of enterprise innovation by reducing the information asymmetry and uncertainty of innovation, so as to improve enterprise performance [36]. In other words, responsible innovation conforms to the "triple bottom line" principle: taking sustainable development as the ideal result of innovation, promoting the integration of responsibility ethics and core business, and innovating achievements that cover three dimensions—economy, environment and society [7,9,26,52].

Specifically, enterprises include different stakeholders and the public at the outset of innovation activities to establish a forward-looking model of responsibility, thus increasing the likelihood of anticipating and discerning how innovation can benefit society and prevent any negative consequences from occurring [21,53]. Stakeholder pressure can promote better learning and decision-making of enterprises [54], which not only encourages enterprises to critically examine the social, environmental, political and moral impacts brought by innovation [55], but also urges enterprises to rethink the relationship between innovation and social needs [7]. Enterprises take actions and adjust according to new knowledge, new ideas, new perceptions and new norms emerging in the innovation process, so as to make innovation adapt to changes and meet new demands [56], and ensure the ethical appropriateness of enterprise products, and the acceptability of relevant performance and quality [9,57,58]. This process not only helps enterprises to create benefits, but also helps enterprises to organize resources and guide innovation in the direction of protecting the natural environment and increasing social welfare as quickly as possible [5,59].

In summary, this study believes that enterprises establish a continuous, transparent and interactive innovation process consistent with social values, needs and expectations through responsible innovation [12]. The process can help enterprises anticipate and respond to ethical, social and environmental concerns, thus not only responding to the pressure of stakeholder expectations but also balancing economic efficiency gains with the need for social values. This measure takes into account the needs of enterprises' economic development and social ethical responsibilities, and will create environmental and social performance while improving the efficiency and benefits of enterprises' innovation, that is, improve corporate sustainability performance. Therefore, this paper proposes the following hypothesis:

Hypothesis 2 (H2). *Stakeholder pressure influences corporate sustainability performance through the mediating role of responsible innovation.*

2.4. The Moderating Effect of Flexible Routine Replication

Organizational routine is repetitive, identifiable and interdependent patterns of behavior involving multiple actors [60,61], and are divided into two categories based on a capability perspective: conventional routine and flexible routine [62]. Conventional routine refers to the general competence patterns of organizations, which contain stable, explicit, continuous and solidified knowledge, while flexible routine emphasizes the dynamic capabilities of enterprises, which contain more complex, implicit and diverse knowledge [20]. In an unstable environment, flexible routines not only help to adjust the original knowledge templates but also promote exploratory learning and searching for heterogeneous knowledge to optimize the allocation of resources and expand organizational boundaries [63]. In this situation, flexible routines will exhibit a high level of replication [20,64]. Flexible routine replication is a new means for enterprises to create problem-solving that can help them break old knowledge coupling, generate new knowledge combinations and create value [19].

Responsible innovation focuses on the interaction between innovation structures and stakeholders, which requires enterprises to be able to respond quickly to new ideas, knowledge and norms emerging in the interaction, and the ever-changing external environment, to make responsible decisions that allow innovation to adapt to change and meet new needs [7,12]. On the one hand, enterprises with a high degree of flexible routine replication can quickly respond to dynamic changes in the environment, capture complex and changing knowledge needs, and then conduct exploratory organizational learning and extensive knowledge search [65]. On the other hand, enterprises promote knowledge transfer and knowledge creation through the splitting and reorganization of existing knowledge modules and the reallocation of organizational resources [66] to improve the efficiency of enterprise innovation model transformation [67]. The development and deployment of flexible routines help improve the firm's capacity for technological change and flexible adaptation. Such dynamic capabilities provide the knowledge, resources and foundation to respond quickly to changing needs, facilitate the inclusion of stakeholders in a deliberative innovation model form of governance and address the opportunities and challenges presented by stakeholder pressure. In addition, enterprises with a high degree of flexible routines replication are more likely to develop a flexible, risk-taking, innovative organizational climate and learning culture. When facing the demands of stakeholders, this type of enterprise is more innovative and proactive and tends to take actions to meet the challenges. Therefore, enterprises with a high degree of flexible routine replication are more inclined to adopt a responsible innovation approach to solve the dilemma of economic benefit, social prosperity and environmental protection. Therefore, this paper proposes the following hypothesis:

Hypothesis 3 (H3). *Flexible routine replication would positively moderate the relationship between stakeholder pressure and responsible innovation.*

Based on the above assumptions of mediating and moderating effects, this study further proposes a moderated mediating effect model. Corporate sustainability means that enterprises must place sustainability goals at the core, rather than enhancing their success "through additional social and environmental goals as a form of responsive corporate social responsibility" [68]. This requires enterprises to have the ability and knowledge to change their existing innovation mode, and at the same time, pioneering independent attempts and efforts are needed to adapt to the special and constantly changing external environment [69]. Enterprises with a high degree of flexible routine replication have low obstacles and resistance to the acquisition, generation, integration and replacement of new knowledge, which enables enterprises to have strong adaptability and fast organizational knowledge update, and focus on the long-term development of enterprises [66]. This means that enterprises have the ability to acquire heterogeneous knowledge through exploratory learning, and adjust their innovation model by integrating existing resource allocation and knowledge reserve, so as to provide an execution basis for meeting the pressure from stakeholders to balance economic, environmental and social performance. In summary, enterprises with high levels of flexible routine replication are more likely to catalyze responsible innovation when faced with stakeholder pressure, which in turn enhances corporate sustainability performance. Therefore, this paper proposes the following hypothesis:

Hypothesis 4 (H4). *Flexible routine replication would positively moderate the mediating role of responsible innovation between stakeholder pressure and corporate sustainability performance.*

The theoretical model diagram of this study is shown in Figure 1.

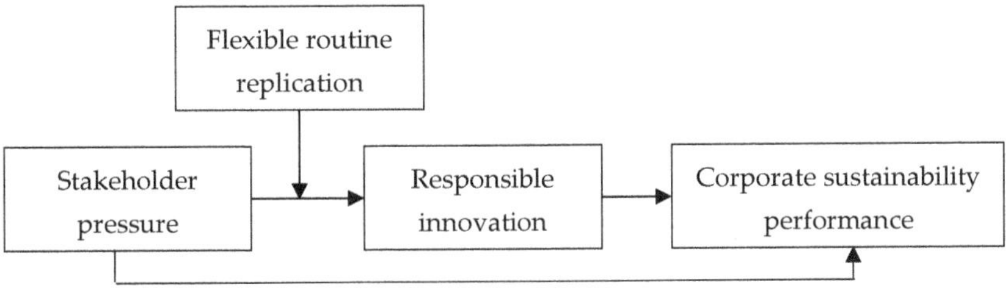

Figure 1. Theoretical model.

3. Methodology

3.1. Sample Selection and Data Collection

This study covers technology-based enterprises in the Yangtze River Delta region, the Pearl River Delta region and the Northeast region of China. The Yangtze River Delta region and the Pearl River Delta region have high innovation activity and strong R&D foundations [70,71]. These two regions are the main gathering places of science and technology enterprises. The Northeast region of China used to be famous as an old industrial base in China, with strong scientific and technological strength and profound industrial deposits. There are also numerous technology-based enterprises. Therefore, these three representative regions were selected as data sources in this study. Influenced by COVID-19, online and offline data collection methods were adopted in this study. To ensure that the research respondents have a clear and comprehensive understanding and knowledge of their companies, the study invited the chairman, president and managers in charge of R&D to fill in the answers based on the actual situation of their companies in the past three years. In China, the COVID-19 epidemic started in late 2019 and lasted for nearly a year and a half by the time the questionnaire was sent out. The three-year data range of 2019, 2020 and 2021 investigated in this study can adequately cover the whole process from the emergence of the epidemic to the outbreak and then to the long-term existence of the epidemic. Before the start of the research, the project team clarified the research intention, purpose, confidentiality measures and precautions to the respondents, emphasizing that the research was conducted anonymously and the questionnaire was only used for scientific research and no personal or corporate information would be disclosed. The questionnaire distribution of this study began in early March 2021 and ended in late April 2021. A total of 600 questionnaires were distributed in this study, and after deleting questionnaires with incomplete or regular responses, 306 valid questionnaires were recovered, with a valid recovery rate of 51.0%. The results of the descriptive statistics of the sample are as follows: in terms of enterprise age, 39.54% are 5 years or less, 42.81% are 6–10 years, and 17.65% are 11 years or more. In terms of enterprise size: 39.21% for 100 persons and below, 33.01% for 101–300 persons, and 27.78% for more than 300 persons. Enterprise nature: state-owned/collective accounted for 24.51%, private 57.84%, foreign/joint venture 17.65%.

3.2. Measures

To ensure the reliability and validity of the questionnaire, well-established scales published in international mainstream academic journals were selected for the measurement of each variable. In this study, a translation team including doctoral students majoring in business management and English was established to form a Chinese questionnaire according to the standard translation–back translation procedure. Before the questionnaire was distributed, the study asked professors in business management to review the questionnaire to ensure its relevance in the Chinese context. The questionnaire was scored on a Likert7 scale, from 1 to 7, indicating "strongly disagree" to "strongly agree".

Depending on the degree of influence on the firm, stakeholders are divided into primary stakeholders (including shareholders, investors, employees, customers and government), which are critical to the firm's survival, and secondary stakeholders (media and nonprofit organizations), which can influence public opinion and thus damage or enhance the firm's reputation [6]. Given the greater influence of primary stakeholders on corporate strategies and decisions in the Chinese context, this study focused on the role of primary stakeholder pressure. Helmig et al.'s [6] 10-item scale for measuring key stakeholder pressure was selected for this study, with representative items such as "Our customers' purchasing habits are changing to support responsible corporations (e.g., fair trade coffee)". Responsible innovation is based on the four-item scale selected by Stilgoe et al. [5] and Cao et al. [23] in which the representative questions include "In the early stage of innovation activities, companies can conduct a forward-looking analysis of the future impact of innovation activities, so as to guide them in an ethically acceptable and socially satisfactory direction, and achieve controlled risks in innovation activities". Flexible routine replication is based on the study of Wei and Dang [65] and a four-item scale was selected, which is representative of questions such as "Firms are able to quickly promote and apply new organizational norms to meet internal and external challenges". Corporate sustainability performance is based on Li et al.'s [36] study, an 11-item scale was selected, including 4 items for environmental performance, 4 items for economic performance, and 3 items for social performance, with representative items such as "Our company has reduced consumption of hazardous and toxic substances", "Our company develops community economic activities and provides more employment opportunities". The control variables were selected as firm age, firm size and firm nature. Among them, the age of the enterprise is expressed by the number of years of establishment, the size of the enterprise is measured by the number of people in the enterprise, and the nature of the enterprise is divided into state-owned enterprises, foreign-funded enterprises, joint ventures and private enterprises.

4. Results and Analysis

4.1. Reliability and Validity

This study used SPSS 23.0 to conduct reliability and validity tests. The results are shown in Table 1. The Cronbach's α coefficients of stakeholder pressure, responsible innovation, flexible routine replication and corporate sustainability performance were all greater than 0.7. The composite reliability of each construct was greater than the recommended level of 0.7, indicating that the questionnaire had good reliability. In terms of validity, this study used the double-blind translation method and appropriately adjusted and modified the relevant questions according to the Chinese scenario, with good content validity. AVE was all greater than the recommended 0.5 level, indicating good convergent validity.

Table 1. Reliability and validity test results.

Variables	Cronbach's α	AVE	CR	KMO	Variance Interpretation
Stakeholder pressure	0.839	0.535	0.911	0.849	66.763%
Responsible Innovation	0.789	0.614	0.864	0.782	61.372%
Flexible Routine Replication	0.802	0.629	0.871	0.791	62.936%
Corporate sustainability performance	0.915	0.508	0.917	0.906	70.681%

4.2. Analysis and Results

Table 2 shows the means, standard deviations and correlation matrix of the variables. Stakeholder pressure was significantly correlated with responsible innovation (r = 0.593, $p < 0.01$), stakeholder pressure was significantly correlated with corporate sustainability performance (r = 0.608, $p < 0.01$) and responsible innovation was significantly correlated with corporate sustainability performance (r = 0.540, $p < 0.01$). These results initially validate the hypotheses of this study, which were further tested by using regression analysis. Furthermore, from the AVE values in Table 1, it can be concluded that the square root of AVE for stakeholder pressure, responsible innovation, flexible routine replication and corporate sustainability performance are 0.731, 0.784, 0.793 and 0.713. When the AVE square root value of the factor is greater than the correlation value between the factor and other factors, it can indicate that it has good discriminative validity. Therefore, the discriminant validity of the variables in this study is good.

4.3. Hypotheses Testing

In this study, multiple linear regression methods are used to test each hypothesis, and the results are presented in Table 3. This study first centralizes the variables used and constructs the interaction term of stakeholder pressure and flexible routine replication after centralization to reduce the multi-collinearity between the variables. M1 is the effect of control variables on responsible innovation, M2 is the effect of independent variables on responsible innovation and M4 is the effect of the interaction term of stakeholder pressure and flexible routine replication on responsible innovation. M5 is the effect of control variables on corporate sustainability performance, M6 is the effect of independent variables on corporate sustainability performance and M7 is the effect of independent and mediating variables on corporate sustainability performance. All models are significant except for models M1 and M5.

Table 2. Descriptive statistical analysis.

	1	2	3	4	5	6	7
1. Firm age	-						
2. Firm size	0.225 **	-					
3. Nature	0.241 **	0.079	-				
4. Stakeholder pressure	−0.018	−0.051	−0.100	-			
5. Responsible innovation	0.045	−0.025	−0.077	0.593 **	-		
6. Flexible routine replication	−0.001	−0.034	−0.086	0.083	0.140 *	-	
7. Corporate sustainability performance	−0.014	0.016	−0.113 *	0.608 **	0.540 **	0.032	-
Mean	1.781	1.886	1.931	4.360	4.275	4.184	4.307
S.D.	0.725	0.812	0.647	0.500	0.742	0.749	0.645

Note: * $p < 0.05$, ** $p < 0.01$ (two-tailed).

Table 3. Results of regression analysis.

Variables	Responsible Innovation				Corporate Sustainability Performance		
	M1	M2	M3	M4	M5	M6	M7
Firm age	0.075	0.065	0.063	0.071	0.009	−0.002	−0.020
Firm size	−0.035	−0.007	−0.004	−0.008	0.023	0.051	0.053
Firm nature	−0.092	−0.033	−0.025	−0.019	−0.117 *	−0.056	−0.047
Stakeholder pressure		0.590 ***	0.584 ***	0.553 ***		0.605 ***	0.441 ***
Flexible routine replication			0.090	0.077			
Stakeholder pressure × Flexible routine replication				0.098 *			
Responsible innovation							0.277 ***
R2	0.011	0.355	0.363	0.372	0.013	0.375	0.424
ΔR2	0.002	0.347	0.353	0.359	0.004	0.366	0.414
F	1.157	41.481 ***	34.239 ***	29.477 ***	1.368	45.091 ***	44.183 ***

Note: * $p < 0.05$, *** $p < 0.001$ (two-tailed); The sample size is 306.

In M6, stakeholder pressure has a significant positive effect on corporate sustainability performance ($\beta = 0.605$, $p < 0.001$), and hypothesis H1 is supported. M5 shows that firm nature has a significant impact on corporate sustainability performance. Therefore, in this study, further tests were conducted by grouping according to firm nature. The total number of samples is 306. After grouping the enterprises according to their nature, the sample size is 75 for state-owned/collective enterprises, 177 for private enterprises, and only 54 for foreign-funded/joint ventures. First, the LSD pairwise t-test was used for comparison, and the results are shown in Table 4. Through data comparison, it is found that the corporate sustainability performance of state-owned/collective enterprises is more outstanding than that of private enterprises. Next, the main hypothesis test was conducted according to enterprises with different natures. The results are shown in Table 5. The corporate sustainability performance of state-owned/collective enterprises and private enterprises are affected by stakeholder pressure, and the regression coefficient of state-owned/collective enterprises is higher. This finding is consistent with the current development in China that state-owned/collective enterprises will take on more corporate social responsibility and respond to stakeholder demands than private enterprises, resulting in a more significant improvement in corporate sustainability performance. The reason for the insignificance of foreign/joint ventures may be due to the small sample size as the ratio of the number of foreign/joint ventures to the number of variables after grouping does not reach 15:1 [72].

Table 4. LSD analysis results for different firm natures.

Variables	Firm Nature	Firm Nature	Mean Difference	Sig.
Corporate sustainability performance	state-owned/collective	private	0.222 *	0.012
	state-owned/collective	foreign/joint	0.202	0.078
	private	foreign/joint	−0.020	0.840

Note: * $p < 0.05$.

Table 5. The results of grouping main hypothesis test for different firm natures.

Variables	Corporate Sustainability Performance					
	State-Owned/ Collective Enterprises		Private Enterprises		Foreign/Joint Venture	
	M8	M9	M10	M11	M12	M13
Firm age	0.016	0.197	−0.043	−0.075	0.077	0.071
Firm size	0.157	0.081	−0.098	0.005	0.260	0.288
Stakeholder pressure		0.697 ***		0.692 ***		−0.122
R2	0.027	0.486	0.012	0.479	0.085	0.099
ΔR2	0.000	0.464	0.001	0.470	0.049	0.045
F	0.997	22.334 ***	1.049	53.012 ***	2.356	1.829
Observations	75	75	177	177	54	54

Note: *** $p < 0.001$ (two-tailed).

M2 in Table 3 shows that stakeholder pressure is a good predictor of responsible innovation ($\beta = 0.590$, $p < 0.001$). M7 builds on M6 by including responsible innovation in the regression equation, and responsible innovation has a positive effect on corporate sustainability performance ($\beta = 0.277$, $p < 0.001$), and the effect of stakeholder pressure on corporate sustainability performance remains significant but decreases ($\beta = 0.441$, $p < 0.001$), assuming that H2 is supported.

This study further examined the mediating effect by Bootstrap method [73,74], and the total effect of stakeholder pressure on corporate sustainability performance was 0.605, the direct effect was 0.442 and the indirect effect was 0.163 (95% confidence interval is [0.059, 0.293]), indicating that responsible innovation plays a partial mediating role.

M4 includes the interaction term between stakeholder pressure and flexible routine replication in the regression equation with responsible innovation as the dependent variable, and the interaction term is significant ($\beta = 0.098$, $p < 0.05$), indicating that flexible routine replication plays a moderating role between stakeholder pressure and responsible innovation. This study further verified the moderating effect by dividing the data into two groups, high and low, by adding and subtracting one standard deviation from the mean value of flexible routine replication, which is shown in Figure 2. The results show that the higher the level of flexible routine replication, the stronger the effect of stakeholder pressure on responsible innovation. Therefore, flexible routine replication plays a positive moderating role between stakeholder pressure and responsible innovation. Therefore, H3 is supported.

This study used the PROCESS procedure to test the mediated moderation model. The results are shown in Table 6. When responsible innovation is the mediator, flexible routine replication moderates the indirect effect of stakeholder pressure on corporate sustainability performance with an INDEX of 0.034 (95% CI = [0.006, 0.198]). Specifically, the moderating effect of flexible routine replication on the indirect effect is insignificant when flexible practice replication takes the mean minus one standard deviation (95% CI = [−0.007, 0.215]), while the moderating effect of flexible practice replication on the indirect effect is significant when flexible practice replication takes the mean plus one standard deviation (95% CI = [0.067, 0.431]); therefore, H4 is supported.

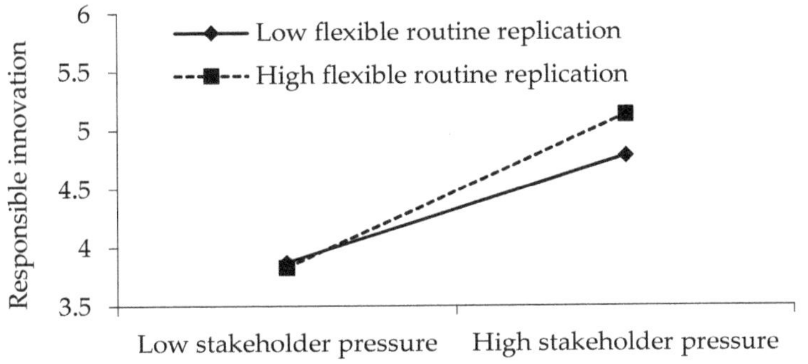

Figure 2. Diagram of regulating role.

Table 6. Results of the mediated moderation model.

	Indirect Effects	BootSE	[BootLLCI, BootULCI]
−1 SD	0.119	0.057	[−0.007, 0.215]
0	0.153	0.058	[0.054, 0.281]
+1 SD	0.187	0.092	[0.067, 0.431]

5. Discussion

This study explores the important role of responsible innovation in dealing with the challenges of stakeholder pressure, and how to transform stakeholder pressure into a driving force for corporate sustainability performance. Based on stakeholder theory, this study constructs a logical framework of "stakeholder pressure–responsible innovation– corporate sustainability performance". Under the boundary condition of flexible routine replication, we investigate the impact of stakeholder pressure on responsible innovation and its effect on corporate sustainability performance. The main finding is that stakeholder pressure has a positive impact on corporate sustainability performance and that responsible innovation plays a partially mediating role in the relationship. Flexible routine replication not only positively moderates the relationship between stakeholder pressure and responsible innovation, but also mediates the role of responsible innovation in mediating the relationship between stakeholder pressure and corporate sustainability performance.

This study explores the effectiveness of responsible innovation in balancing interests and ethics. On the one hand, the important role of responsible innovation in dealing with the challenge of stakeholder pressure and transforming the pressure into the driving force of sustainable development is revealed and empirically tested in this study. When an enterprise actively responds to the demands of stakeholders and takes responsible innovation, this action helps the enterprise find new development opportunities in the challenges, and promote the formation of a mutually beneficial and win–win strategic partnership with stakeholders, so as to achieve value co-creation and improve the corporate sustainability performance. This study responds to the call of Lubberink et al. to study responsible innovation in the business context [7]. In addition, although some scholars have paid attention to the close relationship between stakeholders and responsible innovation (e.g., [10,12]), this study further composes and empirically tests the relationship between the two.

On the other hand, this study regards responsible innovation as a kind of corporate management paradigm, which is an active and long-term strategic choice of enterprises [12], rather than a response under critical circumstances. The content of this study shows that even if the epidemic crisis has a profound impact on the business environment [75], enterprises' actions of actively responding to the pressure from stakeholders and taking responsible innovation will still show effectiveness. This study echoes and extends He and Harris' observation that "the COVID-19 pandemic offers a great opportunity for companies to contribute to addressing global social and environmental challenges" [76]. Responsible innovation can not only help enterprises promote social prosperity and environmental protection, but also guarantees the survival and development of enterprises, and effectively improves the ability of enterprises to resist risks in critical situations.

5.1. Theory Contributions

First, responsible innovation is introduced into the field of corporate strategic management research as a new innovation management paradigm for enterprises to solve the problem of harmonious coexistence of profit and ethics and promote sustainable development. The existing responsible innovation mainly focuses on the policy level, and the theoretical research lags behind and mainly adopts qualitative methods (e.g., [8,10,68]). Few scholars have discussed the applicability and effectiveness of responsible innovation in the context of Chinese organizations (e.g., [23]). This study quantitatively clarifies the positive role of responsible innovation in responding to stakeholder demands, balancing economic, environmental and social values, and enhancing sustainable corporate performance in China. The findings of this study provide a reference for promoting deeper theoretical research on responsible innovation and helps guide enterprises to properly handle the relationship with stakeholders, inspire value co-creation between enterprises and stakeholders, and turn pressure into motivation to improve sustainable performance [8,52].

Second, it expands the intersection study of stakeholder theory and corporate innovation management. The atomic innovation governance of a single subject has revealed its limitations in the new economic development, and innovation governance urgently needs to be transformed to innovation co-governance with the joint participation of multiple subjects. Different from social innovation [77], green innovation and other innovation modes [78] that focus on specific stakeholders and solve specific problems, responsible innovation can broadly absorb the value demands of multi-stakeholders and make it possible for multi-stakeholders to co-govern [7]. Therefore, this study provides a general governance framework for enterprises to balance responsibility and innovation through the study of responsible innovation, which helps to promote the integration of stakeholder pressure and corporate innovation management and strengthen the continuous optimization and multi-subject co-governance of the whole innovation process.

Third, the factors of knowledge and ability are extended to the research framework of corporate social responsibility and business ethics that provide a new theoretical perspective for the research in this field. Existing studies mostly focus on business ethics from the perspectives of corporate values, culture and leadership style, etc. (e.g., [79–81]), while this study focuses on competency factors. By combining capability factors with responsible innovation, this study clarifies the catalytic role of flexible routine replication in the path of responsible innovation, and makes clear that dynamic capabilities and knowledge resources are one of the operational foundations for enterprises to successfully respond to new ideas, new norms and rapidly changing external environments. The conclusions of this study provide a new way of thinking for improving the effectiveness of responsible innovation and corporate social responsibility strategies, and solving the problem of decoupling-related policy formulation and implementation results of business ethics.

5.2. Practice Contributions

First, it provides ideas for solving the dilemma between enterprise benefit growth and social responsibility fulfillment. In recent years, China's industrial structure has shifted from a stage of rapid growth to a stage of high-quality development. At the same time, the government has emphasized the development of a circular economy and an environment-friendly economic model. However, environmental pollution problems still persist. At the same time, some enterprises take responsible behavior to gain legitimacy, but it brings a huge cost to enterprises. As an innovative behavior pattern that can not only produce economic benefits but also sustainable social values, responsible innovation can effectively solve the problem of "the difference between justice and benefit" and the disconnection between "responsibility" and "innovation", and guide enterprise innovation to develop in a morally acceptable, socially desirable and sustainable direction. Therefore, governments and enterprises in China and other countries can learn from and promote responsible innovation models that embed business ethics into the business process. Just as the Chinese traditional culture mentioned, "Justice to generate profits, profits to enrich the people", and then achieve high-quality economic development.

Second, a collaborative innovation and governance system should be created with enterprises as the main body and a wide range of stakeholders involved. On the one hand, enterprises should increase communication links with stakeholders interactively and openly, improve the transparency of information related to technological innovation, and reduce the possibility of conflicting value claims arising from information asymmetry. Moreover, enterprises should proactively understand and grasp the needs of stakeholders and promote a cooperative business model to achieve complementary resources, knowledge sharing and value creation between enterprises and stakeholders, thereby jointly creating economic and social value. On the other hand, enterprises should keep track of the dynamic changes of laws, social situations, science and technology and other factors that can significantly affect the enterprise innovation environment in real-time. These measures can help enterprises to keenly capture the problems that will threaten social and environmental sustainability, and to consider and avoid the potential impact of these problems on the development of society and enterprises.

Third, it provides practical inspiration for improving the effectiveness of responsible innovation from the perspective of ability. Adequate knowledge and resources are the basic elements to form responsible innovation, and flexible routine replication is one of the important guarantees for enterprises to organize and manage knowledge flexibly and respond to the pressure of stakeholders. Therefore, enterprises should increase the investment in the knowledge base and innovation management, improve the ability of searching, absorbing and integrating heterogeneous knowledge, and gradually increase the stock of enterprise knowledge. In addition, enterprises should create an open, interactive, transformational organizational atmosphere and an innovative, learning-oriented organizational culture. Enterprise training, intelligence introduction and other measures enhance the divergent innovative thinking and stimulate the subjective initiative of employees. In this way, enterprises are encouraged to break the subjective cognitive limitations, reduce excessive reliance on existing conventions and knowledge, and improve the operability of the implementation of responsible innovation.

5.3. Limitations and Future Research

First, the cross-sectional data collection method is adopted in this study, which cannot reflect the long-term and dynamic impact of responsible innovation on corporate sustainability performance. In the future, the tracking research method can be used to explore the continuous impact of responsible innovation on corporate sustainability performance. Second, in terms of sample selection, samples in this study are from Chinese science and technology enterprises, with strong pertinence. For different industries in different emerging economies, the business environment for enterprises is very different. Therefore, future research can be extended to different industries and different countries to further explore the effectiveness of responsible innovation, so as to enhance the universality and practical value of the research. Finally, this study only studies the formation mechanism of responsible innovation from the perspective of stakeholders. In practice, responsible innovation may also be affected by institutional environment, corporate culture and other factors. Therefore, future research needs to combine a variety of theoretical perspectives to deepen the theoretical framework of responsible innovation.

6. Conclusions

The focus of this study is on how to solve the problem of "justice and interest debate", aiming to guide enterprises not only to improve their ability to resist risks but also to promote sustainable development while paying attention to social values and environmental protection. To be specific, this study takes Chinese science and technology enterprises as the research object and discusses the following three issues: First, how to effectively deal with the pressure from stakeholders to facilitate corporate sustainability performance. The second is how responsible innovation balances economic growth and social value creation in order to promote corporate sustainability performance. The third is to discuss when responsible innovation can more effectively promote corporate sustainability performance. This study further promotes the theoretical research of responsible innovation in the business context. In terms of practice, enterprises in China and other countries can get practical inspiration from this paper to reasonably balance interests and ethics and promote high-quality development. It also provides ideas for enterprises to promote corporate sustainability performance in times of crisis.

Author Contributions: H.T. and J.T. contributed to conceptualization, formal analysis, investigation, methodology, and writing and editing of the original draft. Both authors have read and agreed to the published version of the manuscript.

Funding: This research was funded by the National Social Science Foundation of China, grant number 20FGLB039 and the Social Science Foundation of Jilin Province, grant number 2020B068.

Institutional Review Board Statement: Not applicable.

Informed Consent Statement: Not applicable.

Data Availability Statement: Data sharing not applicable.

Conflicts of Interest: The authors declare no conflict of interest.

References

1. Yuan, B.L.; Zhang, Y. Flexible environmental policy, technological innovation and sustainable development of China's industry: The moderating effect of environment regulatory enforcement of the article. *J. Clean. Prod.* **2020**, *243*, 118543–118560. [CrossRef]
2. Weber, J. Making worlds: Epistemological, ontological and political dimensions of technoscience of the article. *Poiesis Praxis* **2010**, *7*, 17–36. [CrossRef]
3. Owen, R.; Macnaghten, P.; Stilgoe, J. Responsible research and innovation: From science in society to science for society, with society of the article. *Sci. Public Policy* **2012**, *39*, 751–760. [CrossRef]
4. Owen, R.; Pansera, M.; Macnaghten, P.; Randles, S. Organisational institutionalisation of responsible innovation of the article. *Res. Policy* **2021**, *50*, 104132–104144. [CrossRef]
5. Stilgoe, J.; Owen, R.; Macnaghten, P. Developing a framework for responsible innovation of the article. *Res. Policy* **2013**, *42*, 1568–1580. [CrossRef]
6. Halme, M.; Korpela, M. Responsible Innovation Toward Sustainable Development in Small and Medium-Sized Enterprises: A Resource Perspective of the article. *Bus. Strategy Environ.* **2014**, *23*, 547–566. [CrossRef]
7. Lubberink, R.; Blok, V.; van Ophem, J.; Omta, O. Lessons for Responsible Innovation in the Business Context: A Systematic Literature Review of Responsible, Social and Sustainable Innovation Practices of the article. *Sustainability* **2017**, *9*, 721. [CrossRef]
8. Voegtlin, C.; Scherer, A.G. Responsible Innovation and the Innovation of Responsibility: Governing Sustainable Development in a Globalized World of the article. *J. Bus. Ethics* **2017**, *143*, 227–243. [CrossRef]
9. Stahl, B.C.; Chatfield, K.; Ten Holter, C.; Brem, A. Ethics in corporate research and development: Can responsible research and innovation approaches aid sustainability? of the article. *J. Clean. Prod.* **2019**, *239*, 118044–118059. [CrossRef]
10. Silva, L.M.D.; Bitencourt, C.C.; Faccin, K.; Iakovleva, T. The role of stakeholders in the context of responsible innovation: A meta-synthesis of the article. *Sustainability* **2019**, *11*, 1766. [CrossRef]
11. Hemphill, T.A. Responsible innovation in industry: A cautionary note on corporate social responsibility of the article. *J. Responsible Innov.* **2016**, *3*, 81–87. [CrossRef]
12. Gonzales-Gemio, C.; Cruz-Cazares, C.; Parmentier, M.J. Responsible Innovation in SMEs: A Systematic Literature Review for a Conceptual Model of the article. *Sustainability* **2020**, *12*, 10232. [CrossRef]
13. Lehoux, P.; Silva, H.P.; Oliveira, R.R.; Rivard, L. The responsible innovation in health tool and the need to reconcile formative and summative ends in RRI tools for business of the article. *J. Responsible Innov.* **2020**, *7*, 646–671. [CrossRef]
14. Jones, T.M. Instrumental stakeholder theory—A synthesis of ethics and economics of the article. *Acad. Manag. Rev.* **1995**, *20*, 404–437. [CrossRef]
15. Freeman, R.E. The Politics of Stakeholder Theory: Some Future Directions of the article. *Bus. Ethics Q.* **1994**, *4*, 409–421. [CrossRef]
16. Lee, D.D.; Faff, R.W. Corporate sustainability performance and idiosyncratic risk: A global perspective of the article. *Fin. Rev.* **2009**, *44*, 213–237. [CrossRef]
17. Antolin-Lopez, R.; Delgado-Ceballos, J.; Montiel, I. Deconstructing corporate sustainability: A comparison of different stakeholder metrics of the article. *J. Clean. Prod.* **2016**, *136*, 5–17. [CrossRef]
18. Eikelenboom, M.; de Jong, G. The impact of dynamic capabilities on the sustainability performance of SMEs of the article. *J. Clean Prod.* **2019**, *235*, 1360–1370. [CrossRef]
19. Jonsson, A.; Foss, N.J. International expansion through flexible replication: Learning from the internationalization experience of IKEA of the article. *J. Int. Bus. Stud.* **2011**, *42*, 1079–1102. [CrossRef]
20. Jin, Y.; Shao, Y.F.; Wu, Y.B. Routine replication and breakthrough innovation: The moderating role of knowledge power of the article. *Technol. Anal. Strateg. Manag.* **2021**, *33*, 426–438. [CrossRef]
21. Burget, M.; Bardone, E.; Pedaste, M. Definitions and Conceptual Dimensions of Responsible Research and Innovation: A Literature Review of the article. *Sci. Eng. Ethics* **2017**, *23*, 1–19. [CrossRef]

22. Bauer, A.; Bogner, A.; Fuchs, D. Rethinking societal engagement under the heading of Responsible Research and Innovation: (novel) requirements and challenges of the article. *J. Responsible Innov.* **2020**. [CrossRef]
23. Cao, X.; Lv, D.; Xing, Z.Y. Innovative Resources, Promotion Focus and Responsible Innovation: The Moderating Roles of Adaptive Governance of the article. *Sustainability* **2020**, *12*, 2860. [CrossRef]
24. Themsen, T.N.; Skaerbaek, P. The performativity of risk management frameworks and technologies: The translation of uncertainties into pure and impure risks of the article. *Account. Organ. Soc.* **2018**, *67*, 20–33. [CrossRef]
25. Porter, M.E.; Kramer, M.R. Strategy and society of the article. *Harv. Bus. Rev.* **2006**, *84*, 78–92.
26. Scherer, A.G.; Voegtlin, C. Corporate governance for responsible innovation: Approaches to corporate governance and their implications for sustainable development of the article. *Acad. Manag. Perspect.* **2020**, *34*, 182–208. [CrossRef]
27. van Lente, H.; Swierstra, T.; Joly, P.B. Responsible innovation as a critique of technology assessment of the article. *J. Responsible Innov.* **2017**, *4*, 254–261. [CrossRef]
28. Hadj, T.B. Effects of corporate social responsibility towards stakeholders and environmental management on responsible innovation and competitiveness of the article. *J. Clean. Prod.* **2020**, *250*, 119490–119499. [CrossRef]
29. Gurzawska, A. Responsible Innovation in Business: Perceptions, Evaluation Practices and Lessons Learnt of the article. *Sustainability* **2021**, *13*, 1826. [CrossRef]
30. Elkington, J. Towards the sustainable corporation—Win-win-win business strategies for sustainable developmenT of the article. *Calif. Manag. Rev.* **1994**, *36*, 90–100. [CrossRef]
31. Bansal, P. Evolving sustainably: A longitudinal study of corporate sustainable development of the article. *Strateg. Manag. J.* **2005**, *26*, 197–218. [CrossRef]
32. Artiach, T.; Lee, D.; Nelson, D.; Walker, J. The determinants of corporate sustainability performance of the article. *Account. Financ.* **2010**, *50*, 31–51. [CrossRef]
33. Bartolacci, F.; Caputo, A.; Soverchia, M. Sustainability and financial performance of small and medium sized enterprises: A bibliometric and systematic literature review of the article. *Bus. Strategy Environ.* **2020**, *29*, 1297–1309. [CrossRef]
34. Goyal, P.; Rahman, Z.; Kazmi, A.A. Corporate sustainability performance and firm performance research Literature review and future research agenda of the article. *Manag. Decis.* **2013**, *51*, 361–379. [CrossRef]
35. Qu, Y.; Liu, Y.K.; Nayak, R.R.; Li, M.R. Sustainable development of eco-industrial parks in China: Effects of managers' environmental awareness on the relationships between practice and performance of the article. *J. Clean. Prod.* **2015**, *87*, 328–338. [CrossRef]
36. Li, L.; Msaad, H.; Sun, H.P.; Tan, M.X.; Lu, Y.Q.; Lau, A.K.W. Green Innovation and Business Sustainability: New Evidence from Energy Intensive Industry in China of the article. *Int. J. Environ. Res. Public Health* **2020**, *17*, 7826. [CrossRef]
37. Dey, P.K.; Malesios, C.; De, D.; Chowdhury, S.; Ben Abdelaziz, F. The Impact of Lean Management Practices and Sustainably-Oriented Innovation on Sustainability Performance of Small and Medium-Sized Enterprises: Empirical Evidence from the UK of the article. *Brit. J. Manag.* **2020**, *31*, 141–161. [CrossRef]
38. Horisch, J.; Freeman, R.E.; Schaltegger, S. Applying Stakeholder Theory in Sustainability Management: Links, Similarities, Dissimilarities, and a Conceptual Framework of the article. *Organ. Environ.* **2014**, *27*, 328–346. [CrossRef]
39. Rudyanto, A.; Siregar, S.V. The effect of stakeholder pressure and corporate governance on the sustainability report quality of the article. *Int. J. Ethics Syst.* **2018**, *34*, 233–249. [CrossRef]
40. Bai, C.; Sarkis, J.; Dou, Y. Corporate sustainability development in china: Review and analysis of the article. *Ind. Manag. Data Syst.* **2014**, *115*, 5–40. [CrossRef]
41. Wijethilake, C. Proactive sustainability strategy and corporate sustainability performance: The mediating effect of sustainability control systems of the article. *J. Environ. Manag.* **2017**, *196*, 569–582. [CrossRef]
42. Journeault, M.; Perron, A.; Vallieres, L. The collaborative roles of stakeholders in supporting the adoption of sustainability in SMEs of the article. *J. Environ. Manag.* **2021**, *287*, 112349–112361. [CrossRef]
43. Leonidou, E.; Christofi, M.; Vrontis, D.; Thrassou, A. An integrative framework of stakeholder engagement for innovation management and entrepreneurship development of the article. *J. Bus. Res.* **2020**, *119*, 245–258. [CrossRef]
44. Jakhar, S.K.; Mangla, S.K.; Luthra, S.; Kusi-Sarpong, S. When stakeholder pressure drives the circular economy Measuring the mediating role of innovation capabilities of the article. *Manag. Decis.* **2019**, *57*, 904–920. [CrossRef]
45. Harrison, J.S.; Bosse, D.A.; Phillips, R.A. Managing for stakeholders, stakeholder utility functions, and competitive advantage of the article. *Strateg. Manag. J.* **2010**, *31*, 58–74. [CrossRef]
46. Lobschat, L.; Mueller, B.; Eggers, F.; Brandimarte, L.; Diefenbach, S.; Kroschke, M.; Wirtz, J. Corporate digital responsibility of the article. *J. Bus. Res.* **2021**, *122*, 875–888. [CrossRef]
47. Broadstock, D.C.; Matousek, R.; Meyer, M.; Tzeremes, N.G. Does corporate social responsibility impact firms' innovation capacity? The indirect link between environmental & social governance implementation and innovation performance of the article. *J. Bus. Res.* **2020**, *119*, 99–110.
48. Palazzo, M.; Vollero, A.; Siano, A. From strategic corporate social responsibility to value creation: An analysis of corporate website communication in the banking sector of the article. *Int. J. Bank Mark.* **2020**, *38*, 1529–1552. [CrossRef]
49. Manning, B.; Braam, G.; Reimsbach, D. Corporate governance and sustainable business conduct-Effects of board monitoring effectiveness and stakeholder engagement on corporate sustainability performance and disclosure choices of the article. *Corp. Soc. Responsib. Environ. Manag.* **2019**, *26*, 351–366. [CrossRef]

50. Inigo, E.A.; Blok, V. Strengthening the socio-ethical foundations of the circular economy: Lessons from responsible research and innovation of the article. *J. Clean. Prod.* **2019**, *233*, 280–291. [CrossRef]
51. Waldron, T.L.; Navis, C.; Karam, E.P.; Markman, G.D. Toward a Theory of Activist-Driven Responsible Innovation: How Activists Pressure Firms to Adopt More Responsible Practices of the article. *J. Manag. Stud.* **2019**. [CrossRef]
52. Auer, A.; Jarmai, K. Implementing Responsible Research and Innovation Practices in SMEs: Insights into Drivers and Barriers from the Austrian Medical Device Sector of the article. *Sustainability* **2018**, *10*, 17. [CrossRef]
53. Jarmai, K.; Vogel-Poschl, H. Meaningful collaboration for responsible innovation of the article. *J. Responsible Innov.* **2020**, *7*, 138–143. [CrossRef]
54. Rivard, L.; Lehoux, P. When desirability and feasibility go hand in hand: Innovators' perspectives on what is and is not responsible innovation in health of the article. *J. Responsible Innov.* **2020**, *7*, 76–95. [CrossRef]
55. Boons, F.; Montalvo, C.; Quist, J.; Wagner, M. Sustainable innovation, business models and economic performance: An overview of the article. *J. Clean. Prod.* **2013**, *45*, 1–8. [CrossRef]
56. van de Poel, I.; Asveld, L.; Flipse, S.; Klaassen, P.; Scholten, V.; Yaghmaei, E. Company Strategies for Responsible Research and Innovation (RRI): A Conceptual Model of the article. *Sustainability* **2017**, *9*, 2045. [CrossRef]
57. Long, T.B.; Blok, V.; Dorrestijn, S.; Macnaghten, P. The design and testing of a tool for developing responsible innovation in start-up enterprises of the article. *J. Responsible Innov.* **2020**, *7*, 45–75. [CrossRef]
58. Ranabahu, N. 'Wicked' solutions for 'wicked' problems: Responsible innovations in social enterprises for sustainable development of the article. *J. Manag. Organ.* **2020**, *26*, 995–1013. [CrossRef]
59. Brand, T.; Blok, V. Responsible innovation in business: A critical reflection on deliberative engagement as a central governance mechanism of the article. *J. Responsible Innov.* **2019**, *6*, 4–24. [CrossRef]
60. Feldman, M.S.; Pentland, B.T. Reconceptualizing organizational routines as a source of flexibility and change of the article. *Adm. Sci. Q.* **2003**, *48*, 94–118. [CrossRef]
61. Gao, D.H.; Squazzoni, F.; Deng, X.Q. The Intertwining Impact of Intraorganizational and Routine Networks on Routine Replication Dynamics: An Agent-Based Model of the article. *Complexity* **2018**. [CrossRef]
62. Ma, Y.; Zhang, Q.; Yin, Q.Y. Influence of Environmental Management on Green Process Innovation: Comparison of Multiple Mediating Effects Based on Routine Replication of the article. *Int. J. Environ. Res. Public Health* **2019**, *16*, 4346. [CrossRef] [PubMed]
63. Davies, A.; Frederiksen, L.; Cacciatori, E.; Hartmann, A. The long and winding road: Routine creation and replication in multi-site organizations of the article. *Res. Policy* **2018**, *47*, 1403–1417. [CrossRef]
64. Howard-Grenville, J.A. The persistence of flexible organizational routines: The role of agency and organizational context of the article. *Organ Sci.* **2005**, *16*, 618–636. [CrossRef]
65. Wei, L.; Dang, X.H. Impact of routine replication on bootleg innovation: The moderating effect of network closure and knowledge base of the article. *Manag. Res. Sci.* **2020**, *41*, 32–41.
66. Chen, Y.L.; Gao, C. Study on Replication of Routines in Organizations Based on Organization Ambidexterity Competence of the article. *China Ind. Econ.* **2014**, *28*, 147–159.
67. Santoro, G.; Bresciani, S.; Papa, A. Collaborative modes with Cultural and Creative Industries and innovation performance: The moderating role of heterogeneous sources of knowledge and absorptive capacity of the article. *Technovation* **2020**, *92–93*, 102040–102049. [CrossRef]
68. Imaz, O.; Eizagirre, A. Responsible Innovation for Sustainable Development Goals in Business: An Agenda for Cooperative Firms of the article. *Sustainability* **2020**, *12*, 6948. [CrossRef]
69. Szymanski, E.A.; Smith, R.D.J.; Calvert, J. Responsible research and innovation meets multispecies studies: Why RRI needs to be a more-than-human exercise of the article. *J. Responsible Innov.* **2021**. [CrossRef]
70. Raźniak, P.; Dorocki, S.; Winiarczyk-Raźniak, A. Innovative Industry Sectors in World Economic Centers. In Proceedings of the 5th International Conference IMES, Prague, Czech Republic, 25–26 May 2017; pp. 810–820.
71. Dorocki, S.; Raźniak, P.; Winiarczyk-Raźniak, A.; Boguś, M. The Role of Global Cities in Creation of Innovative Industry Sectors. Case Study—Life Sciences Sector. In Proceedings of the 5th International Conference IMES, Prague, Czech Republic, 25–26 May 2017; pp. 136–146.
72. Pedhazur, E.J. *Multiple Regression in Behavioral Research: Explanation and Prediction*; Harcourt Brace College Publishers: Fort Worth, TX, USA, 1997; p. 207.
73. Preacher, K.J.; Hayes, A.F. Asymptotic and resampling strategies for assessing and comparing indirect effects in multiple mediator models of the article. *Behav. Res. Methods* **2008**, *40*, 879–891. [CrossRef]
74. Zhao, X.; Lynch, J.G., Jr.; Chen, Q. Reconsidering Baron and Kenny: Myths and truths about mediation analysis of the article. *J. Consum. Res.* **2010**, *37*, 197–206. [CrossRef]
75. Brammer, S.; Branicki, L.; Linnenluecke, M.K. COVID-19, societalization, and the future of business in society of the article. *Acad. Manag. Perspect.* **2020**, *34*, 493–507. [CrossRef]
76. He, H.W.; Harris, L. The impact of Covid-19 pandemic on corporate social responsibility and marketing philosophy of the article. *J. Bus. Res.* **2020**, *116*, 176–182. [CrossRef]
77. van der Have, R.P.; Rubalcaba, L. Social innovation research: An emerging area of innovation studies? of the article. *Res. Policy* **2016**, *45*, 1923–1935. [CrossRef]

78. Adams, R.; Jeanrenaud, S.; Bessant, J.; Denyer, D.; Overy, P. Sustainability-oriented Innovation: A Systematic Review of the article. *Int. J. Manag. Rev.* **2016**, *18*, 180–205. [CrossRef]
79. Jamali, D.; Karam, C. Corporate Social Responsibility in Developing Countries as an Emerging Field of Study of the article. *Int. J. Manag. Rev.* **2018**, *20*, 32–61. [CrossRef]
80. Schaltegger, S.; Burritt, R. Business Cases and Corporate Engagement with Sustainability: Differentiating Ethical Motivations of the article. *J. Bus. Ethics* **2018**, *147*, 241–259. [CrossRef]
81. Kolk, A. The social responsibility of international business: From ethics and the environment to CSR and sustainable development of the article. *J. World Bus.* **2016**, *51*, 23–34. [CrossRef]

International Journal of
Environmental Research and Public Health

MDPI

Article

The Moderating Role of Corporate Social Responsibility in the Association of Internal Corporate Governance and Profitability; Evidence from Pakistan

Jihai Lu [1,2], Sohail Ahmad Javeed [2,*], Rashid Latief [3], Tao Jiang [2] and Tze San Ong [4]

1 College of Education, Zhejiang University, Hangzhou 310058, China; mreastlu@163.com
2 Hangzhou College of Commerce, Zhejiang Gongshang University, Hangzhou 311500, China; jtao@263.net
3 School of Finance and Economics, Jiangsu University, Zhenjiang 212013, China; rashidlatief@ujs.edu.cn
4 School of Business and Economics, Universiti Putra Malaysia, Serdang 43400, Malaysia; tzesan@upm.edu.my
* Correspondence: sohailahmaduaf@yahoo.com

Abstract: At present, climate and other environmental problems are arising because of the development of the industrial sector at a large level. The industrial sector is supposed to be a major cause of climate change problems that lead to global warming. Therefore, corporate social responsibility (CSR) with the help of corporate governance is an imperative approach to control these social problems. Consequently, in the context of the organizational and management theory, agency theory, and the stakeholder theory, this study focuses on important factors of internal corporate governance such as chief executive officer (CEO) power, the board size, independence, ownership concentration, managerial ownership, and audit quality for improving the profitability of firms. Moreover, this study considers corporate social responsibility as a controlling and moderating factor for firm performance and internal corporate governance. We employed ordinary least square (OLS) for endogeneity testing, fixed effect (FE), generalized method of moments (GMM), and feasible generalized least square (FGLS) on data of Pakistani firms for the period of 2010–2019. The results of this study demonstrate the following outcomes: firstly, all internal corporate governance factors are positively linked with firm performance; secondly, corporate social responsibility (CSR) is the most valuable tool for improving profitability. Importantly, this study suggests that all internal corporate governance factors are positively linked with firm performance because of the interactive role of corporate social responsibility (CSR). This study practically contributes to the literature by suggesting the imperative role of corporate social responsibility (CSR) for internal corporate governance, which may help to reduce climate and social problems.

Keywords: corporate social responsibility (CSR); internal corporate governance; firm performance; manufacturing firms

1. Introduction

At present, the world is suffering severe environmental glitches and the problem getting worse over time; therefore, institutions and governments are working to minimize or remove these environmental problems [1]. Previous researchers reported that the industrial sector is highly responsible for these environmental and social problems, especially the firms of developing economies [2]. Therefore, corporate social responsibility (CSR) is measured as a major tool to motivate insider corporate governance for social actions [3]. CSR practices normally engaged firm-level governance to participate in social and environmental activities [4]. The internal corporate governance (ICG) is an imperative body to control and monitor corporate social practices. Generally, profit maximization is a major motive of every business or firm. Therefore, corporate governance adopts various techniques to increase the firm profit. The majority of studies revealed that inside corporate governance is highly important for firm profitability and other actions [5,6].

On the other hand, few researchers disclosed the negative or insignificant connection of corporate governance with firm profitability [7,8]. However, no prior study specifically described the reason for this positive, negative, or insignificant affiliation between corporate governance and profitability. Before this, most studies inspected only a single or few dimensions of internal corporate governance. Therefore, this study considers various internal corporate governance elements. Additionally, this study proposes that CSR investigates the reason for this positive, negative, or insignificant relationship, because corporate social responsibility is supposed to be an effective tool for internal corporate governance and has a positive relationship [9]. Besides, Wu, et al. [10] stated that information disclosure serves as an important tool to control the information asymmetry between internal corporate governance and other stakeholders. CSR enhances the firm reputation and, therefore, corporate governance may involve social practices [11].

However, this study has discovered various corporate governance factors according to the guidelines of the Securities and Exchange Commission of Pakistan (SECP) [12]. For instance, the chief executive officer (CEO) and supervisory board, which consists of board independence and size. Moreover, we use an ownership structure that consists of ownership concentration and managerial ownership because it plays an imperative part in internal corporate governance. Similarly, audit quality is also a very important factor of internal corporate governance. For firm performance, this study uses economic value added (EVA) and sustainable growth rate (SGR). To support this study, firstly, the organization and management theory supported the role of CEO power [13]. Secondly, the agency theory supported board structure, ownership structure, and audit committee [14]. Thirdly, the stakeholder theory supported the role of CSR as moderating factor for the link between firm performance and internal corporate governance [15].

This study applied multiple statistical methods for empirical investigation. Firstly, we employed ordinary least squares (OLS) to discover the endogeneity. Secondly, we employed the fixed effect technique to overcome the unobservable heterogeneity. Thirdly, we employed the generalized method of moments (GMM) for correcting the endogeneity issues from our data. Lastly, for the robustness test, feasible generalized least square (FGLS) has been employed to overcome the overall heterogeneity. Our results reported that internal corporate governance factors are positively linked with firm performance. Secondly, our results discovered that CSR is positively connected with firm performance. Importantly, this study highlights that CSR is the highly valuable moderating factor for the positive connection between internal corporate governance factors and firm performance.

The outcomes of our study have various suggestions for policymakers, shareholders, owners, investors, institutes, and governments. This study recommended the role of corporate social responsibility to control and monitor internal corporate governance. Thus the Government of Pakistan (GOP) must tighten these regulations for controlling internal corporate governance and enhancement of profitability. Additionally, this study provides directions for GOP and other institutes for developing corporate social practices. The conclusion of this study is highly valuable for the firms of developing and developed economies to control and monitor the internal corporate governance factors for better outcomes.

The rest of the sections of this paper are categorized into the following parts. Section 2 explains the theoretical and literature framework for hypothesis development. Section 3 reveals the sample selection, data collection, contextual analysis of social and corporate governance practices in Pakistan, variables' construction, and empirical methods. Section 4 sheds light on the empirical findings with a discussion. The last section reveals the conclusion and policy implications. Figure 1 represents the conceptual framework of the study.

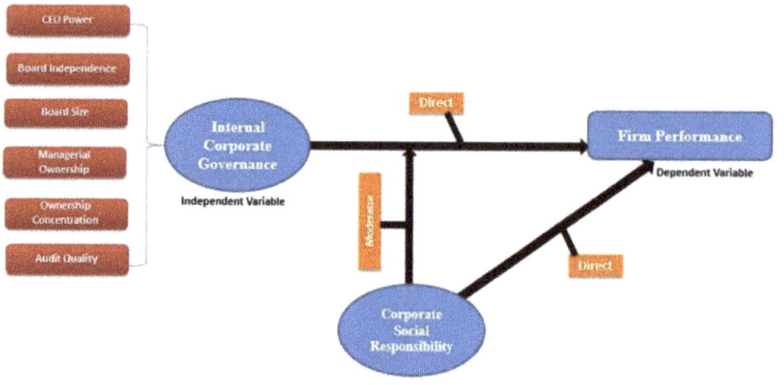

Figure 1. Conceptual Roadmap. CEO: chief executive officer.

2. Theoretical Analysis

Theoretically, various theories shed light on the imperative role of the internal corporate governance factors for firm performance. CEO power as compensation has a significant role in firm performance. In this context, firstly, the organization and management theory stated that a powerful CEO may properly implement their decisions [13]. This theory sheds light on the imperative of the powerful CEO to reduce the managerial unnecessary expenses. A powerful CEO controls and monitors investment decisions that minimize the chances of managerial personal use. Therefore, this theory encouraged firms to have a powerful and strong CEO for the improvement of firm performance.

Furthermore, the firm board has an imperative role in firm performance. In this support, the agency theory exposed that board members endow with monitoring and organizing function on managers actions [14]. Agency theory supported the role of board size in firm performance. The involvement of all board members may create fairness in decision making that builds the firm trust level and attracts more investors. Besides, agency theory also sheds light on the auditing practices for reducing agency costs. The audit committee is a valuable approach to minimize the information asymmetry between owners and management because an independent audit committee focuses on the organization's transparent actions that build confidence between owners and managers [16]. Generally, the audit committee is accountable for making independent audits and monitors both internal and external auditors for transparency. The agency theory also reveals the imperative role of dividend policy in firm performance. This theory focuses on the difference of opinion between principals and agents [14]. The connection between the agent and principal is intrinsically covered with, firstly, the information asymmetry that exists between principal and agent, more on the dispute of interest between them [17]. The timely dividend payment discourages managers from overinvesting and enhances shareholders' confidence.

Thirdly, stakeholder theory supported the role of corporate social responsibility for firm performance [15]. Internal corporate governance always looks for means to enhance firm profit and, therefore, they considered CSR to improve the firm image, which automatically enhances the firm profit [18]. Stakeholder theory also supported the moderating role of CSR because internal corporate governance uses effective ways for saving the interest of the firm stakeholders with the help of CSR [9,19]. CSR puts pressure on the firm internal corporate governance to work for firm performance and a positive firm image in the market. The concern of stakeholders is highly important for corporate governance practices and CSR practices assure all stakeholders [20].

3. Literature Review and Hypothesis Development

3.1. Internal Corporate Governance Factors and Firm Performance

This study divided internal corporate governance into five categories by following the securities and exchange commission of Pakistan [12]. Firstly, this study considers senior executives or top executives as the major decision bodies in the firm. The senior executives consist of the chief executive officer (CEO) power as compensation. Secondly, this study considers board structure or composition, which includes board members, board independence, and remuneration committee. Thirdly, this study considers the structure of ownership, which is further classified as managerial and concentrated ownership. Fourthly, this study focuses on auditing practices as internal corporate governance.

Berger, et al. [21] reported firms' innovational activities normally depend upon the CEO's decision-making. Papadakis [22] reported that shareholders consider the CEO as a leader to enhance firm value. Coles, et al. [23] investigated the industrial tournament incentives as a CEO power with financial elements of investment, value, policies, and risk. They highlighted that a powerful CEO is highly valuable for the above financial elements. Moreover, the CEO is assumed as the most powerful in developing countries such as Pakistan, where this position is mainly held by the family member [24]. The CEO is generally supposed to the most powerful member of the organization [25]. Most of the prior literature supported the role of the CEO for firm financial performance. Moreover, Daily and Johnson [25] also found that a powerful CEO not only works for the enhancement of profit, but also for the long-run survival of the organization. In addition, they have measured CEO power in four different ways and reported that a powerful CEO in all terms is valuable for the improvement of firm profit. Furthermore, Garcia-Sanchez, et al. [26] have investigated the connection of CEO power with integrated reporting. After applying logistic regression on 10,819 observations, they demonstrated that a powerful CEO is valuable for transparency, which leads to creation of firm value. In this aspect, Busco, et al. [27] also supported the role of a powerful CEO for information disclosure. Muttakin, et al. [28] concluded that CEO power is highly valuable for information disclosure, which leads to higher profit.

Besides, board composition is an imperative internal corporate governance factor for firm performance. Raheja and analysis [29] emphasized that board composition and size are functions of the firm major decisions making, and automatically affect the firm performance. Both of these factors of internal corporate governance have much importance for firm performance [30]. Previous scholars believe that expert and adept members on a board can play a vital role in the enhancement of firm performance [31]. Ansari, et al. [32] selected the Pakistani automobile sector to explore the link between firm performance and board size. Their results also suggested positive connections. A study conducted in Hong Kong reported that board independence plays a positive part in the improvement of profitability [33].

Thirdly, this study considers ownership structure as internal corporate governance, which includes ownership concentration and managerial ownership [24]. Generally, ownership structure involves policy-making for the improvement of industrial activities. The Pakistani markets are extremely concentrated owing to family ownership. Abbas, et al. [34] stated that ownership concentration in Pakistan has a significant role in enhancing firm performance. Besides, Yasser and Mamun [35] also inspected the connection between concentrated ownership and firm performance in Pakistan. They discovered a positive relationship. Similarly, multiple studies provided evidence of positivity about the association between firm performance and managerial ownership [24,36]. Kapopoulos and Lazaretou [37] stated that ownership structure is entirely important for the improvement of firm performance. Demsetz and economics [38] also supported the role of large shareholders in firm performance because large shareholders are always interested in the long-run profitability of the firm. Moreover, Raimo, et al. [39] suggested that integrated reporting is an interesting tool for firm short-, medium-, and long-run survival. Thus, after the probe of 152 international firms, they reported that institutional ownership is imperative for integrated reporting, while managerial ownership, state, and concentrated ownership are negatively linked with integrated reporting.

Fourthly, this study focus on auditing practices as an internal corporate governance factor. According to Waweru [40], the audit is an internal part of firm corporate governance. Furthermore, Masood, et al. [41] exposed that audit is an internal governance tool to improve and correct the firm financial affairs, which have huge importance for government and private industries. Matoke, et al. [42] probed the impact of audit quality on firm performance. They established that audit quality is helpful to improve firm performance. Besides, Al Ani, et al. [43] and Sattar, et al. [44] also supported the role of auditing practices for the improvement of firm performance. By following theoretical and empirical analysis, this study has developed various hypotheses:

Hypothesis 1: *Top executives have a positive association with firm performance.*

Hypothesis 2: *Board composition has a positive association with firm performance.*

Hypothesis 3: *Ownership structure has a positive association with firm performance.*

Hypothesis 4: *Audit quality has a positive association with firm performance.*

3.2. Corporate Social Responsibility (CSR) and Firm Performance

In recent years, there has been huge debate related to CSR owing to the higher demands from shareholders and communities. Shareholders and societies considered firms' irresponsible social actions as costly [45]. Moreover, the trust level between shareholders and management is poor in emerging markets; therefore, this external control can improve this trust level. This external verification control works as a strong external corporate governance mechanism [46]. There is mixed evidence available for the association between CSR and firm performance, as some studies reveal positive effects, some reveal negative effects, and some reveal no effect [47–49].

Such uncertain outcomes generate a research space, permitting various scholars to probe the actual and satisfying outcomes. There is a proper theoretical foundation available that suggests the importance of CSR for firm performance. Similarly, Oeyono, et al. [50] stated that firms, by having social activities, can satisfy communities and enhance the relationship with other stakeholders. Thus, CSR is assumed as a strong external corporate governance factor for firm performance. Furthermore, Aerts, et al. [51] also found that firms with CSR actions have better relations with their stakeholders, which lead to higher profit. Besides, multiple studies proved that CSR is a key factor to improve relations with societies and other stakeholders, which automatically lead to higher profitability [24].

Kong, et al. [52] have reviewed various past published research papers on corporate social responsibility and business outcomes. They finally concluded that corporate social practices are valuable for positive business outcomes. Naseem, et al. [53] also highlighted the corporate social practices for business performance in the context of Asia. Their outcomes show that business performance is enhanced when a firm participates in corporate social practices because it wins the shareholders' confidence. Hence, this study has developed the following hypothesis:

Hypothesis 5: *Corporate social responsibility (CSR) has a positive linkage with firm performance.*

3.3. The Moderating Role of CSR

This study used CSR as an imperative tool to control and monitor the internal corporate governance practices for the maximization of profit [9]. Internal corporate governance is always interested in investing in CSR actions for the improvement of firm reputation in the market [54]. Besides, they reported that a strong corporate governance mechanism can overcome the conflicts between agents and owners by using the actual meaning of CSR practices. Board monitoring is a beneficial tool to control and monitor corporate over-investing [55]. Moreover, stakeholder theory stated that a firm does not only have the sole purpose to earn a profit, but also to satisfy its shareholders [15]. Shareholders consider those firms that engage in social practices as more responsible. This practice enhances the long-term value of a firm.

Internal corporate governance always looking for means to enhance the firm profit and therefore they considered CSR to improve the firm image which automatically enhances the firm profit [56]. Besides, Khan, et al. [57] stated that the majority of the internal corporate governance elements are positively connected with CSR in an emerging economy. Jamali, et al. [58] reported that CSR serves as an important controlling mechanism to motivate the corporate governance factors for participation in social practices. Said, et al. [59] exposed that corporate governance as the audit committee and Government ownership has positive effects on the corporate social practices in Malaysia. Furthermore, Zhuang, et al. [60] highlighted that CSR practices automatically enhance the worth of board composition by disclosing the information about board members. Board size and independence significantly improve the CSR practices and firm performance [61].

Besides, Lone, et al. [62] proposed that corporate governance practices are entirely important for CSR activities in Pakistan. Moreover, internal corporate governance has impressive results related to CSR practices in Pakistan [63]. Majeed, et al. [64] investigated the internal corporate governance elements as, board member independence, the board size, ownership structure, and firm size related to the CSR activities in Pakistan. Their finding supported the role of internal corporate governance for CSR practices as having a positive relationship between them. Gul, et al. [65] also demonstrated that CSR practices play an imperative role to control and motivate the internal corporate governance elements. Corporate governance internal characteristics are very important for CSR practices in Pakistan and enhance shareholders' wealth [66]. Furthermore, Javeed and Lefen [24] found that CSR and firm performance have a positive connection in Pakistan. They majorly concluded that internal corporate governance as CEO power, concentrated and managerial ownership are the key factors to improve the corporate social practices which directly enhances firm profit as well.

Cong and Freedman [67] discovered that corporate governance has a positive connection with environmental disclosure practices. Besides, Li, et al. [68] explained that a powerful CEO is beneficial for environmental practices and firm profitability. They concluded that environmental disclosure is positively associated with the firm internal governance factor CEO. CEO considered social practices as an opportunity for earning management [69]. Kock, et al. [70] explained that environmental performance is entirely associated with internal corporate governance as, the board of directors, managerial incentives, auditor, and corporate control. Environmental regulations push corporate governance to perform social action for the sake of society in Pakistan [71]. Major element of corporate governance-CEO can improve firm sustainable and environmental practices.

Environmental regulations force the CEO to adopt environmental practices for the improvement of the firm image and which leads to higher profit [72]. Javeed and Lefen [24] concluded that corporate governance internal elements CEO, ownership concentration, and managerial ownership have an advantageous role in the implementation of corporate social practices in Pakistan. They further reported that these social practices are also valuable for firm performance. Corporate social activities are generally performed by good governance [73]. A better corporate governance system is always interested to perform environmental and social practices for the sake of a better image in the eyes of stakeholders which automatically enhances profitability [74].

On the other hand, various studies showed that board characteristics are also valuable for corporate environmental practices and disclosure [75,76]. Besides, Rabi [77] inspected the connection between board characteristics (board size, ownership, size) and environmental disclosure in Jordan. They found that all these board characteristics and environmental disclosure are positively linked. Moreover, Uwuigbe [78] highlighted that firms with managerial ownership are more willing to participate in social practices. Similarly, ownership concentration and board independence are important tools to enhance the firm disclosure practices which automatically forces firms to participate in social and environmental actions [79].

Ownership concentration have a positive association with social practices [80]. Besides, corporate social practices are very important for auditing because auditing reveals that what firms spending on environmental practices [81]. There is mixed literature available which supported that CSR serves as an external control for internal corporate governance for example CSR and CEO power, concentrated and managerial ownership [24], CSR and board independence, size [82,83], and CSR and audit quality [84]. This study has made the following hypothesis:

Hypothesis 6: *Corporate social responsibility (CSR) positively influences the association between internal corporate governance factors and firm performance.*

Here, internal corporate governance includes all factors such as CEO power, board members, board independence, managerial ownership, ownership concentration, and audit committee.

4. Research Approach

4.1. Description of the Sample

We employed secondary data (panel data) as choosing Pakistani firms. This article used various firms from various sub-sectors, for example, the textile sector which consists of weaving, woolen, spinning, and composite. Specifically, the chemical, cement, oil and gas exploration, fertilizer, pharmaceutical, oil and gas marketing, synthetic and rayon, refinery, engineering, automobile parts and accessories, automobile assembler, transport, glass and ceramics, cable and electrical goods, leather and tanneries, food and personal care products, technology and communication, paper and board, sugar and allied industries power generation and distribution have been used to complete this study.

These sectors include a total of 475 firms which covers 87% of the Pakistan Stock market. This study selected a sample on multiple objectives firstly firms that disclose social practices in annual reports are part of this probe. Secondly, firms with data missing or declared defaulter by the Pakistan Stock Exchange (PSX) are excluded from the sample [24,85]. Therefore, 136 defaulting and non-disclosed data firms dropped from the sample. Finally, this study used 339 firms for this probe. There are multiple sources used to gather the secondary data reported by [24,71] such as the State Bank of Pakistan (SBP), the Pakistan Stock Exchange (PSX), the SECP, sustainability, and annual reports of the firms for 2010–2019.

4.2. CSR and Corporate Governance Practices in Pakistan

The corporate governance connection with firm performance is extremely important for developing economies. Corporate governance plays an imperative role for firm performance which leads to the economic development of the states. The code of corporate governance in Pakistan was established in 2002, and this code extended with further important amendments in 2012 [86]. Therefore, the corporate governance idea in Pakistan has not long passed history because it was developed just one decade ago. Normally, firms of developing countries like Pakistan, India, and Bangladesh are not much involved in the improvement of corporate governance activities. These countries strictly bear economic problems, safety, and health issues at the workplace, low level of environmental and employee safety, violation of human rights in the form of child labor [24].

Moreover, Pakistan is a country that is suffering from various issues such as unbalanced political and economic conditions, health environment, moreover industrial and energy disasters, communal divergence, extensive corruption, and an inadequate controlling outline [71]. On a big platform, overall these issues have repercussions for the industries. Generally, Pakistan's industrial structure has the majority of family ownership. According to Cheema and Din [87], 60% of firms in Pakistan are controlled by family ownership, and only 40% are controlled by other ownership. In addition to this, according to Gamerschlag, et al. [88], corporate governance activities are not much developed in

Pakistan. Concerning this, the SECP is highly committed to implement better corporate governance and social practices for improved performance [89]. There is a lack of work for corporate governance and its other factors in developing countries [90]. Researchers believed that better corporate governance is an alternative model to improve the firm performance and economic conditions of the country. Pakistan Stock Exchange is an emerging market [91].

Despite facing all these issues, Pakistan is a law-abiding country that sturdily focuses on the protection and safety of shareholders the development of the stock market [71]. Pakistan has important capital and financial market have numerous social and political practices as a comparison to other developed economies [92]. Additionally, the world is facing global warming threats and scholars believed that the industrial sector is the major cause of environmental problems [93]. Therefore, this study presents corporate social responsibility's importance in corporate governance for improving profitability and reducing environmental problems. Focusing on the above circumstance, there is an intense need to explore corporate governance and social activities in Pakistan.

4.3. Variable Measurement

Table 1 reveals the measurements of the variables.

Table 1. Variables' construction.

Dependent Variables	Abbreviations	Measures
Economic Value Added	EVA	Net operational profit after tax minus cost of capital into the capital invested [94].
Sustainable Growth Rate	SGR	$PM \times (1 - D) \times (1 + L)/(T - (PM \times (1 - D) \times (1 + L)))$ [1] [24].
Independent Variables		
Chief Executive Officer Power	CEO Power	CEO annual compensations/ Whole board of directors compensations [68].
Board Independence	BI	Independent directors on board/Total number of board of directors on board [95].
Board Size	BS	The total member of board members on the board [96].
Ownership Concentration	OC	The major shareholding portion or Top 5 shareholders [24].
Managerial Ownership	MO	The portion of shares held by the management [24].
Audit Quality	AQ	The statutory audit fees to the number of sales [97].
Corporate Social Responsibility	CSR	The addition of Earning Per Share (EPS), total taxes, staff salaries, interests, and public expenses minus social cost divided by total equity [24].
Control Variables		
Property, Plant, and Equipment	PPE	The ratio of property, plant, and equipment to total sales [71].
Firm Size	LNTA	The natural log of total assets [71].
Asset turnover	ATO	The ratio of total sales to total asset [71].
Environmental Awareness	EA	The ratio of an average green investment divided by No. of employees [71].

[1] PM shows profit margin (existing and target), D indicates dividend payout ratio, L indicates target total debt to total equity ratio, and T indicates ratio of total assets to sales.

4.4. Analysis Techniques

4.4.1. Panel Data Issues

Prior studies revealed that panel data normally carries endogeneity issues. While using panel data for empirical evaluation, the endogeneity issue normally occurs because error terms correlate with explanatory variables, which produces unreliable and biased outcomes [71]. Similarly, econometrics exposed that endogeneity issues happen with the connection between error term and explanatory variables. Nonetheless, these issues available for every field like economics, finance, etc. For example, endogeneity issue highlighted in few prior studies about corporate governance [95], compensation of executives [98], board composition and managerial ownership [99,100], firm control [101], and financial and investment policies [102]. However, most researchers have not mentioned the endogeneity concerns in their studies as Antonakis, et al. [103] and Hamilton and Nickerson [104] exposed that 90 percent of published articles did not highlight the endogeneity concern.

Besides, panel data also carries heteroskedasticity issue, which normally occurs when the variables' standard errors have observation over a particular amount of time, which is not constant [105]. Heteroskedasticity generally occurs in two circumstances, conditional and unconditional situations. The conditional situation is explained as the variable volatility available which leads to the future time of low and high volatility which cannot be recognized. Unconditional situation refers to a position where the future time of low and high volatility can be recognized.

4.4.2. Solution for Panel Data Issues

Moreover, Li [106] presented numerous procedures to overcome the endogeneity issues from panel data. For example, the third-factor effect, instrumental variable method, and the lagged dependent variable can overcome endogeneity such as the effect of control variables. But, his findings highly suggested the use of the GMM model for covering endogeneity. Additionally, the fixed-effect model is considered the best approach for the unobservable time-invariant. After the evaluation of all methods majority of the scholars reported that 2SLS and GMM methods are the most impressive and significant approaches to deal with and control the endogeneity from panel data [68,106–111].

This study used firm-level panel data, therefore, it is a need to control the heteroskedasticity and autocorrelation problem. According to Wooldridge [112] and Baltagi [113] firstly conducted the test for serial autocorrelation between the residuals over the specified period with the use of the FGLS model. Moreover, they suggested that the FGLS model can robust the autocorrelation to evaluate the parameter in the equation. Greene [114] exposed that the FGLS model is best to reduce the possible heteroskedasticity from the panel and cross-sectional data. Furthermore, multiple studies recommended that autocorrelation and heteroskedasticity problems can be overcome with the use of FGLS [113,115–117].

4.5. Empirical Estimation Procedure

Generally, OLS regression is a valuable technique to find the relationship between dependent and independent variables. Thus, we firstly employed OLS regression for each equation to identify the endogeneity by using the Durbin-Wu-Hausman experiment [111,118,119]. Secondly, a fixed-effect model has been employed to cover the inaudible heterogeneity based on the Hausman test [111,119]. The Hausman results permitted us to employ a fixed-effect model instead of a random effect model.

Thirdly, for more accuracy, this study has been used the generalized method of moments (GMM) for solving the endogeneity issues. Prior researchers strongly believed that the use of GMM is the most suitable approach for correcting endogeneity compared to other methods [71,109,110]. Finally, this study employed the FGLS model as a robustness test based on the Hausman test to investigate, the heteroscedasticity and autocorrelation from panel data [113,115–117].

4.5.1. Model Construction

ICG and Firm Performance

Various scholars have developed the econometric equation for the investigation of internal corporate governance association with firm performance [120–123]. Similarly, we have developed the following equation for internal corporate governance and firm performance.

$$Y_{i,t} = \alpha_1 + \beta_1 X_{1i,t} + \beta_2 X_{2i,t} + \beta_3 X_{3i,t} + \beta_4 X_{4i,t} + \beta_5 X_{5i,t} + \beta_6 X_{6i,t} + \gamma_1 Z_{i,t} + \mu_{i,t} \quad (1)$$

In the Equation (1), $Y_{i,t}$: the firm performance (EVA, SGR) of firms i at year t, creating two sub equations for each index; chief executive officer (CEO) power; $X_{1i,t}$: board independence (BI); $X_{2i,t}$: board size (BS); $X_{3i,t}$ managerial ownership (MO); $X_{4i,t}$: ownership concentration (OC); $X_{5i,t}$: audit quality (AQ); $X_{6i,t}$: control variables of firm i at year t; $\mu_{i,t}$: error term; α_n: constant term, $n = 1$; β_m, γ_n: coefficients to be estimated; $m = 1, 2, 3, 4, 5, 6$.

CSR and Firm Performance

Multiple researchers have formed the econometric equation for the evaluation between corporate social responsibility and firm performance, such as [124,125]. Therefore, we have developed the following econometric equation:

$$Y_{i,t} = \alpha_1 + \beta_1 X_{1i,t} + \gamma_1 Z_{i,t} + \mu_{i,t} \quad (2)$$

In the Equation (2), $Y_{i,t}$: the firm performance (EVA, SGR) of firms i at year t, creating two sub equations for each index; $X_{1i,t}$: corporate social responsibility (CSR): control variables of firm i at year t; $\mu_{i,t}$: error term; α_n: constant term, n = 1; β_m, γ_n: coefficients to be estimated; m = 1.

The Moderating Role of CSR

This study used various internal corporate governance factors. To find the relationship between internal corporate governance and firm performance, this study applies corporate social responsibility as a moderating factor. Therefore, this study developed the following equation:

$$Y_{i,t} = \alpha_1 + \beta_1 X_{1i,t} + \beta_2 X_{2i,t} + \beta_3 X_{1i,t} \times X_{2i,t} + \gamma_1 Z_{i,t} + \mu_{i,t} \quad (3)$$

In the Equation (3), $Y_{i,t}$: the firm performance (EVA, SGR) of firms i at year t, creating two sub equations for each index; $X_{1i,t}$: internal corporate governance (ICG_{af}); $X_{2i,t}$: corporate social responsibility (CSR); $X_{1i,t} \times X_{2i,t}$: the interaction between internal corporate governance factors and CSR of firm i at year t; $Z_{i,t}$; control variables of firm i at year t; $\mu_{i,t}$: error term; α_n: constant term, n = 1; β_m, γ_n: coefficients to be estimated; m = 1, 2, 3. In this equation, internal corporate governance (ICG_{af}) represents all internal factors such as CEO power, board independence, board size, managerial ownership, ownership concentration, and audit quality.

5. Results and Discussion

5.1. Results

This study conducted descriptive statistics and correlation tests before testing the hypothesis. Table 2 reveals the mean and standard deviation of all independent and dependent variables. A total of 3950 observations were used for 10 years' firm-level data. Moreover, Table 2 also shows the correlations of all variables.

Afterwards, this study conducted an endogeneity test because panel data has been used to probe the connection between internal corporate governance and firm performance with the moderating role of CSR. Thus, panel data normally caries endogeneity issues for empirical studies [71,126]. Therefore, we applied OLS regression to conduct the test for the detection of endogeneity in our panel data.

The use of OLS regression normally occurred to find the upshot of independent variables on the dependent variables. Our main equations have two dependent variables such as EVA, and SGR, but we used each independent variables (CEO POWER, BS, BI, OC, MO, AQ, and CSR) as dependent variable one by one to find the endogeneity bias (Beiner et al. (2006); Schultz et al. (2010); and Wintoki et al. (2012)).

Table 2. Variables' construction.

Variables	M	SD	1	2	3	4	5	6	7	8	9	10	11	12	13
1. EVA	0.27	0.5	1												
2. SGR	0.68	0.13	1.00 ***	1											
3. CEO POWER	3.38	4.21	0.78 ***	0.79 ***	1										
4. BI	2.43	5.01	0.98 ***	0.98 ***	0.77 ***	1									
5. BS	0.2	0.37	0.52 ***	0.53 ***	0.71 ***	0.50 ***	1								
6. MO	5.36	3.54	0.45 ***	0.44 ***	0.33 ***	0.47 ***	0.28 ***	1							
7. OC	1.24	1.64	0.73 ***	0.74 ***	0.92 ***	0.70 ***	0.66 ***	0.25 ***	1						
8. AQ	0.92	1.72	0.99 ***	0.97 ***	0.79 ***	0.99 ***	0.53 ***	0.46 ***	0.73 ***	1					
9. CSR	0.97	1.36	0.74 ***	0.73 ***	0.92 ***	0.72 ***	0.68 ***	0.30 ***	0.86 ***	0.73 ***	1				
10. ATO	−0.71	0.59	−0.44 ***	−0.63 ***	−0.32 ***	−0.46 ***	−0.17 ***	−0.43 ***	−0.27 ***	−0.47 ***	−0.20 ***	1			
11. EA	0.29	0.4	0.06 ***	0.02 ***	0.29 ***	0.09 ***	0.24 ***	0.42 ***	0.21 ***	0.07 ***	0.21 ***	−0.25 ***	1		
12. LNTA	0.11	0.13	0.25 ***	0.24 ***	0.29 ***	0.28 ***	0.22 ***	0.66 ***	0.24 ***	0.26 ***	0.18 ***	−0.49 ***	0.72 ***	1	
13. PPE	1.77	4.18	0.76 ***	0.75 ***	0.86 ***	0.79 ***	0.62 ***	0.53 ***	0.74 ***	0.78 ***	0.76 ***	−0.47 ***	0.45 ***	0.51 ***	1

Significance level *** $p < 0.01$.

The Durbin–Wu–Hausman test is conducted using OLS regression and the results are explained in the Table 3. The significant values of F statistics reveal that our independent variables are endogenous. Furthermore, these results show that there is a correlation between residuals and independent variables. Thus, if there are endogenous variables in the model then there is a need to employ an appropriate techniques to cover the endogeneity issues [120]. Table 3 presents the endogeneity test for internal corporate governance variables.

Table 3. Endogeneity test.

Independent Variables	Model 1	Model 2	Model 3	Model 4	Model 5	Model 6	Model 7
CEO POWER	0.625 ***						
BI		1.288 ***					
BS			2.862 ***				
MO				0.051 **			
OC					0.261 ***		
AQ						1.423 **	
CSR							2.635 **
ATO							
EA							
LNTA							
PPE	10.827 **	6.429 ***	12.651 ***	7.956 **	13.733 **	9.617 ***	11.388 **
Constant	0.698 **	2.577 ***	0.737 ***	0.764 ***	1.492 **	0.468 ***	2.815 **
R^2	0.8741	0.9216	0.8563	0.7889	0.9350	0.8819	0.8931
Durbin–Wu–Hausman	25.78 ***	31.57 ***	27.41 ***	28.74 ***	36.65 ***	33.44 ***	32.94 ***

Significance levels *** $p < 0.01$, ** $p < 0.05$.

Finally, Table 4 shows the outcomes of the link between all internal corporate governance variables and firm performance. For instance, model 1 highlights the results of all internal corporate governance variables CEO POWER, BI, BS, MO, OC, and AQ with EVA using FE (β = 0.004, p = 0.01, β = 0.015, p = 0.01, β = 0.008, p = 0.01, β = 0.006, p = 0.01, β = 0.012, p = 0.01, β = 0.240, p = 0.01). Model 2 highlights the results of all internal corporate governance variables CEO POWER, BI, BS, MO, OC, and AQ with EVA using GMM (β = 0.005, p = 0.01, β = 0.018, p = 0.01, β = 0.004, p = 0.01 β = 0.005, p = 0.01 β = 0.009, p = 0.01, β = 0.237, p = 0.01). The Hausman test value supported the employment of fixed effect model, as (β = 58.56, p = 0.01).

Table 4. Results on ICG and FP.

Dependent Variables	Model 1		Model 2	
	EVA		SGR	
Independent Variables	FE	GMM	FE	GMM
CEO POWER	0.004 ***	0.005 ***	0.001 ***	0.011 ***
BI	0.015 ***	0.018 ***	0.003 ***	0.004 ***
BS	0.008 ***	0.004 **	0.002 ***	0.001 **
MO	0.006 ***	0.005 ***	0.001 ***	0.002 ***
OC	0.012 ***	0.009 ***	0.003 ***	0.003 ***
AQ	0.240 ***	0.237 ***	0.060 ***	0.059 ***
ATO	−0.004 ***	−0.005 **	−0.001	−0.002 **
EA	−0.007	−0.003	−0.015	−0.008
LNTA	−0.004	0.006	−0.002	−0.001
PPE	0.009 ***	−0.010 ***	−0.002 ***	−0.003 ***
Constant	−0.033 ***	−0.025 ***	−0.008 ***	−0.006 ***
R^2	0.9920		0.9921	
F	31.54 ***		31.54 ***	
N	3686	2891	3686	2891
Hausman Test	58.86 ***		56.87 ***	
Wald Chi^2		381,653.42 ***		382,654.44 ***

Significance levels *** $p < 0.01$, ** $p < 0.05$.

Furthermore, Table 4 explains model 2, which reveals the outcomes of all internal corporate governance variables CEO POWER, BI, BS, MO, OC, and AQ with SGR using FE such as (β = 0.001, p = 0.01, β = 0.003, p = 0.01, β = 0.002, p = 0.01, β = 0.001, p = 0.01, β = 0.003, p = 0.01, β = 0.060, p = 0.01). Model 4 reveals the outcomes of all internal corporate governance variables CEO POWER, BI, BS, MO, OC, and AQ with SGR using GMM such as (β = 0.011, p = 0.01, β = 0.004, p = 0.01, β = 0.001, p = 0.01, β = 0.002, p = 0.01, β = 0.003, p = 0.01, β = 0.059, p = 0.01). Similarly, the Hausman test value also supported the employment of fixed effect model as (β = 56.87, p = 0.01). Hence, our results proved that all internal corporate governance variables are positively linked with firm performance.

Moreover, Table 5 displays the outcomes of the link between all CSR variables and firm performance. Model 3 reveals the outcomes of CSR with EVA using FE and GMM, respectively, such as (β = 0.155, p = 0.01 and β = 0.144, p = 0.01). The Hausman test value confirmed the employment of the fixed-effect model as (β = 83.86, p = 0.01). Model 4 highlights the outcomes of CSR with SGR using FE and GMM, respectively, such as (β = 0.038, p = 0.01 and β = 0.035, p = 0.01). Likewise, the Hausman test value confirmed the employment of the fixed-effect model as (β = 13.54, p = 0.01). Our results stated that CSR and firm performance are positively linked.

Table 5. Results on CSR and FP.

Dependent Variables	Model 3		Model 4	
Independent Variables	EVA		SGR	
	FE	GMM	FE	GMM
CSR	0.155 ***	0.144 ***	0.038 ***	0.035 ***
ATO	0.011	−0.009	0.002	−0.003
EA	−0.840 ***	−1.092 ***	−0.209 ***	−0.272 ***
LNTA	0.749 ***	0.655 ***	0.188 ***	0.164 ***
PPE	0.052 ***	0.054 ***	0.012 ***	0.013 ***
Constant	0.126 ***	0.229 ***	0.051 ***	0.058 ***
R^2	0.6355		0.6412	
F	13.42 ***		13.54 ***	
N	3686	2891	3686	2891
Hausman Test	83.86 ***		84.85 ***	
Wald Chi^2		4657.13 ***		4655.14 ***

Significance levels *** $p < 0.01$.

Lastly, Table 6 shows the results of the moderating role of CSR on the link between internal corporate governance variables and firm performance. Model 5 reveals the outcomes of all internal corporate governance variables with the interaction of CSR such as CEOPOWER × CSR, BI × CSR, BS × CSR, MO × CSR, OC × CSR, and AQ × CSR with EVA using FE such as (β = 0.001, p = 0.01, β = 0.471, p = 0.01, β = 0.856, p = 0.01, β = 2.153, p = 0.01, β = 1.935, p = 0.01, β = 10.88, p = 0.01). Model 5 also reveals the outcomes of all internal corporate governance variables with the interaction of CSR such as CEOPOWER × CSR, BI × CSR, BS × CSR, MO × CSR, OC × CSR, and AQ × CSR with EVA using GMM such as (β = 0.002, p = 0.01, β = 0.524, p = 0.01, β = 0.875, p = 0.01, β = 1.976, p = 0.01, β = 1.760, p = 0.01, β = 11.87, p = 0.01). The Hausman test value allowed to use of fixed effect model as (β = 44.03, p = 0.01). In addition, model 6 reveals the outcomes of all internal corporate governance variables with the interaction of CSR such as CEOPOWER × CSR, BI × CSR, BS × CSR, MO × CSR, OC × CSR, and AQ × CSR with SGR using FE such as (β = 0.009, p = 0.01, β = 0.117, p = 0.01, β = 0.214, p = 0.01, β = 0.538, p = 0.01, β = 0.483, p = 0.01, β = 2.722, p = 0.01). Model 6 also reveals the outcomes of all internal corporate governance variables with the interaction of CSR such as CEOPOWER × CSR, BI × CSR, BS × CSR, MO × CSR, OC × CSR, and AQ × CSR with SGR using GMM such as (β = 0.002, p = 0.01, β = 0.131, p = 0.01, β = 0.218, p = 0.01, β = 0.494, p = 0.01, β = 0.440, p = 0.01, β= 2.968, p = 0.01). Likewise, the Hausman test value allowed to use of fixed effect model as (β = 45.44, p = 0.01). Finally, our results supported our hypothesis, which reveals that all internal corporate governance variables are positively linked with firm performance with the moderating role of CSR.

5.2. Additional Test

This study applied the fixed feasible generalized least square (FGLS) as an additional test for further robustness of the results. Table 7 reveals the results of ICG association with FP, CSR with FP, and the association between ICG and FP with the moderating role of CSR as a robustness test. These robustness results with the FGLS model confirmed the results of the previous models. Furthermore, these robustness results support the previous findings.

Table 6. Results of the impact of ICG on FP with the moderating role of CSR.

Dependent Variables	Model 5		Model 6	
Independent Variables	EVA		SGR	
	FE	GMM	FE	GMM
CEO POWER	0.002 ***	0.003 ***	0.006 ***	0.007 ***
BI	−0.008 ***	−0.007 ***	−0.002 ***	−0.003 ***
BS	0.004	0.005 **	0.001	0.004
MO	0.005 ***	0.004 ***	0.002 ***	0.001 ***
OC	0.008 ***	0.008 ***	0.001 ***	0.002 ***
AQ	0.050 ***	0.052 ***	0.012 ***	0.013 ***
CSR	−0.006 ***	−0.007 ***	−0.001 ***	−0.001 ***
CEO POWER × CSR	0.001 ***	0.002 **	0.009 ***	0.002 ***
BI × CSR	0.471 ***	0.524 ***	0.117 ***	0.131 ***
BS × CSR	0.856 ***	0.875 ***	0.214 ***	0.218 ***
MO × CSR	2.153 ***	1.976 ***	0.538 ***	0.494 ***
OC × CSR	1.935 ***	1.760 ***	0.483 ***	0.440 ***
AQ × CSR	10.88 ***	11.87 ***	2.722 ***	2.968 ***
ATO	−0.001	−0.003	-0.004	−0.007
EA	−0.002	−0.002 *	−0.006 ***	−0.009 ***
LNTA	−0.006 ***	−0.007 **	−0.001 **	−0.007 **
PPE	−0.001 ***	−0.001 ***	−0.003 ***	−0.004 ***
Constant	−0.008 **	−0.005	−0.002	−0.002
R^2	0.9999		0.9998	
F	25.38 ***		26.37 ***	
N	3686	2891	3686	2891
Hausman Test	44.03 ***		45.44 ***	
Wald Chi^2		29,303.31 ***		35,768.19 ***

Significance levels *** $p < 0.01$, ** $p < 0.05$, * $p < 0.10$.

5.3. Discussion

The results of relationship between ICG (CEO POWER, BI, BS, MO, OC, and AQ) and firm performance (EVA and SGR) showed various outcomes after employing fixed effect, GMM, and FGLS models. Firstly, our results confirmed that a powerful CEO in the term of compensations have a significant and positive role for firm performance. Javeed and Lefen [24] also supported that a powerful CEO is highly beneficial for firm performance in Pakistan. Various other studies also confirmed these results [121–123]. Theoretically, the organizational and management theory provided evidence for the positive relationship between CEO Power and firm performance [124].

Secondly, our findings exposed that BI and BS have a positive linkage with internal and external firm performance measures. The board structure has a significant role in firm performance in Pakistan [120]. Multiple scholars supported this evidence [127,128]. Independent board can make decisions for good governance without the pressure of owners which leads to higher profitability. Besides, various previous studies provided evidence to support the connection of BS and firm performance [129–132]. Pearce and Zahra [133] exposed that adept members on the board are imperative for firm performance. In addition to this, agency theory supported this positive connection, because agency cost can be reduced with expert board members [14].

Table 7. Robustness results of ICG and FP, CSR and FP, and ICG and FP with the moderating role of CSR.

Dependent Variables	Model 1	Model 2	Model 3	Model 4	Model 5	Model 6
Independent Variables	EVA	SGR	EVA	SGR	EVA	SGR
	FGLS	FGLS	FGLS	FGLS	FGLS	FGLS
CEO POWER	0.009 ***	0.002 ***			0.003 ***	0.008 ***
BI	0.007 ***	0.001 ***			−0.006 ***	−0.001 ***
BS	0.003 ***	0.002 ***			0.001	0.002
MO	0.002 **	0.0001 **			0.002 ***	0.004 ***
OC	0.001 ***	0.004 ***			−0.003 **	−0.005 **
AQ	0.264 ***	0.066 ***			0.036 ***	0.009 ***
CSR			0.141 ***	0.035 ***	−0.001 ***	−0.001 ***
CEO POWER × CSR					0.003 ***	0.004 ***
BI × CSR					0.304 ***	0.076 ***
BS × CSR					0.626 ***	0.156 ***
MO × CSR					2.761 ***	0.691 ***
OC × CSR					3.148 ***	0.787 ***
AQ × CSR					9.272 ***	2.318 ***
ATO	−0.002 ***	0.001 ***	−0.072 ***	−0.018 ***	−0.001 ***	−0.001 ***
EA	−0.005 ***	−0.012 ***	−0.356 ***	−0.090 ***	0.006 ***	0.002 ***
LNTA	−0.027 ***	0.006 ***	0.314 ***	0.078 ***	0.005 ***	−0.005 ***
PPE	0.011 ***	−0.002 ***	0.070 ***	0.017 ***	−0.001 ***	0.004 ***
Constant	−0.001 ***	−0.003 ***	0.025 ***	0.006 ***	−0.009 ***	−0.002 ***
N	3686	3686	3686	3686	3686	3686
Wald Chi^2	972,427 ***	98,403.85 ***	52,988.46 ***	21,598.47 ***	63,849.06 ***	224,869.16 ***

Significance levels *** $p < 0.01$, ** $p < 0.05$.

Thirdly, our results presented that MO and OC are positively linked with internal and external firm performance. To support these outcomes, Javeed and Lefen [24] discovered that ownership structure and firm performance in the Pakistani market have a positive connection. Additionally, these findings are similar to many previous scholars such as [133–135]. Kim, et al. [136] found that MO is an imperative means for improving firm performance in developing countries. In addition to this, to support the association between OC and firm performance different researchers provided evidence [137–139]. Furthermore, agency theory also supported that ownership structure can minimize the agency cost which may gain higher profit [14]. Pakistani market has higher family ownership and therefore managers and other shareholder's involvement in the ownership may reduce agency conflict. These practices enhance international shareholder's confidence as well.

Fourthly, the findings of this study reported that AQ and firm performance have a positive connection. In this context, Sattar, Javeed and Latief [44] discovered that the quality of audit is highly beneficial for firm performance in Pakistan. Bonazzi and Islam [140] discovered that agency cost can be minimized by appointing a quality auditor, which highlights every financial and non-financial aspect of a firm clearly and truly. Multiple researchers provided evidence to support these results [141,142]. Seventhly, our outcomes reported that firm performance and dividend payment have a positive association. In this support, Farrukh, et al. [143] found a positive linkage between dividend policy and firm performance in Pakistan. Various studies suggested the positive connection between dividend payment and firm performance [144,145].

On the other side, our results discovered that corporate social responsibility and firm performance are positively linked. For the Pakistani market, Javeed and Lefen [24] supported the role of CSR for firm performance. Furthermore, multiple scholars have provided evidence for the positive association between CSR and firm performance [48,144]. Stakeholder theory supported these results as CSR is an imperative means to improve shareholder wealth and motivate more stakeholders for social actions [15].

Most importantly, the results of our study confirmed that all internal corporate governance factors (CEO POWER, BI, BS, MO, OC, AQ) have positive effects on firm performance with the moderating role of CSR. CSR is a valuable tool that controls, monitors, and publishes internal corporate governance activities [9]. Reputation is a major thing for the long-run survival of the firms, therefore, internal corporate governance factors focus on the social activities for the improvement of the firm image in the market [54]. Theoretically, stakeholder theory supports these findings as the internal corporate governance uses effective ways for saving the interest of the firm stakeholders with the help of CSR [9,19]. CSR put pressure on the firm internal corporate governance to work for firm performance and firm positive image in the market. Pakistani market already has a lack of trust of stakeholders, therefore, CSR serves as a strong tool to boost the relationship between corporate governance and shareholders.

6. Conclusions

Corporate social responsibility has great importance for the industrial sector and it may control the industrial negative environmental impacts. Therefore, the object of this study is to evaluate the relationship between internal corporate governance and firm performance. Before this study, no study has used all of these internal corporate governance factors together. Secondly, this study examines the role of corporate social responsibility for firm performance. Importantly, we used corporate social responsibility as a moderating factor to find out the reason for the positive, negative, or insignificant relationship between internal corporate governance factors and firm performance. For this investigation, this study selected 339 Pakistani firms from 2010 to 2019, which covers 10 years, and developed 3950 observations. Multiple sources have been used to collect the data such as the Pakistan Stock Exchange (PSX), the State Bank of Pakistan (SBP), the Securities and Exchange Commission of Pakistan (SECP), sustainability reports, and the companies' annual reports from their respective websites. This study applied various statistical techniques, such as OLS, FE, 2SLS, GMM, and FGLS, and concluded various outcomes.

The empirical results demonstrated that firm performance can be enhanced with a powerful CEO. Moreover, board independence has a significant and positive association with firm performance. Board size has a significant and positive influence on firm performance. Besides, managerial ownership and firm performance also presented significant and positive relationships with each other. Furthermore, ownership concentration and firm performance have also significant and positive connections. Furthermore, this study's results revealed that audit quality and firm performance have a significant and positive relationship. Besides, our findings discovered that CSR have a positive and significant relationship with firm performance.

Imperatively, this study applied corporate social responsibility as a moderating factor to inspect the association between internal corporate governance and firm performance. Our findings revealed that all internal corporate governance factors such as CEO power, BI, BS, OC, MO, and AQ positively influence firm performance with the moderating role of corporate social responsibility. Based on these results, we can suggest that the moderating role of corporate social responsibility plays an important role in the positive relationship between internal corporate governance and firm performance.

6.1. Policy Implications

In light of these outcomes, this study has numerous suggestions and policy implications for policymakers, owners, investors, shareholders, and governments of both developing and developed economies to improve corporate governance and social activities. The following are important implications of this study: First, firms should abide by the guidance of regulatory bodies for the improvement of corporate governance and social practices. Second, firms should identify and implement the proper actors of corporate governance for the improvement of firm performance. Third, the corporate governance main bodies such as CEOs, board members, and ownership structure have a superior role to follow and implement the corporate governance activities. While making corporate strategies, the present study sheds light on the important role of the executives, managers, ownership structure, regulatory bodies, and corporate social aspects to execute the strategies for the sake of shareholders' interests. Furthermore, managers are warned of the reality that their actions are being watched and supervised by the top executives and committees, thus they are accountable for their activities.

Fourth, firms should also focus on corporate social responsibility for the improvement of firm performance and internal corporate governance practices. Fifth, the Government of Pakistan (GOP) should formulate strict regulations of corporate social practices that monitor the actions of internal corporate governance. This study suggests that Pakistani regulatory bodies, for focusing on corporate social responsibility, should control the internal corporate governance in the firms where family ownership and unstable political conditions exist. Sixth, the GOP should present awards and benefits to those firms that are properly publishing information about corporate governance and social practices. Importantly, the whole world is suffering from environmental issues that lead to global warming, and researchers believe that industrial sectors are major sources of those environmental problems. Thus, governments and regulatory authorities should focus on corporate social responsibility for firms, which may reduce those industrial negative impacts on the environment. Thus, the findings of this study are helpful for governments and policymakers to form stringent regulations that can ultimately improve the performance of industrial sectors. Firms of developing countries are the major source of environmental problems; thus, this study proposes that proper implementation of corporate social practices may reduce these problems.

6.2. Limitation and Future Research Directions

This study is limited to a single country for the investigation of the association between corporate governance and firm performance. Moreover, this study used data for 10 years because of data availability; therefore, this study period could be extended for future research. Because of data constraints, this study used few variables for internal and external firm performance. Additionally, the role of women is highly important for organizational performance and it is also the main agenda of corporate social aspects [146]. Therefore, the role of women on board is being enhanced for the improvement of profitability and firm social practices. Even, the United Nations (UN) 2030 plan also focuses on the role of women on board and firm top management [147].

Furthermore, for future research, this study can be extended by focusing on the role of women on the board and other corporate governance variables. Financing configuration and organization structure can be considered in future research. Besides, these governance variables can be used as a moderator in the future to prove their impact on firm performance. A study on corporate governance practices in multiple countries can also be conducted in the future.

Author Contributions: Conceptualization, Writing—Original Draft Preparation, J.L. and S.A.J.; Methodology, Writing—Review and Editing, R.L.; Supervision, T.J.; Formal Analysis, T.S.O. All authors have read and agreed to the published version of the manuscript.

Funding: This research is funded by Hangzhou College of Commerce, Zhejiang Gongshang University, Hangzhou, China.

Institutional Review Board Statement: Not applicable.

Informed Consent Statement: Not applicable.

Data Availability Statement: Not applicable.

Acknowledgments: The authors would like to acknowledge the comments and suggestions given by anonymous reviewers that have significantly improved the quality of our work.

Conflicts of Interest: The authors declare no conflict of interest.

References

1. Liao, Z. Market orientation and FIRMS' environmental innovation: The moderating role of environmental attitude. *Bus. Strat. Environ.* **2018**, *27*, 117–127. [CrossRef]
2. Song, M.; Zhang, L.; An, Q.; Wang, Z.; Li, Z. Statistical analysis and combination forecasting of environmental efficiency and its influential factors since China entered the WTO: 2002–2010–2012. *J. Clean. Prod.* **2013**, *42*, 42–51. [CrossRef]
3. Adnan, S.M.; Hay, D.; van Staden, C.J. The influence of culture and corporate governance on corporate social responsibility disclosure: A cross country analysis. *J. Clean. Prod.* **2018**, *198*, 820–832. [CrossRef]
4. Contrafatto, M.; Ferguson, J.; Power, D.; Stevenson, L.; Collison, D. Understanding power-related strategies and initiatives. *Account. Audit. Acc. J.* **2019**, *33*, 559–587. [CrossRef]
5. Bhagat, S.; Bolton, B. Corporate governance and firm performance. *Sequel* **2019**, *58*, 142–168.
6. Bhatt, P.R.; Bhatt, R.R. Corporate governance and firm performance in Malaysia. *Corp. Gov. Int. J. Bus. Soc.* **2017**, *17*, 896–912. [CrossRef]

7. Hutchinson, M.; Gul, F.A. Investment opportunity set, corporate governance practices and firm performance. *J. Corp. Financ.* **2004**, *10*, 595–614. [CrossRef]
8. Prevost, A.K.; Rao, R.P.; Hossain, M. Determinants of board composition in New Zealand: A simultaneous equations approach. *J. Empir. Financ.* **2002**, *9*, 373–397. [CrossRef]
9. Jo, H.; Harjoto, M.A. Corporate Governance and Firm Value: The Impact of Corporate Social Responsibility. *J. Bus. Ethic.* **2011**, *103*, 351–383. [CrossRef]
10. Wu, S.; Quan, X.; Xu, L. CEO power, disclosure quality and the variability of firm performance. *Nankai Bus. Rev. Int.* **2011**, *2*, 79–97. [CrossRef]
11. Bolourian, S.; Angus, A.; Alinaghian, L. The impact of corporate governance on corporate social responsibility at the board-level: A critical assessment. *J. Clean. Prod.* **2021**, *291*, 125752. [CrossRef]
12. SECP. *Rules and Regulations for Firms*; Pakistan Stock Exchange: Islamabad, Pakistan, 2017.
13. Sah, R.K.; Stiglitz, J. The Architecture of Economic Systems: Hierarchies and Polyarchies. *Archit. Econ. Syst. Hierarchies Polyarchies* **1984**, 716–727. [CrossRef]
14. Jensen, M.C.; Meckling, W.H. Theory of the firm: Managerial behavior, agency costs and ownership structure. *J. Financ. Econ.* **1976**, *3*, 305–360. [CrossRef]
15. Freeman, R. *Strategic Management: A Stakeholder Perspective*; Pitman: Boston, MA, USA, 1984.
16. Wiseman, R.M.; Cuevas-Rodríguez, G.; Gomez-Mejia, L.R. Towards a social theory of agency. *J. Manag. Stud.* **2012**, *49*, 202–222. [CrossRef]
17. Hill, C.W.; Jones, T.M. Stakeholder-agency theory. *J. Manag. Stud.* **1992**, *29*, 131–154. [CrossRef]
18. Jizi, M.; Nehme, R. Board monitoring and audit fees: The moderating role of CEO/chair dual roles. *Manag. Audit. J.* **2018**, *33*, 217–243. [CrossRef]
19. Calton, J.M.; Payne, S.L. Coping with paradox: Multistakeholder learning dialogue as a pluralist sensemaking process for addressing messy problems. *Bus. Soc.* **2003**, *42*, 7–42. [CrossRef]
20. Brown, J.A.; Forster, W.R. CSR and stakeholder theory. *Tale Adam Smith* **2013**, *112*, 301–312.
21. Berger, R.; Dutta, S.; Raffel, T.; Samuels, G. *Innovating at the Top: How Global CEOs Drive Innovation for Growth and Profit*; Springer: Berlin/Heidelberg, Germany, 2008.
22. Papadakis, V.M. Do CEOs shape the process of making strategic decisions? Evidence from Greece. *Manag. Decis.* **2006**, *44*, 367–394. [CrossRef]
23. Coles, J.L.; Li, Z.; Wang, A.Y. Industry tournament incentives. *Rev. Financ. Stud.* **2017**, *31*, 1418–1459. [CrossRef]
24. Javeed, S.A.; Lefen, L. An Analysis of Corporate Social Responsibility and Firm Performance with Moderating Effects of CEO Power and Ownership Structure: A Case Study of the Manufacturing Sector of Pakistan. *Sustainability* **2019**, *11*, 248. [CrossRef]
25. Daily, C.M.; Johnson, J.L. Sources of CEO power and firm financial performance. *Longitud. Assess.* **1997**, *23*, 97–117.
26. Garcia-Sanchez, I.-M.; Raimo, N.; Vitolla, F. CEO power and integrated reporting. *Meditari Acc. Res.* **2020**. [CrossRef]
27. Busco, C.; Frigo, M.L.; Quattrone, P.; Riccaboni, A. Towards Integrated Reporting: Concepts, Elements and Principles. In *Integrated Reporting*; Springer: Berlin/Heidelberg, Germany, 2013; pp. 3–18.
28. Muttakin, M.B.; Khan, A.; Mihret, D.G. The Effect of Board Capital and CEO Power on Corporate Social Responsibility Disclosures. *J. Bus. Ethics* **2016**, *150*, 41–56. [CrossRef]
29. Raheja, C.G. Determinants of board size and composition: A theory of corporate boards. *J. Financ. Quant. Anal.* **2005**, *40*, 283–306. [CrossRef]
30. Bennedsen, M.; Kongsted, H.C.; Nielsen, K.M. The causal effect of board size in the performance of small and medium-sized firms. *J. Bank. Financ.* **2008**, *32*, 1098–1109. [CrossRef]
31. Pearce, J.A.; Zahra, S.A. Board Composition from a strategic contingency perspective. *J. Manag. Stud.* **1992**, *29*, 411–438. [CrossRef]
32. Ansari, B.; Gul, K.; Ahmad, N. Corporate Governance and Firm Performance: Automobile Assemblers Listed in Pakistan Stock Exchange (Psx). *J. Bus. Strateg.* **2017**, *11*, 125–140.
33. Leung, S.; Richardson, G.; Jaggi, B. Corporate board and board committee independence, firm performance, and family ownership concentration: An analysis based on Hong Kong firms. *J. Contemp. Acc. Econ.* **2014**, *10*, 16–31. [CrossRef]
34. Abbas, A.; Naqvi, H.A.; Mirza, H.H. Impact of large ownership on firm performance: A case of non-financial listed companies of Pakistan. *World Appl. Sci. J.* **2013**, *21*, 1141–1152.
35. Yasser, Q.R.; Mamun, A.A. The impact of ownership concentration on firm performance: Evidence from an emerging market. *Emerg. Econ. Stud.* **2017**, *3*, 34–53. [CrossRef]
36. Leung, S.C.M.; Horwitz, B. Corporate governance and firm value during a financial crisis. *Rev. Quant. Financ. Acc.* **2009**, *34*, 459–481. [CrossRef]
37. Kapopoulos, P.; Lazaretou, S. Corporate Ownership Structure and Firm Performance: Evidence from Greek firms. *Corp. Gov. Int. Rev.* **2007**, *15*, 144–158. [CrossRef]
38. Demsetz, H. The structure of ownership and the theory of the firm. *J. Law Econ.* **1983**, *26*, 375–390. [CrossRef]
39. Raimo, N.; Vitolla, F.; Marrone, A.; Rubino, M. The role of ownership structure in integrated reporting policies. *Bus. Strat. Environ.* **2020**, *29*, 2238–2250. [CrossRef]
40. Waweru, N. Determinants of quality corporate governance in Sub-Saharan Africa: Evidence from Kenya and South Africa. *Manag. Audit. J.* **2014**, *29*, 455–485. [CrossRef]

41. Masood, A.; Afzal, M. Determinants of Audit Quality in Pakistan. *J. Qual. Technol. Manag.* **2016**, *12*, 25–49.
42. Matoke, V.; Omwenga, J. Audit Quality and Financial Performance of Companies Listed in Nairobi Securities Exchange. *Int. J. Sci. Res. Publ.* **2016**, *6*, 372–381.
43. Al Ani, M.K.; Mohammed, Z.O. Auditor quality and firm performance: Omani experience. *Eur. J. Econ. Financ. Adm. Sci.* **2015**, *74*, 13–23.
44. Sattar, U.; Javeed, S.A.; Latief, R. How Audit Quality Affects the Firm Performance with the Moderating Role of the Product Market Competition: Empirical Evidence from Pakistani Manufacturing Firms. *Sustainability* **2020**, *12*, 4153. [CrossRef]
45. Jacoby, G.; Liu, M.; Wang, Y.; Wu, Z.; Zhang, Y. Corporate governance, external control, and environmental information transparency: Evidence from emerging markets. *J. Int. Financ. Mark. Inst. Money* **2019**, *58*, 269–283. [CrossRef]
46. King, A.A.; Lenox, M.J.; Terlaak, A. The Strategic Use of Decentralized Institutions: Exploring Certification with the ISO 14001 Management Standard. *Acad. Manag. J.* **2005**, *48*, 1091–1106. [CrossRef]
47. Alexander, G.J.; Buchholz, R.A. Corporate social responsibility and stock market performance. *Acad. Manag. J.* **1978**, *21*, 479–486. [CrossRef]
48. Orlitzky, M.; Schmidt, F.L.; Rynes, S.L. Corporate Social and Financial Performance: A Meta-Analysis. *Organ. Stud.* **2003**, *24*, 403–441. [CrossRef]
49. Turban, D.B.; Greening, D.W. Corporate social performance and organizational attractiveness to prospective employees. *Acad. Manag. J.* **1997**, *40*, 658–672.
50. Oeyono, J.; Samy, M.; Bampton, R. An examination of corporate social responsibility and financial performance. *J. Glob. Responsib.* **2011**, *2*, 100–112. [CrossRef]
51. Aerts, W.; Cormier, D.; Magnan, M. Corporate environmental disclosure, financial markets and the media: An international perspective. *Ecol. Econ.* **2008**, *64*, 643–659. [CrossRef]
52. Kong, Y.; Antwi-Adjei, A.; Bawuah, J. A systematic review of the business case for corporate social responsibility and firm performance. *Corp. Soc. Responsib. Environ. Manag.* **2020**, *27*, 444–454. [CrossRef]
53. Naseem, T.; Shahzad, F.; Asim, G.A.; Rehman, I.U.; Nawaz, F. Corporate social responsibility engagement and firm performance in Asia Pacific: The role of enterprise risk management. *Corp. Soc. Responsib. Environ. Manag.* **2020**, *27*, 501–513. [CrossRef]
54. Barnea, A.; Rubin, A.J. Corporate social responsibility as a conflict between shareholders. *J. Bus. Ethics* **2010**, *97*, 71–86. [CrossRef]
55. Fama, E.F.; Jensen, M.C. Separation of ownership and control. *J. Law Econ.* **1983**, *26*, 301–325. [CrossRef]
56. Jizi, M.I.; Salama, A.; Dixon, R.; Stratling, R. Corporate governance and corporate social responsibility disclosure: Evidence from the US banking sector. *J. Bus. Ethics* **2014**, *125*, 601–615. [CrossRef]
57. Khan, A.; Muttakin, M.B.; Siddiqui, J. Corporate governance and corporate social responsibility disclosures: Evidence from an emerging economy. *J. Bus. Ethics* **2013**, *114*, 207–223. [CrossRef]
58. Jamali, D.; Safieddine, A.M.; Rabbath, M. Corporate Governance and Corporate Social Responsibility Synergies and Interrelationships. *Corp. Gov. Int. Rev.* **2008**, *16*, 443–459. [CrossRef]
59. Said, R.; Zainuddin, Y.H.; Haron, H. The relationship between corporate social responsibility disclosure and corporate governance characteristics in Malaysian public listed companies. *Soc. Responsib. J.* **2009**, *5*, 212–226. [CrossRef]
60. Zhuang, Y.; Chang, X.; Lee, Y. Board Composition and Corporate Social Responsibility Performance: Evidence from Chinese Public Firms. *Sustainability* **2018**, *10*, 2752. [CrossRef]
61. Guerrero-Villegas, J.; Pérez-Calero, L.; Hurtado-González, J.M.; Giráldez-Puig, P. Board Attributes and Corporate Social Responsibility Disclosure: A Meta-Analysis. *Sustainability* **2018**, *10*, 4808. [CrossRef]
62. Lone, E.J.; Ali, A.; Khan, I. Corporate governance and corporate social responsibility disclosure: Evidence from Pakistan. *Corp. Gov. Int. J. Bus. Soc.* **2016**, *16*, 785–797. [CrossRef]
63. Sharif, M.; Rashid, K. Corporate governance and corporate social responsibility (CSR) reporting: An empirical evidence from commercial banks (CB) of Pakistan. *Qual. Quant.* **2013**, *48*, 2501–2521. [CrossRef]
64. Majeed, S.; Aziz, T.; Saleem, S. The Effect of Corporate Governance Elements on Corporate Social Responsibility (CSR) Disclosure: An Empirical Evidence from Listed Companies at KSE Pakistan. *Int. J. Financ. Stud.* **2015**, *3*, 530–556. [CrossRef]
65. Gul, S.; Muhammad, F.; Rashid, A. Corporate governance and corporate social responsibility: The case of small, medium, and large firms. *Pak. J. Commer. Soc. Sci.* **2017**, *11*, 1–34.
66. Naseem, M.A.; Rehman, R.U.; Ikram, A.; Malik, F. Impact of board characteristics on corporate social responsibility disclosure. *J. Appl. Bus. Res.* **2017**, *33*, 801–810.
67. Cong, Y.; Freedman, M. Corporate governance and environmental performance and disclosures. *Adv. Acc.* **2011**, *27*, 223–232. [CrossRef]
68. Li, Y.; Gong, M.; Zhang, X.-Y.; Koh, L. The impact of environmental, social, and governance disclosure on firm value: The role of CEO power. *Br. Acc. Rev.* **2018**, *50*, 60–75. [CrossRef]
69. Freedman, M.; Park, J.D.; Romero, J. Recognizing Environmental Liabilities Surrounding CEO Turnovers. In *Managing Reality: Accountability and the Miasma of Private and Public Domains*; Emerald Group Publishing Limited: Bingley, UK, 2014.
70. Kock, C.J.; Santaló, J.; Diestre, L. Corporate Governance and the Environment: What Type of Governance Creates Greener Companies? *J. Manag. Stud.* **2011**, *49*, 492–514. [CrossRef]
71. Javeed, S.A.; Latief, R.; Lefen, L. An analysis of relationship between environmental regulations and firm performance with moderating effects of product market competition: Empirical evidence from Pakistan. *J. Clean. Prod.* **2020**, *254*, 120197. [CrossRef]

72. Shahab, Y.; Ntim, C.G.; Chen, Y.; Ullah, F.; Li, H.-X.; Ye, Z. CEO Attributes, Sustainable Performance, Environmental Performance, and Environmental Reporting: New Insights from Upper Echelons Perspective. *SSRN Electron. J.* **2019**. [CrossRef]
73. Welford, R. Corporate governance and corporate social responsibility: Issues for Asia. *Corp. Soc. Responsib. Environ. Manag.* **2007**, *14*, 42–51. [CrossRef]
74. Lenssen, G.; Blagov, Y.; Bevan, D.; Peters, S.; Miller, M.; Kusyk, S. How Relevant is Corporate Governance and Corporate Social Responsibility in Emerging Markets? Available online: https://www.emerald.com/insight/content/doi/10.1108/14720701111159262/full/html?queryID=57%2F5412077 (accessed on 28 May 2021).
75. Odoemelam, N.; Ofoegbu, G. Corporate Board Characteristics and Environmental Disclosure Quantity: A Comparative Analysis of Traditional and Integrated Reporting Evidence. *Preprints* **2018**. [CrossRef]
76. Osazuwa, N.P.; Che-Ahmad, A.; Che-Adam, N. Political Connection, Board Characteristics and Environmental Disclosure in Nigeria. *Adv. Sci. Lett.* **2017**, *23*, 9356–9361. [CrossRef]
77. Rabi, A.M. Board Characteristics and Environmental Disclosure: Evidence from Jordan. *Int. J. Bus. Manag.* **2019**, *14*, 57. [CrossRef]
78. Uwuigbe, U. An examination of the relationship between management ownership and corporate social responsibility disclosure: A study of selected firms in Nigeria. *Res. J. Financ. Account.* **2011**, *2*, 23–30.
79. García-Meca, E.; Sánchez-Ballesta, J.P. The Association of Board Independence and Ownership Concentration with Voluntary Disclosure: A Meta-analysis. *Eur. Acc. Rev.* **2010**, *19*, 603–627. [CrossRef]
80. Sufian, M.A.; Zahan, M. Ownership structure and corporate social responsibility disclosure in Bangladesh. *Int. J. Econ. Financ. Issues* **2013**, *3*, 901–909.
81. Power, M. Expertise and the construction of relevance: Accountants and environmental audit. *Account. Organ. Soc.* **1997**, *22*, 123–146. [CrossRef]
82. Ahmad, N.B.J.; Rashid, A.; Gow, F. Board independence and corporate social responsibility (CSR) reporting in Malaysia. *Australas. Account. Bus. Financ. J.* **2017**, *11*, 61–85. [CrossRef]
83. Chang, Y.K.; Oh, W.-Y.; Park, J.H.; Jang, M.G. Exploring the Relationship Between Board Characteristics and CSR: Empirical Evidence from Korea. *J. Bus. Ethics* **2017**, *140*, 225–242. [CrossRef]
84. Dewi, K.; Monalisa, M. Effect of Corporate Social Responsibility Disclosure on Financial Performance with Audit Quality as a Moderating Variable. *Binus. Bus. Rev.* **2016**, *7*, 149. [CrossRef]
85. Tamimi, N.; Sebastianelli, R. Transparency among S&P 500 companies: An analysis of ESG disclosure scores. *Manag. Decis.* **2017**, *55*, 1660–1680. [CrossRef]
86. SECP. Corporate Social Responsibility Voluntary Guidelines. 2013. Available online: http://www.secp.gov.pk/notification/pdf/2013/VoluntaryGuidelinesforCSR_2013.pdf (accessed on 10 July 2013).
87. Cheema, K.U.R.; Din, M.S. Impact of corporate governance on performance of firms: A case study of cement industry in Pakistan. *J. Bus. Manage. Sci.* **2013**, *4*, 44–46.
88. Gamerschlag, R.; Möller, K.; Verbeeten, F. Determinants of voluntary CSR disclosure: Empirical evidence from Germany. *Rev. Manag. Sci.* **2011**, *5*, 233–262. [CrossRef]
89. Ahmad, N.; Taiba, S.; Kazmi, S.M.A.; Ali, H.N. Concept and Elements of Corporate Social Responsibility (CSR) and its Islamic Perspective: Mainstream Business Management Concern in Pakistan. *Pak. J. Soc. Sci.* **2015**, *35*, 925–934.
90. Ali, W.; Frynas, J.G. The Role of Normative CSR-Promoting Institutions in Stimulating CSR Disclosures in Developing Countries. *Corp. Soc. Responsib. Environ. Manag.* **2018**, *25*, 373–390. [CrossRef]
91. Dawn. Pakistan Stock Exchange. *Dawn Newspaper*. Available online: https://www.dawn.com/ (accessed on 25 June 2020).
92. Yusuf, F.; Yousaf, A.; Saeed, A. Rethinking agency theory in developing countries: A case study of Pakistan. *Acc. Forum* **2018**, 281–292. [CrossRef]
93. Liao, Z. Is environmental innovation conducive to corporate financing? The moderating role of advertising expenditures. *Bus. Strategy Environ.* **2020**, *29*, 954–961. [CrossRef]
94. Kramer, J.K. Peters An Interindustry Analysis of Economic Value Added as a Proxy for Market Value Added. Available online: http://www.cunyspsc.org/files/papers_o/p_ECO_2001_jaf5899650_o.pdf (accessed on 19 May 2021).
95. Zaid, M.A.; Abuhijleh, S.T.; Pucheta-Martínez, M.C. Ownership structure, stakeholder engagement, and corporate social responsibility policies: The moderating effect of board independence. *Corp. Soc. Responsib. Environ. Manag.* **2020**, *27*, 1344–1360. [CrossRef]
96. Vitolla, F.; Raimo, N.; Rubino, M. Board characteristics and integrated reporting quality: An agency theory perspective. *Corp. Soc. Responsib. Environ. Manag.* **2020**, *27*, 1152–1163. [CrossRef]
97. Sun, J.; Wang, J.; Kent, P.; Qi, B. Does sharing the same network auditor in group affiliated firms affect audit quality? *J. Acc. Public Policy* **2020**, *39*, 106711. [CrossRef]
98. Hubbard, R.; Palia, D. Executive pay and performance Evidence from the U.S. banking industry. *J. Financ. Econ.* **1995**, *39*, 105–130. [CrossRef]
99. Hermalin, B.E.; Weisbach, M.S. The Effects of Board Composition and Direct Incentives on Firm Performance. *Financ. Manag.* **1991**, *20*, 101. [CrossRef]
100. Demsetz, H.; Lehn, K. The Structure of Corporate Ownership: Causes and Consequences. *J. Polit. Econ.* **1985**, *93*, 1155–1177. [CrossRef]

101. Boone, A.L.; Field, L.C.; Karpoff, J.M.; Raheja, C.G. The determinants of corporate board size and composition: An empirical analysis. *J. Financ. Econ.* **2007**, *85*, 66–101. [CrossRef]
102. DeAngelo, H.; DeAngelo, L.; Whited, T.M. Capital structure dynamics and transitory debt. *J. Financ. Econ.* **2011**, *99*, 235–261. [CrossRef]
103. Antonakis, J.; Bendahan, S.; Jacquart, P.; Lalive, R. On making causal claims: A review and recommendations. *Lead. Q.* **2010**, *21*, 1086–1120. [CrossRef]
104. Hamilton, B.H.; Nickerson, J.A. Correcting for Endogeneity in Strategic Management Research. *Strat. Organ.* **2003**, *1*, 51–78. [CrossRef]
105. Aitken, A.C., IV. On Least Squares and Linear Combination of Observations. In *Proceedings of the Royal Society of Edinburgh*; Cambridge University Press (CUP): Cambridge, UK, 1936.
106. Li, F. Endogeneity in CEO power: A survey and experiment. *Invest. Anal. J.* **2016**, *45*, 149–162. [CrossRef]
107. Arellano, M.; Bond, S. Some Tests of Specification for Panel Data: Monte Carlo Evidence and an Application to Employment Equations. *Rev. Econ. Stud.* **1991**, *58*, 277. [CrossRef]
108. Blundell, R.; Griffiths, R.; Van Reenen, J. Market Share, Market Value and Innovation in a Panel of British Manufacturing Firms. *Rev. Econ. Stud.* **1999**, *66*, 529–554. [CrossRef]
109. Feng, Y.; Chen, H.H.; Tang, J. The Impacts of Social Responsibility and Ownership Structure on Sustainable Financial Development of China's Energy Industry. *Sustainability* **2018**, *10*, 301. [CrossRef]
110. Ullah, S.; Akhtar, P.; Zaefarian, G. Dealing with endogeneity bias: The generalized method of moments (GMM) for panel data. *Ind. Mark. Manag.* **2018**, *71*, 69–78. [CrossRef]
111. Wintoki, M.B.; Linck, J.S.; Netter, J.M. Endogeneity and the dynamics of internal corporate governance. *J. Financ. Econ.* **2012**, *105*, 581–606. [CrossRef]
112. Wooldridge, J.M. Inverse probability weighted M-estimators for sample selection, attrition, and stratification. *Port. Econ. J.* **2002**, *1*, 117–139. [CrossRef]
113. Baltagi, B. *Econometric Analysis of Panel Data*; John Wiley & Sons: Hoboken, NJ, USA, 2008.
114. Greene, W.H. *Heteroscedasticity. Econometric Analysis*, 4th ed.; Upper Saddle River, Prentice-Hall Inc.: Hoboken, NJ, USA, 2000; pp. 499–524.
115. Mayur, M.; Saravanan, P. Performance implications of board size, composition and activity: Empirical evidence from the Indian banking sector. *Corp. Gov. Int. J. Bus. Soc.* **2017**, *17*, 466–489. [CrossRef]
116. Singh, S.; Guha, M. Experiential learning: Analyzing success and failures in Indian telecom sector. *Benchmarking Int. J.* **2018**, *25*, 3702–3719. [CrossRef]
117. Chen, H.; Li, X.; Zeng, S.; Ma, H.; Lin, H. Does state capitalism matter in firm internationalization? Pace, rhythm, location choice, and product diversity. *Manag. Decis.* **2016**, *54*, 1320–1342. [CrossRef]
118. Beiner, S.; Drobetz, W.; Schmid, M.M.; Zimmermann, H. An integrated framework of corporate governance and firm valuation. *Eur. Financ. Manag.* **2006**, *12*, 249–283. [CrossRef]
119. Schultz, E.L.; Tan, D.T.; Walsh, K.D. Endogeneity and the corporate governance performance relation. *Aust. J. Manag.* **2010**, *35*, 145–163. [CrossRef]
120. Gujarati, D.N. *Basic Econometrics*; Tata McGraw-Hill Education: New York, NY, USA, 2009.
121. Weisbach, M.S. Outside directors and CEO turnover. *J. Financ. Econ.* **1988**, *20*, 431–460. [CrossRef]
122. Brickley, J.A.; Coles, J.L.; Jarrell, G. Leadership structure: Separating the CEO and Chairman of the Board. *J. Corp. Financ.* **1997**, *3*, 189–220. [CrossRef]
123. Cotter, J.F.; Shivdasani, A.; Zenner, M. Do independent directors enhance target shareholder wealth during tender offers? *J. Financ. Econ.* **1997**, *43*, 195–218. [CrossRef]
124. Sah, R.K.; Stiglitz, J.E. The architecture of economic systems: Hierarchies and polyarchies. *Am. Econ. Rev.* **1986**. [CrossRef]
125. Malik, M.; Wan, D.; Ahmad, M.I.; Naseem, M.A.; Rehman, R.U. Role of Board Size in Corporate Governance and Firm Performance Applying Pareto Approach, Is It Cultural Phenomena? *J. Appl. Bus. Res.* **2014**, *30*, 1395. [CrossRef]
126. Bhagat, S.; Bolton, B. Corporate governance and firm performance. *J. Corp. Financ.* **2008**, *14*, 257–273. [CrossRef]
127. Liu, Y.; Miletkov, M.K.; Wei, Z.; Yang, T. Board independence and firm performance in China. *J. Corp. Financ.* **2015**, *30*, 223–244. [CrossRef]
128. Nazir, M.S.; Afza, T. Does managerial behavior of managing earnings mitigate the relationship between corporate governance and firm value? Evidence from an emerging market. *Futur. Bus. J.* **2018**, *4*, 139–156. [CrossRef]
129. Adhikary, B.; Huynh, L.; Hoang, G. Board structure and firm performance in emerging economies: Evidence from Vietnam. *Ruhuna J. Manag. Financ.* **2014**, *1*, 53–72.
130. Coles, J.L.; Daniel, N.D.; Naveen, L. Boards: Does one size fit all? *J. Financ. Econ.* **2008**, *87*, 329–356. [CrossRef]
131. Fauzi, F.; Locke, S. Board structure, ownership structure and firm performance: A study of New Zealand listed-firms. *Manag. J. Account. Financ.* **2012**, *8*, 43–67.
132. Jackling, B.; Johl, S. Board structure and firm performance: Evidence from India's top companies. *Corp. Gov. Int. Rev.* **2009**, *17*, 492–509. [CrossRef]
133. Li, D.; Moshirian, F.; Nguyen, P.; Tan, L.-W. Managerial ownership and firm performance: Evidence from China's privatizations. *Res. Int. Bus. Financ.* **2007**, *21*, 396–413. [CrossRef]

134. Chen, C.R.; Guo, W.; Mande, V. Managerial ownership and firm valuation: Evidence from Japanese firms. *Pac. Basin Financ. J.* **2003**, *11*, 267–283. [CrossRef]
135. Uwuigbe, U.; Olusanmi, O. An Empirical Examination of the Relationship between Ownership Structure and the Performance of Firms in Nigeria. *Int. Bus. Res.* **2011**, *5*, 208. [CrossRef]
136. Kim, K.A.; Kitsabunnarat, P.; Nofsinger, J.R. Ownership and operating performance in an emerging market: Evidence from Thai IPO firms. *J. Corp. Financ.* **2004**, *10*, 355–381. [CrossRef]
137. Claessens, S.; Djankov, S.; Pohl, G. *Ownership and Corporate Governance: Evidence from the Czech Republic*; World Bank Publications: Washington, DC, USA, 1997; Volume 1737.
138. Hanousek, J.; Kočenda, E.; Svejnar, J. Origin and concentration: Corporate ownership, control and performance in firms after privatization. *Econ. Transit.* **2007**, *15*, 1–31. [CrossRef]
139. Omran, M. Post-privatization corporate governance and firm performance: The role of private ownership concentration, identity and board composition. *J. Comp. Econ.* **2009**, *37*, 658–673. [CrossRef]
140. Bonazzi, L.; Islam, S.M. Agency theory and corporate governance: A study of the effectiveness of board in their monitoring of the CEO. *J. Model. Manag.* **2007**, *2*, 7–23. [CrossRef]
141. Agyemang-Mintah, P. Remuneration Committee governance and firm performance in UK financial firms. *Invest. Manag. Financ. Innov.* **2016**, *13*, 176–190. [CrossRef]
142. Crespi-Cladera, R.; Gispert-Pellicer, C. Board Remuneration, Performance and Corporate Governance in Large Spanish Companies. *SSRN Electron. J.* **1999**. [CrossRef]
143. Farrukh, K.; Irshad, S.; Khakwani, M.S.; Ishaque, S.; Ansari, N.Y. Impact of dividend policy on shareholders wealth and firm performance in Pakistan. *Cogent Bus. Manag.* **2017**, *4*, 1408208. [CrossRef]
144. Arnott, R.D.; Asness, C.S. Surprise! Higher Dividends = Higher Earnings Growth. *Financ. Anal. J.* **2003**, *59*, 70–87. [CrossRef]
145. Ouma, O.P. The relationship between dividend payout and firm performance: A study of listed companies in Kenya. *Eur. Sci. J.* **2012**, *8*, 9.
146. Birindelli, G.; Dell'Atti, S.; Iannuzzi, A.P.; Savioli, M. Composition and activity of the board of directors: Impact on ESG performance in the banking system. *Sustainability* **2018**, *10*, 4699. [CrossRef]
147. Valls Martínez, M.d.C.; Martín Cervantes, P.A.; Cruz Rambaud, S.E. Women on corporate boards and sustainable development in the American and European markets: Is there a limit to gender policies? *JCSR Manag.* **2020**, *27*, 2642–2656. [CrossRef]

International Journal of
Environmental Research and Public Health

MDPI

Article

Exploring the Impact of Corporate Social Responsibility Communication through Social Media on Banking Customer E-WOM and Loyalty in Times of Crisis

Dianxi Zhang [1], Asif Mahmood [2], Antonio Ariza-Montes [3], Alejandro Vega-Muñoz [4], Naveed Ahmad [5], Heesup Han [6,*] and Muhammad Safdar Sial [7]

1 Economics and Management School, Wuhan University, Wuhan 430072, China; dxrache@126.com
2 Department of Business Studies, Namal Institute, Mianwali 42250, Pakistan; asif.mahmood@namal.edu.pk
3 Social Matters Research Group, Universidad Loyola Andalucía, C/Escritor Castilla Aguayo, 4 14004 Córdoba, Spain; ariza@uloyola.es
4 Public Policy Observatory, Universidad Autónoma de Chile, 425 Pedro de Valdivia Avenue, Providencia, Santiago 7500912, Chile; alejandro.vega@uautonoma.cl
5 Faculty of Management Studies, University of Central Punjab, Lahore 54000, Pakistan; naveeddgk2010@gmail.com
6 College of Hospitality and Tourism Management, Sejong University, 98 Gunja-Dong, Gwanjin-Gu, Seoul 143-747, Korea
7 Department of Management Sciences, COMSATS University Islamabad (CUI), Islamabad 44000, Pakistan; safdarsial@comsats.edu.pk
* Correspondence: heesup.han@gmail.com

Abstract: Previous studies have largely explored corporate social responsibility (CSR) for organization-centric outcomes to achieve organizational performance, organizational commitment, or organizational citizenship behavior. However, the importance of CSR to achieve customer-centric outcomes is underexplored to date. Contemporary researchers have recently turned their attention toward CSR from the viewpoint of customer-centric outcomes. Therefore, the present study attempts to test the influence of CSR communication on social media and customer loyalty in the banking sector of a developing economy in times of crisis. This study also investigates the mediating effect of electronic word of mouth (E-WOM) with this relationship. The data of the present study were collected from different banking customers using a self-administered questionnaire. The empirical findings of this study validated that the CSR communication of a bank on social media increases customer loyalty, and E-WOM partially mediates this relationship. This study will be helpful for the banking sector to understand the importance of CSR communication to increase customer loyalty, which is very important for every bank in times of crisis.

Keywords: social media; customer loyalty; positive customer emotions; corporate social responsibility; E-word of mouth; banking customers; times of crisis

1. Introduction

The emergence of social media has facilitated modern business with a digital platform in order to communicate with customers interactively [1]. Social media provides a flexible and interactive forum for businesses in the current age of digitalization [2]. Likewise, social media have revolutionized the field of marketing as the importance of social commerce is being recognized by different contemporary researchers [3,4]. This is perhaps the reason that modern businesses recognize social media as a key player in order to involve different stakeholders, which include involving customers meaningfully with a brand [5]. Social media has brought a substantial change in the field of organizational communication as a new communication medium especially when it takes place from the traditional communication model, which is a one-way model of communication [6]. In the current digital age, the attractiveness of social media is not without logic because its interactive and fast communicability provides an opportunity for businesses to communicate with diverse stakeholders, which is contrary to conventional media [7]. Presently, more than 3.8 billion individuals are already using social media. The attractiveness and acceptability of social media are evident due to the fact that the rate of social media users all over the world is increasing by 7% per year [8].

Contemporary businesses use social media for different communication purposes, which include their corporate social responsibility communication (CSR) [9]. There is a stream of researchers who recognize the importance of communicating CSR through social media (S–CSR) as a building block in order to maintain meaningful relationships with stakeholders [10–12]. This study defines CSR according to the definition from Carroll [13] who states "CSR is the economic, legal, ethical and philanthropic responsibility of a business". The extant literature has long established that through well-planned CSR activities, an organization can achieve multiple benefits that include organizational financial performance [14], brand reputation [15], employees' behavior [16], and organizational commitment [17]. However, how the CSR activities of an organization can generate customer-centric outcomes is an issue that has not received due attention from contemporary CSR researchers thus far. It is quite recent that researchers have turned their attention to investigate the phenomenon of CSR from the perspective of the customers [18–20], but these studies are inconclusive, which highlights that there is a need to conduct more research in this field. With this background, the present study attempts to examine the impact of S–CSR on customer loyalty and proposes electronic word of mouth (E-WOM) as a mediator in this relationship.

The study discovered that the banking sector in Pakistan is a suitable segment to test the proposed relationship. The relevance of the banking sector is important for two reasons. First, the banking sector is labeled as a homogenized sector, in which most of the players offer the same type of standard product/services. However, it is very difficult for a bank to earn loyalty from the customers due to this homogenization issue, because loyalty can be earned through different efforts that include a well-differentiated market offering [21], which is almost nonexistent in a homogenized segment. Second, Pakistan's banking sector is very competitive, which demands some extraordinary and unconventional efforts from a bank to hold its market share. This study argues that the S–CSR of a bank may serve as an extraordinary strategy that can grab the attention of the customers to stay with that bank.

The establishment of a strong brand is critical in services due to service heterogeneity and intangibility [22], and hence, it involves a higher level of purchase risk, compared to physical products [23]. Likewise, service brands possess various touchpoints and customer interactions than brands dealing in the physical product sector [24]. Thus, it is difficult for service brands to portray their image as a socially responsible brand because it is a key strategic touchpoint to develop positive relationships with customers [25]. Hence, the importance to earn an image of a socially responsible brand is increasing for the service sector than ever before [18,26]. Therefore, banks, as one of the players in the service industry, employ various additional strategies to earn a favorable customer attitude [27–30]. However, it is evident in extant literature that the banking sector received little attention from contemporary scholars to explain how CSR activities of a bank can create positive customer outcomes. Although some attempts have been made by extant researchers [31–35], these studies are sparse, especially from the perspective of developing economies. The above discussion highlights that there is a daunting need to conduct more researches in this area. Furthermore, it is also established in the literature that the relationship between CSR and customer loyalty is complex, and explaining this relationship through a direct influence of CSR on loyalty is not sufficient. In fact, in their recent study, Khan and Fatma [36] mentioned that customers' CSR perception of an organization is not enough to explain loyalty. Thus, it is better to explain this relationship through moderators and mediators.

Likewise, there are different important contributions of the present study to the existing literature. First of all, this study adds to the existing CSR literature from the perspective of the customers, whereas the prior studies have largely addressed the relationship of CSR in other domains as opposed to the customers. For example, Barauskaite and Streimikiene [14] investigated CSR in order to enhance the financial performance of an organization. George, Aboobaker, and Edward [17] tested the effect of CSR in order to boost organizational commitment, and Tuan [37] examined CSR from the perspective of employee citizenship behavior. However, the important role of CSR to shape customer emotions and behavior through social media has largely been ignored by contemporary researchers. The present study contends that S–CSR creates an emotional pull (E-WOM) on the part of the customers, which is ultimately translated into a positive customer outcome, i.e., customer loyalty. Lastly, this study is a pioneer to consider the phenomenon of S–CSR in order to achieve marketing-related outcomes, such as customer loyalty and E-WOM, which are very important for every business sector.

2. Theory and Hypotheses

The present study uses the lenses of the social exchange theory [38] and the theory of norm reciprocity [39] as the grounding theories. The theory of social exchange proposes that the behavior of individual results from an exchanged process that intends to maximize benefits and reduce costs. Likewise, the theory of norm reciprocity suggests that when an individual receives some benefit from someone, he or she is urged to return that benefit positively.

Customers make purchase decisions based on their perception of an organizational commitment toward society, the environment, and their analysis of a product/service [40]. When customers see an organization is participating in CSR activities, their positive evaluation of that organization is likely improved [41]. Unfortunately, the idea of CSR has been around for the last two decades in Pakistan, but it is still in the early stages, and the majority of the customers do not have a good level of understanding about the importance of CSR knowledge. The rise of social media is a game-changer from this perspective because it provides an interactive platform for the organizations, which they not only communicate their CSR strategies through with different stakeholders, such as customers, but it also highlights the importance of their CSR initiatives for the community and the environment [42]. Furthermore, CSR initiatives of an organization on social media are also important because of the interactive feature of social media. The customers and the company interactively communicate with each other through social media [43]. This interactive atmosphere of social media plays a key role to build customer confidence for a specific brand, which in turn is translated into increased customers' loyalty [44]. Different researchers hold the same argument in the context of the banking sector that CSR activities of a bank may induce customer loyalty. For instance, Pérez and Rodríguez del Bosque [45] explored the relationship between customer-centric CSR activities and customer loyalty in the commercial banking sector and found a positive relationship. In different instances, other scholars have also produced the same findings [29,46–48].

The customers are more likely to accept products and services from an organization that is a trusted one [49]. The organizations, which are perceived by the customers as socially responsible, are also perceived as trusted organizations. True CSR activities of an organization nurture an environment of transparency, which is very important in order to win customer trust [50]. When customers observe that an organization is contributing positively toward society and the environment through CSR activities, they feel the benefits of CSR overrun the costs, which is in line with the social exchange theory [23]. Likewise, when an organization communicates its CSR activities through social media with the customers, they feel positive and want to reciprocate with the organization positively. Hence, from the perspective of the theory of norm reciprocity [39], S–CSR is expected to earn positive customer outcomes, such as enhanced customer loyalty. As a result, the following hypothesis is postulated.

Hypothesis 1 (H1). *CSR activities of a bank through social media positively relate to banking customer loyalty.*

Word of mouth (WOM) embraces the informal communication of a customer that is directed at other customers about the characteristics and the experiences of a specific product or brand [51]. Sometimes, WOM has also been recognized as a referral, but it is only one facet of it. Referral means the endorsements of customers about a brand to others [52]. In other words, it is an implicit or an explicit form of recommendation. WOM is regarded as an important element in the field of business, in which WOM customers recommend or do not recommend a brand to others [53]. Research has long established that WOM is a strategic enabler to influence customer loyalty [54–56]. E-WOM is the process in which the customers exchange information with each other online about a brand [57]. There have been different researchers in the extant literature, who have acknowledged that E-WOM is positively associated with customer loyalty [58,59]. Prior studies have also established that online communities and forums, customer reviews, and recommendations have transformed digital commerce [60,61].

Organizations participate in CSR activities on social media in order to generate an emotional pull among the customers and earn the image of being a socially responsible organization [62]. When social media customers observe that an organization is positively contributing to society and the environment, they feel appreciation for that organization. Hence, the customers want to reciprocate the organization positively, and they are likely to use positive E-WOM about that brand on social media with other customers [63], which is in line with the theory of norm reciprocity [39].

Incorporating a CSR program increases the organization's visibility, and it encourages more communication with the customers. Therefore, it is expected that an organization's engagement in CSR activities is likely to induce positive WOM on the part of the customers [64]. In the context of the banking sector, Guping et al. [65] validated that CSR activities of a bank help induce WOM for that bank from customers. Similarly, the study of Khan et al. [66] confirmed that CSR activities of a bank are a direct determinant of WOM in the Pakistani banking sector. Different other scholars have also confirmed the positive relationship between CSR activities of a bank and positive WOM [63,67,68].

Customers expect that a responsible organization will provide them with quality products or services without neglecting their social responsibility [69]. The CSR engagement of an organization builds a positive image of the organization [70]. The positive image of an organization that is created by CSR activities leads customers to develop a better perception of the organization through the halo effect. This well-rounded perception of an organization attracts customers to the organization's products and services [71]. As a result, customers often speak positively about the organization that is engaged in CSR initiatives, and they also associate themselves positively with the products and services of the organization.

The role of positive WOM is well recognized among contemporary researchers in order to obtain new customers [72–74]. Furthermore, it has also been recognized by recent researchers that positive WOM influences the customer's positive brand preference [75], perception [76], buying intentions [77], and loyalty [78]. Therefore, WOM is very important for organizations that effectively use WOM in order to increase their sales or have successful promotions. Online media has facilitated WOM online communication with the advent of the internet. Moreover, organizations participate in CSR for several reasons, which include positive WOM [79]. Customers will be more willing to talk about the organization's CSR activities with their peers, family, and partners as a result of CSR involvement [80]. Modern organizations in the present era use social media to communicate their CSR motives with customers and other stakeholders. In a nutshell, the S–CSR of an organization is expected to engage the customers with a brand meaningfully. In response to the CSR activities of an organization, the customers are self-motivated to support that organization among their social media peers by using positive WOM. All of these activities will ultimately take the customers toward a higher level of loyalty. As a result, the authors propose the following set of hypotheses along with the proposed research model, which is shown in Figure 1.

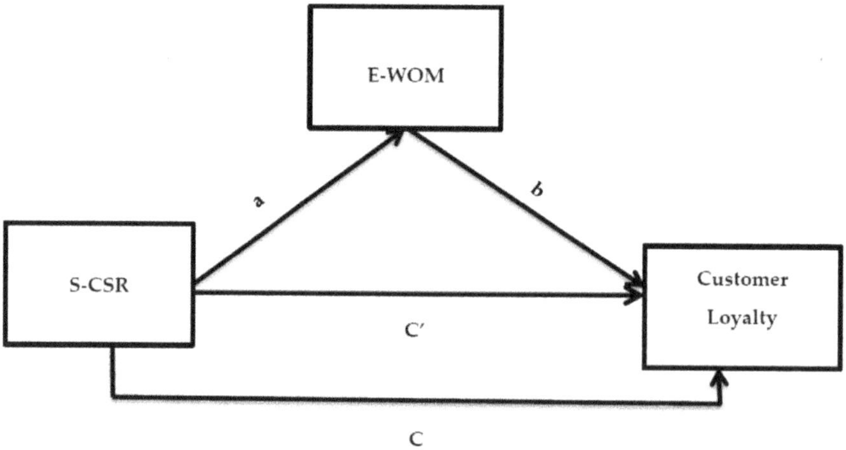

Figure 1. Proposed research model where corporate social responsibility through social media (S–CSR) = the independent variable, customer loyalty = the dependent variable, electronic word of mouth (E-WOM) = the mediating variable, C′ = indirect direct effect of X on Y with the effect of the mediator, and C = direct effect of X on Y without a mediator. a= direct path from S-CSR to E-WOM and b = direct path from E-WOM to customer loyalty.

Hypothesis 2 (H2). *CSR activities of a bank through social media positively relate to E-WOM for a bank.*

Hypothesis 3 (H3). *E-WOM mediates the relationship between S-CSR and customer loyalty in the banking sector.*

3. Methodology

3.1. Population, Sample, and the Handling of Social Desirability

The authors selected Pakistan's banking sector to validate the proposed research model, which is shown in Figure 1. For the data collection procedure, the authors first of all intensively assessed the banks that were actively involved in different CSR activities. Furthermore, the authors also verified either the selected banks use social media, such as Facebook, Twitter, Instagram, or YouTube to communicate with their customers. This initial assessment resulted in the selection of four banks, which included Habib Bank Limited (HBL), United Bank Limited (UBL), National Bank of Pakistan (NBP), and Allied Bank Limited (ABL). Likewise, these four banks contain the major share of the banking customers in Pakistan, and they have a presence in almost every city in the country. The authors collected the data from the cities of Lahore, Islamabad, and Karachi. These are all big cities, and they have multiple branches of the banks that were mentioned above in different locations.

The banking sector of Pakistan uses social media to serve different purposes, including communication with stakeholders during the time of crises. Since banking segment is one of those segments that are highly volatile due to different market situation that causes a crisis, these causes may include an excessive risk-taking attitude of a bank, weakness in finance management, changing external market situation, etc. In these instances, the banking institutions need to communicate effectively with their stakeholders, including customers and creditors, to reassure them that their bank will revive soon and will dispose of any crisis-related situation. In this regard, the role of social media, as an interactive medium of communication cannot be neglected because banks communicate their crisis with stakeholders on social media and also share the possible solution and steps taken by the bank to address a crisis-related situation.

The authors accessed the respondents while they were leaving a particular branch of a bank, or they were found near the ATM premises. Before the collection of the data, the authors received informed consent from each respondent in order to voluntarily participate in the data collection process. Furthermore, the authors also verified that the person who consented to participate in the survey maintained at least one bank account in one of the sample banks mentioned above. Before disseminating the questionnaire among different respondents, they were informed by the authors that they can quit the survey anytime if they feel uncomfortable.

Next, the authors addressed the issue of social desirability by taking different steps. For example, the authors scattered the survey items randomly throughout the questionnaire in order to break any intended sequence of responses regarding answering the questions. Furthermore, this strategy is also helpful to mitigate the impact of any liking or disliking of a specific variable. Likewise, the authors informed the respondents about the importance of genuine response in order to generate the appropriate results from the survey. Additionally, the authors visited different branches of the selected banks during different times; hence, the respondents from all the fields would be included in the survey. The authors distributed 800 surveys among the respondents, and 431 fully completed questionnaires were eventually received, which are included in the final data list. As a result, the response rate of the present survey is 53.87%.

3.2. Measures

In order to address the issue of reliability and validity, the authors used adapted scales to measure all the variables of the present survey. In this regard, the authors borrowed the items of S–CSR from the studies of van Asperen et al. [81] and Eisingerich et al. [82]. This scale contained five items. Similarly, three items that were used to measure E-WOM were taken from the study of Kang and Hustvedt [83]; this scale was also used by Guping et al. [65], in the banking context. Lastly, the three items scale for customer loyalty was adapted from Dagger et al. [84], which is also used by Iglesias et al. [85] in the healthcare insurance context and by Raza et al. [27] in the banking context. A five-point Likert scale was used to record the responses from the different respondents of the present survey. Table 1 illustrates the demographic detail of the respondents. As per the results of Table 1, the gender segment is mainly dominated by males since the majority of the respondents were male who participated in the survey. This dominance is justified in the context of Pakistan, which is a male-dominant society. Likewise, the ages section shows that majority of the respondents were from the age group of 26–30 and 31–40. These insights are also logical and relevant in the context of Pakistan because the first age bracket (20–25) mostly constitute the individuals who are either student or young entrepreneurs at small levels, and they are not frequent bank account users, which is why their portion of frequency is low. One possible reason why the respondents in the last group were low in numbers lies in the logic that the data of the current survey were collected during the period of the COVID-19 crisis in the country, and the majority of the old citizens were not visiting their banks frequently. The detail of all survey items is given in Table 2.

Table 1. Demographic information of the sample.

Demographic	Frequency	%
Gender		
Male	288	66.8
Female	143	33.2
Age		
20–25	73	16.9
26–30	153	35.5
31–40	138	32.1
Above 40	67	15.5
Education		
Intermediate	77	17.9
Graduate	112	26.0
Master	183	42.4
Higher	59	13.7
Total	**431**	**100**

Table 2. Factor loading, convergent validity, and reliability results.

Variable	Statement	Loading	AVE	CR
	I consider this bank a socially responsible bank.	0.71		
	This bank is more beneficial to society's welfare than other banks.	0.74		
S–CSR	This bank contributes something to society.	0.79		
	I share this bank's (CSR) posts on my own Facebook (or other social media) page.	0.83		
	I engage in conversations (CSR) on the Facebook (or other social media) page of this bank.	0.82	0.61	0.88
E-WOM	I am likely to spread positive word of mouth about this bank (on social media).	0.70		
	I would recommend this bank's products/services to my friends (on social media).	0.77		
	If my friends were looking to purchase banking services, I would tell them to try this bank (on social media).	0.72	0.53	0.77
Loyalty	I consider this bank my first choice when I purchase the services they supply.	0.73		
	I am willing to maintain my relationship with this bank	0.72		
	I am loyal to this bank.	0.84	0.59	0.81

Notes: Loadings = factor loadings, CR = composite reliability, AVE = average-variance-extracted, S–CSR = corporate social responsibility through social medial, E-WOM = electronic word of mouth.

4. Results and Analysis

In the data analysis phase, the authors first assessed for the presence of a common method bias (CMB). For this reason, the data for the present survey were collected by the same individual. Hence, the presence of an issue with the CMB is not out of the question. In order to detect a potential issue with the CMB, the authors performed a single-factor analysis according to the guidelines from Harman [86]. In this regard, the authors loaded all the items of variables onto a single factor using IBM-SPSS software version 23. The results of the single-factor analysis validated the absence of any issues with the factors, which shared a total variance of more than 50%. The largest variance shared by a single factor was 39.58%. Therefore, the authors established that there is no issue with the CMB in the present survey. The variance shared by a single factor was 39.58%. Therefore, the authors established that there is no issue with the CMB in the present survey.

Next, the authors performed an exploratory factor analysis (EFA) by conducting a principal component analysis with a varimax rotation in SPSS in order to detect any cross-item loadings or weak-item loadings. The results showed that the item loadings for all the items were above the threshold level of 0.5 [87]. This validates the data appropriate for further analysis. Tables 2 and 3 show different results, which include factor loadings, validity analysis, correlation analysis, reliability analysis, and multicollinearity analysis. In this regard, the results of convergent validity (Table 2) were established on the values of the average variance extracted (AVE) for each variable. Additionally, the standard rule here is if the value of AVE for a variable is greater than 0.5, it is established that the criterion for convergent validity is maintained. According to the results from Table 2, all three variables have AVE values greater than 0.5, and therefore, the authors observed no issues with convergent validity.

Table 3. Correlations and discriminant validity.

Variable	Mean	SD	S–CSR	E-WOM	Loyalty	Skewness	Kurtosis
S–CSR	3.88	0.58	**(0.781)**	0.27 **	0.24 **	−0.56	0.47
E-WOM	4.10	0.61		**(0.728)**	0.31 **	−0.63	0.51
Loyalty	4.28	0.55			**(0.721)**	−0.68	0.44
(χ^2/df = 4.09, RMSEA = 0.068, NFI = 0.924, CFI = 0.929, GFI = 0.925)							

Notes: Bold diagonal = square root of average variance extracted (AVE), ** = values are significant.

The authors also report the discriminant validity results in Table 3, which were obtained by calculating the square root values of AVE for each variable and comparing it with the values of correlation. For instance, the square root value of AVE for the variable loyalty is 0.721, which is larger than the correlation values they were compared to, which are 0.24 ** and 0.31 **. Therefore, it is established that the variables discriminate against each other; hence, the requirement for discriminant validity is fulfilled. The values of composite reliability (CR) were also significant (CR > 0.7). The model fit indices values attained from the confirmatory factor analysis (CFA) are reported in Table 2, (χ^2/df = 4.09, RMSEA = 0.0682, NFI = 0.924, CFI = 0.929, and GFI = 0.925). All the results for the model fit indices were in acceptable ranges, which is confirmation that the data are well fitted to the theoretical model. Lastly, the authors reported the results of data normality as per the suggestions from Brown and Dacin [88], who suggested that the data are normally distributed if the skewness and kurtosis values are between ± 3 and ± 10, which is the case here.

Hypotheses Testing

The authors performed the hypotheses testing for the present study using the structural equation modeling technique (SEM) in IBM-AMOS 21. In this regard, the authors performed the analysis in two steps. In the first step, the authors assessed the results of the direct effect for Hypothesis 1 and Hypothesis 2. The results for the direct effect structural model, which is illustrated in Table 4, revealed that both H1 (H1; β = 0.225 **, LLCI = 0.293, ULCI = 0.537, and $p < 0.05$) and H2 (H2; β = 0.257 **, LLCI = 0.310, ULCI = 0.583, and $p < 0.05$) are significant and true. Hence, the first two hypotheses, which are denoted as H1 and H2, of the present study are accepted. In the second step, the authors tested the mediating effect of E-WOM between CSR and customer loyalty. The authors used the bootstrapping option in AMOS by using a larger bootstrap sample of 2000. The bootstrapping results confirmed that there is a partial mediation effect of E-WOM between CSR and customer loyalty. The authors confirmed this partial mediation of E-WOM by observing the beta value, which is reduced from 0.225 ** to 0.173 ** but remained positive, which showed that the LLCI and the ULCI are nonzero. All these results confirmed the mediating effect of E-WOM between CSR and customer loyalty. Hence, all three hypotheses of the present study are accepted.

Table 4. Results of the hypotheses testing.

Path	Beta Value	S.E	LLCI	ULCI	Decision
The Results of Hypothesis 1 and 2					
S–CSR → Loyalty	0.225 **	0.0442	0.293	0.537	supported
S–CSR → E-WOM	0.257 **	0.0371	0.310	0.583	supported
(χ^2/df = 3.394, RMSEA = 0.0578, NFI = 0.946, CFI = 0.949, and GFI = 0.947) ***					
The Results of Hypothesis 3					
S–CSR → E-WOM → Loyalty	0.173 **	0.021	0.044	0.063	supported
(χ^2/df = 2.98, RMSEA = 0.0486, NFI = 0.952, CFI = 0.958, and GFI = 0.956) ***					

S–CSR, CSR on social media; E-WOM, electronic word of mouth; S.E = standard error, LLCI = lower limit confidence interval, ULCI = upper limit confidence interval, and *** and ** = significant values.

5. Discussion and Implications

This study aimed to test the effect of S–CSR on customer loyalty with the mediating effect of E-WOM in Pakistan's banking sector in times of crisis. In this regard, the empirical findings of the present study confirmed that S–CSR positively influences customer loyalty. The respondents of the present study confirmed that when they are aware of the CSR initiatives of their bank through social media, they have positive feelings, and they want to stay with their bank for a longer time period. The theory of social exchange also justifies this finding since banking customers perceive the CSR practices of a bank in order to create more benefits for society, compared to costs. Hence, they believe that the CSR practices of an organization are helpful to uplift society and the environment. These results revealed that CSR and customer loyalty are positively related. This study is not the first to propose this relationship since various other scholars have also acknowledged that CSR activities of a bank are positively related to banking customer loyalty [29,46–48]. This finding can also be explained in the light of social exchange theory because the CSR activities of a bank are well appreciated by the customers when they observe such information on different social media platforms. In exchange, they are urged to hold a higher level of loyalty to a socially responsible bank. The recent studies from different contemporary CSR researchers also provide support for this relationship [9,18,29,89].

Moreover, the result of the mediating effect of E-WOM between S–CSR and customer loyalty confirmed that there is a mediating role of E-WOM between this relationship. The theory of norm reciprocity is helpful to explain this result because it shows that when banking customers are informed through different social media platforms about CSR activities of their bank, an emotional pull on the part of the customers is created. In response to this type of emotional pull, the customers are self-motivated to reciprocate their bank positively. Hence, they spread positive WOM about their bank in their social media circles. Eventually, the emotional pull, which is E-WOM, that is created by the CSR initiatives of a bank promotes the customers to a higher level of loyalty. The previous studies showed that the responsible moves of an organization are helpful to create positive emotions on the part of the customers, which are illustrated in the studies by Castro-González et al. [19], and Tajvidi et al. [90]. In addition, it is also evident from the extant researchers that the CSR activities of an organization develop an emotional pull among the customers [91]. From the perspective of social media, the study of D'Acunto et al. [92] is a recent study that acknowledges the importance of S–CSR to create positive emotions among the customers. Different other scholars have also confirmed the existence of a positive relationship between CSR activities of a bank and positive WOM [63,67,68].

There are some important theoretical and practical implications for the present study. First, the study at hand enriches the existing CSR literature from the perspective of the customers, which is very important for every organization. However, the majority of the previous studies have not explored the CSR phenomenon well from the context of the customer-related outcomes. Second, the present study adds to the existing literature by arguing that the S–CSR activities of an organization are helpful to create positive emotions among the customers. In this regard, the previous studies have not adequately addressed the important relationship of CSR to create an emotional pull on the part of the customers. Lastly, the present study is an important contribution to the existing literature from the marketing point of view, because the study argues that the CSR strategies on social media are important to induce the customers' loyalty. The extant literature surprisingly has not paid due consideration in this domain because the majority of the previous studies addressed CSR in other contexts, such as organizational performance [14], organizational commitment [17], and citizenship behavior [37].

This study has some important implications for the practitioners of the banking sector. For instance, this study can help policymakers to improve their understanding of CSR from a marketing perspective. In this regard, the policymakers are encouraged to base their marketing strategies close to the CSR phenomenon, because the well-planned CSR initiatives of a bank can be a source of a stable competitive advantage. Likewise, the policymakers need to realize that using CSR activities to shape the behavior of the customers in a positive manner is not without logic. The banking sector needs to realize that they are dealing with an industry that is mostly homogenized by nature and earning customer loyalty in a segment that is homogenized is very difficult. For this reason, CSR strategies are very important since they may be helpful to grab the loyalty of the customers, which is of the utmost importance for every bank. Another practical implication of this study is that it brings to the surface that policymakers from the banking sector are encouraged to use social media intelligently because it provides an interactive and flexible forum to communicate with their customers. A particular bank is likely to receive a positive evaluation from the customers through the effective utilization of S–CSR, and the customers are self-motivated to promote that bank among their social media peers.

Limitations and Direction for Future Research

This study also has some limitations. The first limitation of the current study is that understanding human behavior is a difficult task due to its multidimensionality. Hence, explaining the complex customer behavior, which is similar to loyalty, only from the perspective of S–CSR, is not without concern. Therefore, future researchers are encouraged to include more variables in the proposed research model. In this regard, the authors suggest including customer green behavior, customer commitment for sustainability, and organizational image as independent or mediating variables for a better explanation of customer loyalty in future studies. Similarly, another limitation of the present study lies in the nature of the data, because the data are cross-sectional in nature, which limits the ability of the proposed relation(s) for causality. A remedy to address this limitation for future researchers is to use longitudinal data, which are able to explain the causal relationship in a better way, compared to cross-sectional data. Likewise, the present study only considered the positive effect of E-WOM on social media, but it neglected the negative effect of E-WOM on customer loyalty, which is very important to examine. Hence, future researchers need to examine the negative impact of W-WOM on customer loyalty. Furthermore, the present study deals with social media in a positive context, but the reality is that the emergence of social media also brings some challenges, such as information privacy being an issue in social media. Additionally, other challenges include information credibility and ethical issues. Future researchers need to deal with these types of issues in order to find solutions. Last but not the least, considering e-reputation risk for a bank is also an important variable that is not included in the present study, and hence, future researchers are suggested to consider this limitation in their future studies.

Author Contributions: All of the authors contributed to conceptualization, formal analysis, investigation, methodology, and writing and editing of the original draft equaly. All authors have read and agreed to the published version of the manuscript.

Funding: This research received no external funding.

Institutional Review Board Statement: Due to the observational nature of the study, and the absence of any involvement of therapeutic medication, no formal approval of the Institutional Review Board of the local Ethics Committee was required. Nonetheless, all subjects were informed about the study and participation was fully voluntary. Participants were ensured of confidentiality and anonymity of the information associated with the surveys. The study was conducted according to the guidelines of the Declaration of Helsinki.

Informed Consent Statement: Informed consent has been obtained from all subjects involved in this study to publish this paper.

Data Availability Statement: The datasets used in this research are available upon request from the corresponding author. The data are not publicly available due to restrictions, i.e., privacy or ethics.

Conflicts of Interest: The authors declare no conflict of interest.

References

1. Sharma, S.; Singh, S.; Kujur, F.; Das, G. Social Media Activities and its Influence on Customer-Brand Relationship: An Empirical Study of Apparel Retailers' Activity in India. *J. Theor. Appl. Electron. Commer. Res.* **2020**, *16*, 602–617. [CrossRef]
2. Shahbaznezhad, H.; Dolan, R.; Rashidirad, M. The Role of Social Media Content Format and Platform in Users' Engagement Behavior. *J. Interact. Mark.* **2021**, *53*, 47–65. [CrossRef]
3. Hajli, N. The impact of positive valence and negative valence on social commerce purchase intention. *Inf. Technol. People* **2019**, *33*, 774–791. [CrossRef]
4. Hajli, N.; Featherman, M.S. Social commerce and new development in e-commerce technologies. *Int. J. Inf. Manag.* **2017**, *37*, 177–178. [CrossRef]

5. Ma, L.; Zhang, X.; Ding, X.; Wang, G. How social ties influence customers' involvement and online purchase intentions. *J. Theor. Appl. Electron. Commer. Res.* **2020**, *16*, 395–408. [CrossRef]
6. Chatterjee, S.; Kar, A.K. Why do small and medium enterprises use social media marketing and what is the impact: Empirical insights from India. *Int. J. Inf. Manag.* **2020**, *53*, 102103. [CrossRef]
7. Voorveld, H.A. Brand communication in social media: A research agenda. *J. Advert.* **2019**, *48*, 14–26. [CrossRef]
8. Social, W.A. Digital 2020: 3.8 billion people use social media. *Dostupné* **2020**, *15*, 2020.
9. Ahmad, N.; Naveed, R.T.; Scholz, M.; Irfan, M.; Usman, M.; Ahmad, I. CSR Communication through Social Media: A Litmus Test for Banking Consumers' Loyalty. *Sustainability* **2021**, *13*, 2319. [CrossRef]
10. Wang, R.; Huang, Y. Communicating corporate social responsibility (CSR) on social media. *Corp. Commun. Int. J.* **2018**, *23*, 326–341. [CrossRef]
11. Sreejesh, S.; Sarkar, J.G.; Sarkar, A. CSR through social media: Examining the intervening factors. *Mark. Intell. Plan.* **2019**, *38*, 103–120. [CrossRef]
12. Kucukusta, D.; Perelygina, M.; Lam, W.S. CSR communication strategies and stakeholder engagement of upscale hotels in social media. *Int. J. Contemp. Hosp. Manag.* **2019**, *31*, 2129–2148. [CrossRef]
13. Carroll, A.B. Corporate social responsibility: Evolution of a definitional construct. *Bus. Soc.* **1999**, *38*, 268–295. [CrossRef]
14. Barauskaite, G.; Streimikiene, D. Corporate social responsibility and financial performance of companies: The puzzle of concepts, definitions and assessment methods. *Corp. Soc. Responsib. Environ. Manag.* **2021**, *28*, 278–287. [CrossRef]
15. Mahmood, A.; Bashir, J. How does corporate social responsibility transform brand reputation into brand equity? Economic and noneconomic perspectives of CSR. *Int. J. Eng. Bus. Manag.* **2020**, *12*, 1847979020927547. [CrossRef]
16. Kong, L.; Sial, M.; Ahmad, N.; Sehleanu, M.; Li, Z.; Zia-Ud-Din, M.; Badulescu, D. CSR as a potential motivator to shape employees' view towards nature for a sustainable workplace environment. *Sustainability* **2021**, *13*, 1499. [CrossRef]
17. George, N.A.; Aboobaker, N.; Edward, M. Corporate social responsibility and organizational commitment: Effects of CSR attitude, organizational trust and identification. *Soc. Bus. Rev.* **2020**, *15*, 255–272. [CrossRef]
18. Ahmad, N.; Scholz, M.; Ullah, Z.; Arshad, M.; Sabir, R.; Khan, W. The Nexus of CSR and Co-Creation: A Roadmap towards Consumer Loyalty. *Sustainability* **2021**, *13*, 523. [CrossRef]
19. Castro-González, S.; Bande, B.; Fernández-Ferrín, P.; Kimura, T. Corporate social responsibility and consumer advocacy behaviors: The importance of emotions and moral virtues. *J. Clean. Prod.* **2019**, *231*, 846–855. [CrossRef]
20. Shabib, F.; Ganguli, S. Impact of CSR on consumer behavior of Bahraini women in the cosmetics industry. *World J. Entrep. Manag. Sustain. Dev.* **2017**, *13*, 174–203. [CrossRef]
21. Sousa, B.; Silva, A.; Malheiro, A. Differentiation and market loyalty: An approach to cultural tourism in northern Portugal. In *Crisis Management for Software Development and Knowledge Transfer*; Metzler, J.B., Ed.; Springer: Singapore, 2019; pp. 681–690.
22. Brady, M.K.; Bourdeau, B.L.; Heskel, J. The importance of brand cues in intangible service industries: An application to investment services. *J. Serv. Mark.* **2005**, *19*, 401–410. [CrossRef]
23. Markovic, S.; Iglesias, O.; Singh, J.J.; Sierra, V. How does the perceived ethicality of corporate services brands influence loyalty and positive word-of-mouth? Analyzing the roles of empathy, affective commitment, and perceived quality. *J. Bus. Ethic.* **2015**, *148*, 721–740. [CrossRef]
24. Grönroos, C. Adopting a service logic for marketing. *Mark. Theory* **2006**, *6*, 317–333. [CrossRef]
25. Sierra, V.; Iglesias, O.; Markovic, S.; Singh, J.J. Does ethical image build equity in corporate services brands? The influence of customer perceived ethicality on affect, perceived quality, and equity. *J. Bus. Ethic.* **2015**, *144*, 661–676. [CrossRef]
26. Balmer, J.M.T. The Three virtues and seven deadly sins of corporate brand management. *J. Gen. Manag.* **2001**, *27*, 1–17. [CrossRef]
27. Raza, A.; Saeed, A.; Iqbal, M.K.; Saeed, U.; Sadiq, I.; Faraz, N.A. Linking corporate social responsibility to customer loyalty through co-creation and customer company identification: Exploring sequential mediation mechanism. *Sustainability* **2020**, *12*, 2525. [CrossRef]
28. Sun, H.; Rabbani, M.; Ahmad, N.; Sial, M.; Guping, C.; Zia-Ud-Din, M.; Fu, Q. CSR, co-creation and green consumer loyalty: Are green banking initiatives important? A moderated mediation approach from an emerging economy. *Sustainability* **2020**, *12*, 10688. [CrossRef]
29. Osakwe, C.N.; Yusuf, T.O. CSR: A roadmap towards customer loyalty. *Total Qual. Manag. Bus. Excel.* **2020**, 1–17. [CrossRef]
30. Poolthong, Y.; Mandhachitara, R. Customer expectations of CSR, perceived service quality and brand effect in Thai retail banking. *Int. J. Bank Mark.* **2009**, *27*, 408–427. [CrossRef]
31. McDonald, L.M.; Rundle-Thiele, S. Corporate social responsibility and bank customer satisfaction. *Int. J. Bank Mark.* **2008**, *26*, 170–182. [CrossRef]
32. McDonald, L.M.; Lai, C.H. Impact of corporate social responsibility initiatives on Taiwanese banking customers. *Int. J. Bank Mark.* **2011**, *29*, 50–63. [CrossRef]
33. Ajina, A.S.; Japutra, A.; Nguyen, B.; Alwi, S.F.S.; Al-Hajla, A.H. The importance of CSR initiatives in building customer support and loyalty. *Asia Pac. J. Mark. Logist.* **2019**, *31*, 691–713. [CrossRef]

34. Fatma, M.; Rahman, Z. Consumer responses to CSR in Indian banking sector. *Int. Rev. Public Nonprofit Mark.* **2016**, *13*, 203–222. [CrossRef]
35. Fatma, M.; Rahman, Z. The CSR's influence on customer responses in Indian banking sector. *J. Retail. Consum. Serv.* **2016**, *29*, 49–57. [CrossRef]
36. Khan, I.; Fatma, M. Connecting the dots between CSR and brand loyalty: The mediating role of brand experience and brand trust. *Int. J. Bus. Excell.* **2019**, *17*, 439–455. [CrossRef]
37. Tuan, L.T. Activating tourists' citizenship behavior for the environment: The roles of CSR and frontline employees' citizenship behavior for the environment. *J. Sustain. Tour.* **2018**, *26*, 1178–1203. [CrossRef]
38. Blau, P.M. *Social Exchange Theory*; John Wiley & Sons: New York, NY, USA, 1964; Volume 3, p. 62.
39. Gouldner, A.W. The Norm of Reciprocity: A Preliminary Statement. *Am. Sociol. Rev.* **1960**, *25*, 161. [CrossRef]
40. Jarvis, W.; Ouschan, R.; Burton, H.J.; Soutar, G.; O'Brien, I.M. Customer engagement in CSR: A utility theory model with moderating variables. *J. Serv. Theory Pr.* **2017**, *27*, 833–853. [CrossRef]
41. Fatma, M.; Khan, I.; Rahman, Z. CSR and consumer behavioral responses: The role of customer-company identification. *Asia Pac. J. Mark. Logist.* **2018**, *30*, 460–477. [CrossRef]
42. Badenes-Rocha, A.; Ruiz-Mafé, C.; Bigné, E. Engaging customers through user-and company-generated content on CSR. *Span. J. Mark. ESIC* **2019**, *23*, 339–372. [CrossRef]
43. Engerman, J.A.; Otto, R.F. The shift to digital: Designing for learning from a culturally relevant interactive media perspective. *Educ. Technol. Res. Dev.* **2021**, *69*, 301–305. [CrossRef] [PubMed]
44. Mohammed, A.; Al-Swidi, A. The influence of CSR on perceived value, social media and loyalty in the hotel industry. *Span. J. Mark. ESIC* **2019**, *23*, 373–396. [CrossRef]
45. Pérez, A.; Del Bosque, I.R. Corporate social responsibility and customer loyalty: Exploring the role of identification, satisfaction and type of company. *J. Serv. Mark.* **2015**, *29*, 15–25. [CrossRef]
46. Moisescu, O.-I. From CSR to Customer Loyalty: An Empirical Investigation in the Retail Banking Industry of a Developing Country. *Sci. Ann. Econ. Bus.* **2017**, *64*, 307–323. [CrossRef]
47. Shabbir, M.S.; Shariff, M.N.M.; Yusof, M.S.B.; Salman, R.; Hafeez, S. Corporate social responsibility and customer loyalty in Islamic banks of Pakistan: A mediating role of brand image. *Acad. Account. Financ. Stud. J.* **2018**, *22*, 1–6.
48. Aramburu, I.A.; Pescador, I.G. The effects of corporate social responsibility on customer loyalty: The mediating effect of reputation in cooperative banks versus commercial banks in the Basque country. *J. Bus. Ethic.* **2019**, *154*, 701–719. [CrossRef]
49. Prasad, S.; Garg, A.; Prasad, S. Purchase decision of generation Y in an online environment. *Mark. Intell. Plan.* **2019**, *37*. [CrossRef]
50. Kollat, J.; Farache, F. Achieving consumer trust on Twitter via CSR communication. *J. Consum. Mark.* **2017**, *34*, 505–514. [CrossRef]
51. Nyilasy, G. Word of mouth: What we really know and what we don't. In *Connected Marketing*; Routledge: Abington, UK, 2006; pp. 161–184.
52. Li, C.-Y. How social commerce constructs influence customers' social shopping intention? An empirical study of a social commerce website. *Technol. Forecast. Soc. Chang.* **2019**, *144*, 282–294. [CrossRef]
53. Romero, J.; Ruiz-Equihua, D. Be a part of it: Promoting WOM, eWOM, and content creation through customer identification. *Span. J. Mark. ESIC* **2020**, *24*, 55–72. [CrossRef]
54. Tseng, T.H.; Lee, C.T. Facilitation of consumer loyalty toward branded applications: The dual-route perspective. *Telemat. Inform.* **2018**, *35*, 1297–1309. [CrossRef]
55. Rialti, R.; Zollo, L.; Pellegrini, M.M.; Ciappei, C. Exploring the Antecedents of Brand Loyalty and Electronic Word of Mouth in Social-Media-Based Brand Communities: Do Gender Differences Matter? *J. Glob. Mark.* **2017**, *30*, 147–160. [CrossRef]
56. Ngoma, M.; Ntale, P.D. Word of mouth communication: A mediator of relationship marketing and customer loyalty. *Cogent Bus. Manag.* **2019**, *6*, 1580123. [CrossRef]
57. Ismagilova, E.; Slade, E.L.; Rana, N.P.; Dwivedi, Y.K. The Effect of Electronic Word of Mouth Communications on Intention to Buy: A Meta-Analysis. *Inf. Syst. Front.* **2020**, *22*, 1203–1226. [CrossRef]
58. Alhulail, H.; Dick, M.; Abareshi, A. The Influence of Word of Mouth on Customer Loyalty to Social Commerce Websites: Trust as a Mediator. In *Recent Trends in Data Science and Soft Computing, Proceedings of the 3rd International Conference of Reliable Information and Communication Technology (IRICT 2018), Kuala Lumpur, Malaysia, 23–24 June 2018*; Saeed, F., Gazem, N., Mohammed, F., Busalim, A., Eds.; Springer: Cham, Switzerland, 2018; pp. 1025–1033.
59. Khan, M.M.; Hashmi, H.B.A. Impact of interactivity of electronic word of mouth systems and website quality on customer e-loyalty. *Pak. J. Commer. Soc. Sci. (PJCSS)* **2016**, *10*, 486–504.
60. Hajli, N. Social commerce constructs and consumer's intention to buy. *Int. J. Inf. Manag.* **2015**, *35*, 183–191. [CrossRef]
61. Nadeem, W.; Juntunen, M.; Shirazi, F.; Hajli, N. Consumers' value co-creation in sharing economy: The role of social support, consumers' ethical perceptions and relationship quality. *Technol. Forecast. Soc. Chang.* **2020**, *151*, 119786. [CrossRef]
62. Chu, S.-C.; Chen, H.-T.; Gan, C. Consumers' engagement with corporate social responsibility (CSR) communication in social media: Evidence from China and the United States. *J. Bus. Res.* **2020**, *110*, 260–271. [CrossRef]

63. Fatma, M.; Ruiz, A.P.; Khan, I.; Rahman, Z. The effect of CSR engagement on eWOM on social media. *Int. J. Organ. Anal.* **2020**, *28*, 941–956. [CrossRef]
64. Schaefer, S.D.; Terlutter, R.; Diehl, S. Talking about CSR matters: Employees' perception of and reaction to their company's CSR communication in four different CSR domains. *Int. J. Advert.* **2019**, *39*, 191–212. [CrossRef]
65. Cheng, G.; Cherian, J.; Sial, M.; Mentel, G.; Wan, P.; Álvarez-Otero, S.; Saleem, U. The Relationship between CSR Communication on Social Media, Purchase Intention, and E-WOM in the Banking Sector of an Emerging Economy. *J. Theor. Appl. Electron. Commer. Res.* **2021**, *16*, 1025–1041. [CrossRef]
66. Khan, Z.; Ferguson, D.; Pérez, A. Customer responses to CSR in the Pakistani banking industry. *Int. J. Bank Mark.* **2015**, *33*, 471–493. [CrossRef]
67. Rastini, N.M.; Nurcaya, N. Customers trust mediation: Effect of CSR and service quality towards e-WOM. *Int. Res. J. Manag. IT Soc. Sci.* **2019**, *6*, 169–173. [CrossRef]
68. Abbas, M.; Gao, Y.; Shah, S.S.H. CSR and Customer Outcomes: The Mediating Role of Customer Engagement. *Sustainability* **2018**, *10*, 4243. [CrossRef]
69. Kuokkanen, H.; Sun, W. Companies, Meet Ethical Consumers: Strategic CSR Management to Impact Consumer Choice. *J. Bus. Ethic.* **2020**, *166*, 403–423. [CrossRef]
70. Pang, A.; Lwin, M.O.; Ng, C.S.-M.; Ong, Y.-K.; Chau, S.R.W.-C.; Yeow, K.P.-S. Utilization of CSR to build organizations' corporate image in Asia: Need for an integrative approach. *Asian J. Commun.* **2018**, *28*, 335–359. [CrossRef]
71. Hur, W.M.; Kim, H.; Kim, H.K. Does customer engagement in corporate social responsibility initiatives lead to customer citizenship behaviour? The mediating roles of customer-company identification and affective commitment. *Corp. Soc. Responsib. Environ. Manag.* **2018**, *25*, 1258–1269. [CrossRef]
72. Lacey, R.; Kennett-Hensel, P.A. Longitudinal Effects of Corporate Social Responsibility on Customer Relationships. *J. Bus. Ethic.* **2010**, *97*, 581–597. [CrossRef]
73. Ng, S.; David, M.E.; Dagger, T.S. Generating positive word-of-mouth in the service experience. *Manag. Serv. Qual. Int. J.* **2011**, *19*, 229–242. [CrossRef]
74. Popp, B.; Woratschek, H. Consumer–brand identification revisited: An integrative framework of brand identification, customer satisfaction, and price image and their role for brand loyalty and word of mouth. *J. Brand Manag.* **2017**, *24*, 250–270. [CrossRef]
75. Kudeshia, C.; Kumar, A. Social eWOM: Does it affect the brand attitude and purchase intention of brands? *Manag. Res. Rev.* **2017**, *40*, 310–330. [CrossRef]
76. Karjaluoto, H.; Munnukka, J.; Kiuru, K. Brand love and positive word of mouth: The moderating effects of experience and price. *J. Prod. Brand Manag.* **2016**, *25*, 527–537. [CrossRef]
77. Khan, S.A.; Ramzan, N.; Shoaib, M.; Mohyuddin, A. Impact of word of mouth on consumer purchase intention. *Age* **2015**, *18*, 78.
78. Serra-Cantallops, A.; Ramon-Cardona, J.; Salvi, F. The impact of positive emotional experiences on eWOM generation and loyalty. *Span. J. Mark. ESIC* **2018**, *22*, 142–162. [CrossRef]
79. Chu, S.-C.; Chen, H.-T. Impact of consumers' corporate social responsibility-related activities in social media on brand attitude, electronic word-of-mouth intention, and purchase intention: A study of Chinese consumer behavior. *J. Consum. Behav.* **2019**, *18*, 453–462. [CrossRef]
80. Ogunmokun, O.A.; Timur, S. Effects of the Awareness of University's CSR on Students' Word-of-Mouth Intentions. In Proceedings of the Global Joint Conference on Industrial Engineering and Its Application Areas, Gazimagusa, North Cyprus, 2–3 September 2019; pp. 133–147.
81. Van Asperen, M.; de Rooij, P.; Dijkmans, C. Engagement-based loyalty: The effects of social media engagement on customer loyalty in the travel industry. *Int. J. Hosp. Tour. Adm.* **2018**, *19*, 78–94. [CrossRef]
82. Eisingerich, A.B.; Rubera, G.; Seifert, M.; Bhardwaj, G. Doing Good and Doing Better despite Negative Information?: The Role of Corporate Social Responsibility in Consumer Resistance to Negative Information. *J. Serv. Res.* **2010**, *14*, 60–75. [CrossRef]
83. Kang, J.; Hustvedt, G. Building trust between consumers and corporations: The role of consumer perceptions of transparency and social responsibility. *J. Bus. Ethic.* **2014**, *125*, 253–265. [CrossRef]
84. Dagger, T.S.; David, M.E.; Ng, S. Do relationship benefits and maintenance drive commitment and loyalty? *J. Serv. Mark.* **2011**, *25*, 273–281. [CrossRef]
85. Iglesias, O.; Markovic, S.; Bagherzadeh, M.; Singh, J.J. Co-creation: A key link between corporate social responsibility, customer trust, and customer loyalty. *J. Bus. Ethic.* **2018**, *163*, 151–166. [CrossRef]
86. Harman, H.H. *Modern Factor Analysis*; University of Chicago Press: Chicago, IL, USA, 1976.
87. Fornell, C.; Larcker, D.F. Evaluating structural equation models with unobservable variables and measurement error. *J. Mark. Res.* **1981**, *18*, 39–50. [CrossRef]
88. Brown, T.J.; Dacin, P.A. The company and the product: Corporate associations and consumer product responses. *J. Mark.* **1997**, *61*, 68–84. [CrossRef]
89. Latif, K.F.; Pérez, A.; Sahibzada, U.F. Corporate social responsibility (CSR) and customer loyalty in the hotel industry: A cross-country study. *Int. J. Hosp. Manag.* **2020**, *89*, 102565. [CrossRef]
90. Tajvidi, M.; Wang, Y.; Hajli, N.; Love, P.E. Brand value Co-creation in social commerce: The role of interactivity, social support, and relationship quality. *Comput. Hum. Behav.* **2021**, *115*, 105238. [CrossRef]

91. Han, H.; Al-Ansi, A.; Chi, X.; Baek, H.; Lee, K.-S. Impact of Environmental CSR, Service Quality, Emotional Attachment, and Price Perception on Word-of-Mouth for Full-Service Airlines. *Sustainability* **2020**, *12*, 3974. [CrossRef]
92. D'Acunto, D.; Tuan, A.; Dalli, D.; Viglia, G.; Okumus, F. Do consumers care about CSR in their online reviews? An empirical analysis. *Int. J. Hosp. Manag.* **2020**, *85*, 102342. [CrossRef]

International Journal of
Environmental Research and Public Health

MDPI

Article

The Inter-Relation of Corporate Social Responsibility at Employee Level, Servant Leadership, and Innovative Work Behavior in the Time of Crisis from the Healthcare Sector of Pakistan

Naveed Ahmad [1,*], Miklas Scholz [2,3,4,*], Muhammad Zulqarnain Arshad [5], Syed Khuram Ali Jafri [6], Raja Irfan Sabir [1], Waris Ali Khan [7] and Heesup Han [8]

1 Faculty of Management Studies, University of Central Punjab, Lahore 54000, Pakistan; irfan.sabir@ucp.edu.pk
2 Department of Building and Environmental Technology, Division of Water Resources Engineering, Faculty of Engineering, Lund University, P.O. Box 118, 221 00 Lund, Sweden
3 Department of Civil Engineering Science, Kingsway Campus, School of Civil Engineering and the Built Environment, University of Johannesburg, Aukland Park 2006, Johannesburg PO Box 524, South Africa
4 Department of Town Planning, Engineering Networks and Systems, South Ural State University (National Research University), 76, Lenin prospekt, 454080 Chelyabinsk, Russia
5 Department of Management Sciences, Lahore Garrison University, Lahore 54000, Pakistan; muhammad.zulqarnain11@gmail.com
6 Department of Management Sciences, Bahria University, Lahore 54000, Pakistan; Skhurram.bulc@bahria.edu.pk
7 Faculty of Business, Economics, and Accountancy, Universti Malaysia Sabah, Sabah 88400, Malaysia; warissalikhan@gmail.com
8 College of Hospitality and Tourism Management, Sejong University, 98 Gunja-Dong, Gwanjin-Gu, Seoul 143-747, Korea; heesup.han@gmail.com
* Correspondence: naveeddgk2010@gmail.com (N.A.); miklas.scholz@tvrl.lth.se (M.S.)

Abstract: Organizational crisis can serve as a base to provide an opportunity to an organization for enhancing individuals, organizations, and communities. The healthcare sector is one of those sectors that remains under continuous pressure to provide high-quality service delivery to the patients. Hence, the requirement of innovation for this sector is huge when compared to other sectors. The majority of the previous studies have investigated the phenomenon of CSR at the employee's level (CSR-E) to influence employee behavior positively. However, the importance of CSR-E to enhance the innovative capability of the employees at the workplace is not well-explored in extant literature. Moreover, it is not clear from previous studies how the concept of servant leadership can explain the employee's engagement towards innovative work behavior (EIB). Thus, the current survey aims to test the relationship of CSR-E and EIB in the healthcare sector of Pakistan with the mediating effect of servant leadership. The data of the current study were obtained through a self-administered (paper-pencil) survey and they were analyzed through the structural equation modeling (SEM) technique. The empirical results of SEM analysis revealed that CSR-E and EIB are positively related and servant leadership partially mediates this relationship. The findings of the current study will be helpful for policymakers to improve their understanding towards CSR-E to induce EIB in the time of crisis. At the same time, the current study also highlights the importance of servant leadership to the policymakers in encouraging the employees to display their innovative capability at the workplace to serve their organization during the time of crisis.

Keywords: servant leadership; CSR-E; innovative work behavior; healthcare sector; servant employee

1. Introduction

Corporate social responsibility (CSR) has been of interest not only to the academician but also to business professionals [1]. CSR has become a reality in the industry and caring about the well-being of the environment, and the community has emerged as an important factor in organizational planning [2]. CSR is a strategic decision that an organization takes the environmental issues into account and is accountable to the community, for example, in the form of support and commitment to the local community [3]. Recent CSR approaches have changed the organization's approach to revenue generation and improved their business profiles in terms of environmental, economic, social, legal, regulatory, and organizational objectives [4]. A plethora of previous studies have extensively explored CSR from a macro-level perspective [5–8]. However, the impact of CSR strategies at the level of employees (CSR-E) is not well-explored in previous literature. It is quite recent that research has shifted from the macro-level CSR to the micro-level, highlighting how CSR affects the attitudes and behaviors of employees [9–11]. Micro-CSR is a study of the results and experience of CSR strategies on employees at workplaces evaluated at different levels of individuals [12].

The dynamic business environment in the recent era has forced organizations to quickly adjust their strategies to become more competitive. Innovation is one of the most important strategies for organizations to ensure success [13]. It is worth mentioning here that employees are the real innovators, not the organizations, and perhaps this is the reason that recent research studies are stressing the importance of employees' innovative work behavior (EIB) [14–16]. Successful organizations encourage their employees to display their innovative capabilities at workplaces [17]. EIB is a special form of employee behavior that is important for organizational outcomes including survival and growth [18]. An employee's innovative work behavior is all about the initiation and implementation of an idea, and it is well-differentiated with the concept of creativity that only considers the novelty and usefulness of an idea [19].

Research has considerably established that CSR is helpful to achieve different employee-related outcomes, for example, employee's satisfaction [20,21], employee's psychological capital [22], employee's well-being [23], employee's commitment [24], employee's engagement [25], etcetera. However, when compared to external stakeholders, studies on internal stakeholders (employees in the present case) are still sparse. In this context, few studies have been specifically conducted examining the effects of CSR on employee's attitudes and behavior [26,27]. However, it is not clear from extant literature why CSR motivates employees to the desired behavior and attitudes. It is important to understand how CSR affects employee behavior and performance, as employees are directly involved in the implementation and execution of CSR measures and can consider resources that are related to CSR policy, depending on the impact and duration of this policy [28]. EIB is complex, because, when an employee introduces an idea, he or she has to face different hurdles, for example, insecurity, resistance from other employees, fear of failure, and lack of resources [29]. Therefore, it is even more important to look at the employee's underlying mechanism for EIB.

CSR is an integral part of business strategies and it has a long-lasting impact on the employees to induce their performance [30]. CSR engagement of an organization promotes fairness and honesty at the workplace and employees believe that their organization will reliability and psychological security, where employees can act without fear of consequences and take risks [31]. Thus, CSR promotes a work environment that has a significant impact on employees' innovative capability [32]. Moreover, different research studies have also established that the phenomenon of servant leadership promotes EIB [33–35]. However, it is not known from existing research studies how the concept of servant leadership and CSR-E can encourage the employees to display EIB. Therefore, exploring the relationship of CSR-E and EIB with a mediating effect of servant leadership in the healthcare sector of Pakistan during the time of crisis is the objective of the current survey. The proposed research model is presented in Figure 1.

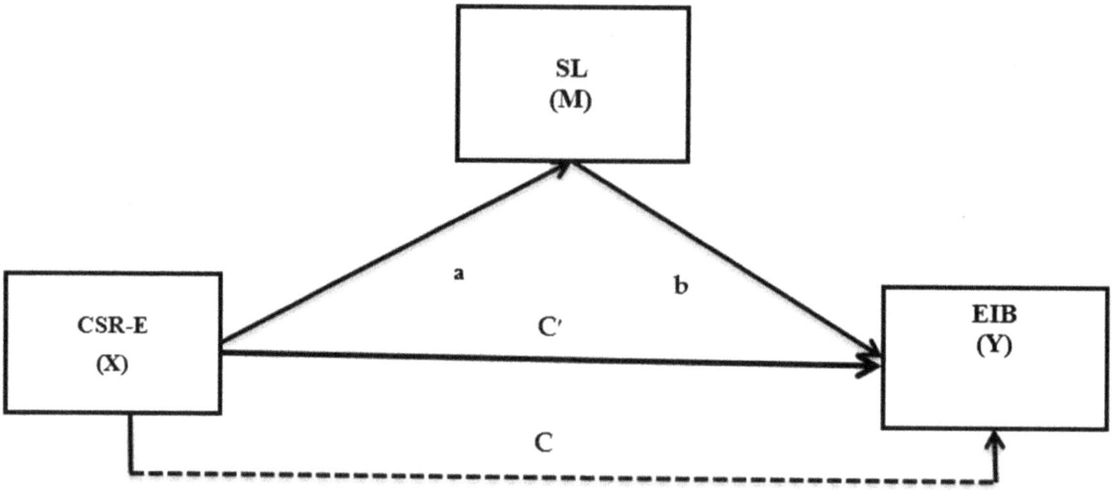

Figure 1. The proposed research model, based on the authors' conception. This model comprises three variables, corporate social responsibility at the employee level (CSR-E) = the independent variable (X), servant leadership (SL) = the mediating variable (M), and employee innovative work behavior (EIB) = the dependent variable (Y).

The healthcare sector of Pakistan was purposefully selected to serve the objectives of the current survey due to some specific reasons. First, the healthcare sector of Pakistan is a kind of service industry that continuously faces a challenge to provide high-quality health-related services to patients. This high-quality service deliverance is only possible when this sector is willing to continuously adapt to new and innovative ways to serve the patients [36,37]. In this regard, the current research study argues that employees are an important source in providing innovative solutions in an organization and, hence, seeking to enhance EIB in healthcare organizations is not without logic. This importance of employees as a source of innovation is also supported by extant researchers [38–40]. Second, the healthcare sector represents a classic case in which the duration of employee–patient interaction is when as compared to other segments as healthcare employees keep in touch with the patients even for several weeks during their stay in a hospital [41,42]. Therefore, they can play an important role in innovation, because, during their interaction with patients, they observe and learn new things to perform a task innovatively. Likewise, they sometimes get new ideas from patients as well, which again highlights the importance of employees as a source of innovation for this sector. Third, the stiff situation of competitiveness in the healthcare sector of Pakistan also demands continuous innovation, because, through innovative ways of doing things, a hospital is capable of overrunning its rivals. Because, as per the findings of Porter [43], in an industry where the level of rivalry is high, innovation is a key strategic enabler that provides a strong competitive advantage to an organization over its rivals.

There are some state-of-the-art contributions of the current survey to extant literature. First of all, the current survey adds to the existing literature of CSR and organizational management by acknowledging the employees as a source of innovation. The majority of the past studies have investigated the impact of CSR to achieve different organizational outcomes [44–48]; however, the relationship of CSR-E to foster EIB is barely addressed by extant researchers. Further, it is not clear from extant studies how servant leadership can be linked with EIB. Although there have been some studies on this topic [49–51], studies have produced mixed findings that highlight that there is more need for research in this area. Finally, the majority of the past studies have explored CSR relationships with employees in other sectors, like hospitality [52,53], banking sector [54], and small and medium-sized enterprises [55]; however, the healthcare sector did not receive due attention. The remainder of this article is composed in the following parts. The coming part discusses the literature review and theoretical support. After this, there comes the methodology part, in which the authors have discussed the sampling and data collection process along with instrument details. The last two parts discuss results and discussion for hypotheses testing, discussion, and implications.

2. Theory and Hypotheses

The current survey uses the lenses of social learning theory [56] and social identity theory [57] to explain the proposed relationship and formulate hypotheses. Social learning theory states that individuals learn different things by observing others. In this regard, when employees observe the helping behavior of their leader (servant leader) at the workplace, they imitate his behavior and practice this on their part. In the context of the current study, the employees are expected to help their organization by performing extra roles. One such extra role is to display the innovative capability of the employees. The servant leaders are likely to set an example of role-model for their employees by helping, promoting, and encouraging the employees at workplaces. Similarly, CSR philosophy also stresses the betterment of different stakeholders, and employees are important internal stakeholders. Thus, an organization that follows CSR principles, is expected to help and support its workers. In response, employees feel an extraordinary motivation to help their organization and, hence, they try their level best to think of new and innovative ways to help their organization. Moreover, social identity theory focuses on the interplay between personal and social identities. This theory attempts to explain and predict different circumstances for which people think of themselves as individuals or as a member of certain groups. In other words, social identity theory states that individuals are expected to categorize others based on some characteristics. In the scenario of the current survey, as the servant leader focuses on the betterment of followers, thus a strong bond of belongingness is developed that encourages motivating the employees to advance their thinking to achieve different organizational goals. Hence, the dyadic relationship between a servant leader and the employee works as a base of motivation for employees to display their innovative capabilities to enhance the overall efficiency of the group that they belong to or they identify themselves (the organization in this case).

Businesses that follow CSR principles focus on remaining profitable, comply with the law, adhere to the code of ethics, protect the environment, and ensure the larger benefit of society [58]. The current research study defines CSR as per the definition of Carroll [59], who described it as the actions taken by organizations to take care of diverse stakeholders, such as the environment, the community, and government agencies. Based on this definition, the organization must work to protect the well-being of the entire community and improve its interests and the preservation and care of nature [60]. Organizations need to publish CSR strategies and inform stakeholders about their genuine efforts to improve society and the environment [28]. It is worth mentioning that earning a positive CSR perception from stakeholders is very important for every organization. This is important because if stakeholders' CSR perception of an organization is not positive, they will feel that the organization's engagement in CSR is only symbolic, which leads to igniting negativity among stakeholders [61]. In this regard, employees are one of the most important stakeholders in an organization, so their CSR perspective is very important [62]. EIB is defined as "the behavior of individuals intended to initiate and deliberately create new and useful ideas or processes at the workplace" [63]. Employees' CSR perceptions of an organization positively influence their behavior [26,64]. Employees are proud to be a member of an organization when they see that the organization is engaged in CSR for the benefit of society and the environment and is ethically responsible [65]. The CSR engagement of an organization creates a sense of confidence and security, where employees can act without fear of consequences and take risks [66]. When employees are risk-takers, they are not inclined to perform routine tasks, rather, they are engaged to invent new ways of doing things at workplaces, which ultimately enhances their innovative capability [17,67].

The atmosphere of the workplace has a significant impact on the innovative capability of employees [68]. In an organization where the safety and mental stability of employees are encouraged, it is likely to expect that employees to come up with new and innovative ideas. A plethora of previous research studies establishes that CSR-E is positively related to EIB [31,53,69,70]. The CSR activities of an organization foster an environment of confidence among the employees and this sense of confidence urges them to take risks and think about innovative ways to induce organizational effectiveness [71]. Employees who see that an organization's CSR efforts are focused on improving the community and the environment have a greater sense of 'meaningful work', which, in turn, improves productivity and creativity [72]. Effective socially responsible organizations provide their employees with open and free employment opportunities to produce innovative solutions for the organization [73]. As a result, an employee's perception of CSR for the organization improves his motivation to try new ideas, and that they can take a step forward in the implementation of these ideas due to a supportive organizational environment [74]. Different researchers in the extant literature have also acknowledged that CSR is positively related to EIB. As an instance, Li, et al. [69], conducted a research study to investigate the impact of CSRE on service innovation performance with EIB as a mediating variable and came out with the results that CSRE directly, and via EIB, enhances EIB in the service sector. Likewise, Li, Zhang, Wu, and Peng [70] verified, in their research study, that CSR-E can foster the innovative behavior of employees at the workplace in Taiwan. Moreover, Ratajczak and Szutowski [75] also confirmed that an organization's CSR activities are directly related to employee's innovation performance. Several other scholars also hold the same argument that CSR is positively related to EIB [76–79].

In line with social identity theory, when employees recognize the social responsibility of the organization in which they work, they positively identify themselves with such organizations and they are urged to enhance the overall progress of their organization by thinking of new ways to perform different organizational tasks. Given the above discussion, it is established that, when an employee realizes that the organization is involved in CSR for the betterment of society and the environment, it may affect work-related behavior such as EIB. Thus, the authors propose the following hypothesis.

Hypothesis 1 (H1). *CSR-E and EIB are positively related.*

Servant leadership is a style of leadership in which corporate leaders serve and help others to achieve different development opportunities, prepare subordinates for their best, and, ultimately, support their organization in achieving organizational success [80]. Servant leadership is a concept that is rooted in the philosophy of "serving others". A servant leader puts the needs and interests of his followers first and is focused on caring for others, including society as a whole [81]. This description reflects the extent to which a servant leader has a deliberate focus on the interests and well-being, relationships with employees, organizational care, and the larger benefit of the community [82]. Serving others comes first in servant leadership. They deliver guidance to the followers for their development and growth and they have a positive impact on their behavior, ethics, and performance [83]. Previous research has confirmed that servant leadership has a positive impact on EIB [35,49,50,84], which, in turn, helps to understand the relationship between employee leadership and EIB.

An important drive of servant leadership is to serve stakeholders and, hence, a servant leader sets an example to the followers to become a "servant employee" who tries to help the organization by engaging himself in innovative activities [50]. Innovation is multi-faceted in that it requires different tasks and individual behavior at each stage, involving the generation, promotion, and implementation of new ideas. During this process, a person first comes up with ideas or solutions to the identified problems. These ideas and solutions can be borrowed from different sources. The later step is to come up with a legitimate approach or solution by seeking the support of the organization [85]. Past literature in the field of organizational ethics has shown that the formation of a strong work ethic creates positive ethics and helping behavior among employees [86,87]. In particular, the innovative capability of employees is closely linked to the ethical context, as the values of "accepted work ethic" grow in the context of "participatory thinking" related to innovation, which is regarded as the ability of employees to evaluate, understanding of the situation, as well as the workplace as a whole [88,89].

By the same token, the concept of CSR also stresses caring for others (society, stakeholders, nature, etc.) and, hence, an organization's engagement in CSR activities inculcates a sense of caring among workers [90]. Employees working for a socially responsible organization are likely to develop a kind of spiritual consciousness that ultimately encourages them towards creativity and innovation [73]. According to the theory of social learning, employees perceive their servant leaders as role models and imitate their helping behavior on their part. Thus, because of the leadership effect of a servant leader, the behavior of employees is also molded, and they want to engage themselves in extra-role behaviors (innovative work behavior) to help their organization to achieve business excellence. Moreover, as per social identity theory, the employees feel positive to identify themselves with a socially responsible organization. Thus, as a member of such an organization, they put every effort to enhance the group image (organizational image). Hence, CSR-E and servant leadership both support employees to be engaged in EIB. The above discussion and theoretical support lead the authors to frame the following hypotheses.

Hypothesis 2 (H2). *Servant leadership is positively related to EIB.*

Hypothesis 3 (H3). *Servant leadership mediates between CSR-E and EIB.*

3. Methodology

The current research study selected the healthcare sector of Pakistan to test the proposed relationships. To do this, the authors selected four large hospitals from the city of Lahore in Pakistan. These four hospitals included Hijaz hospital (HH), Pakistan Kidney and Liver Institute and Research Centre (PKLI), Shaukat Khanum Memorial Cancer Hospital and Research Centre (SKMCH&RC), and Iqraa Medical Complex. There were specific reasons for choosing these hospitals, such as all of these hospitals are engaged in different CSR-related activities. Moreover, these are state-of-the-art hospitals that deal with a large number of patients around the clock and employ thousands of employees. Likewise, these hospitals are actively engaged in arranging different training sessions for their employees for their skill development, which shows they are concerned with employees. Lastly, these hospitals use, up-to-date technology in their procedures that is an indication of their innovation preference. Hence, the selection of these hospitals is not without logic.

Before starting the actual data analysis phase, the authors contacted spokespersons of the selected hospitals to seek their support and permission to collect the data from their staff. The authors also signed an agreement with the ethical bodies of these hospitals to maintain ethical standards in the process of data collection. Further, the authors obtained informed consent from every respondent to participate in the survey voluntarily. The respondents were also given a choice to quit the survey at any stage if they do not feel comfortable. After seeking formal approval from the officials of each hospital, the authors arranged for the data collection process. The wake of Covid-19 posed serious challenges for the authors during the process of data collection and, hence, the authors had to arrange for special protocols in this regard. Thus, the authors had to stay for long hours in hospitals for the sake of data collection. The data were collected from the respondents during January 2021. The authors distributed a total of 900 surveys among the respondents of these four hospitals and received back 431 surveys from different respondents. Hence, the response rate of the current survey was 47.88%. The data were collected in two waves with a time-lagged difference of two weeks. This study followed the ethical guidelines given in Helsinki Declaration. The authors also obtained approval from the ethical committee of PKLI.

Measures and Handling of Social Desirability

The current survey used already established scales to measures the constructs. Thus, the issue of validity and reliability was non-existent here, because adapted scales have their pre-established validity and reliability. The scale of CSR-E was taken from Schaufeli and Bakker [91], which consisted of three items. Similarly, a seven-item scale of servant leadership was taken from the study of Liden, et al. [92]; likewise, the scale of EIB was taken from Hu, et al. [93], and this scale consisted of six items. The authors used a five-point Likert scale for the current survey.

The authors took several measures to address the issue of social desirability. For example, the survey items were randomly scattered throughout the questionnaire. The authors did this in order to break any sequence of answering the responses by the respondents. This step is also helpful in dealing with the likelihood of any liking and disliking for a particular construct. Likewise, the instrument was checked for accuracy and suitability by experts in the field. This step is necessary in order to address any ambiguity or confusion in any item statement due to complex or dual-meaning words. Likewise, the authors requested the respondents for their true response, so that the findings generated by their input may reflect the reality. Different scholars also recommend these steps to mitigate the level of social desirability [10,11,94,95]. Table 1 presents the demographic detail of the sample.

Table 1. Demographic detail.

Demographic	Frequency	%
Gender		
Male	246	57.08
Female	185	42.92
Age-group (Year)		
18–25	56	12.99
26–30	109	25.29
31–35	126	29.23
36–40	77	17.86
Above 40	63	14.62
Experience (Years)		
1–4	66	15.31
5–7	117	27.15
8–10	128	29.70
Above 10	120	27.84
Total	**431**	**100**

4. Results

4.1. Common Method Variance

Since all of the information in the current survey was obtained from the same individual, there is a possibility that the issue of common method variance (CMV) may exist in the dataset. Hence, to validate whether the issue of CMV does exist, the authors performed Harman single-factor-analysis (SFA). The authors allowed all of the items to converge on a single-factor to detect CMV, according to the guidelines of Harman [96]. The general guideline here is that, if the results of SFA confirm the presence of any single-factor that is dominant and explains more than 50% of the total variance, then it is evident that CMV is a potential issue to be addressed by the researchers. In the current scenario, the results of SFA confirmed that there is no such factor that explains more than 50% of the total variance. The largest variance that was explained in the case of the current survey was 44.68% which is less than 50%. Hence, based on the results of SFA it is verified that there is no issue of CMV in the dataset of the current survey.

4.2. Convergent Validity, Factor Loadings, and the Reliability Analyses

The authors started the data analysis phase by performing different tests after validating that there is no issue of CMV in the current survey. The results of these tests are reported in Table 2, which includes the results of convergent validity, reliability analysis, and factor loadings. The convergent validity was assessed on the basis of average-variance-extracted (AVE) values. To achieve this, the authors took the sum of squares of all loadings and dividing by the number of items. For example, the sum of square loadings for CSR-E was 1.81, which was divided by the number of factors (1.81/3) that resulted in 0.60 as AVE value for CSR-E. The general rule for convergent validity is that if the value of AVE for a variable is larger than 0.5 then it is established that the criterion for convergent validity for that variable is fulfilled. Likewise, the authors have also reported the factor loading for each variable in Table 2. To this end, all of the loadings were well above the minimum threshold of 0.40. Lastly, Table 2 also contains the results of reliability that were observed through Cronbach alpha (α) values and composite reliability values (C.R). The α values were obtained through SPSS software whereas, C.R values were calculated using AMOS software during confirmatory factor analysis (CFA). It is to be noted that both reliability values are important to calculate, but Cronbach alpha (α) is an average measure of inter-item consistency that is preferred during exploratory factor analysis. However, calculating and reporting composite reliability is a modern way to conduct reliability analysis and it is more preferred by contemporary researchers. Both types of reliabilities were significant (both α and C.R were > 0.70)

Table 2. Item loadings, convergent validity, and reliability results.

Item	Loadings	Square	S.S	AVE	α	C.R
CSR-E1	0.74	0.55				
CSR-E2	0.78	0.61				
CSR-E3	0.81	0.66	1.81	0.60	0.73	0.75
SL-1	0.69	0.48				
SL-2	0.73	0.53				
SL-3	0.78	0.61				
SL-4	0.71	0.50				
SL-5	0.81	0.66				
SL-6	0.76	0.58				
SL-7	0.77	0.59	3.94	0.56	0.78	0.77
EIB-1	0.66	0.44				
EIB-2	0.74	0.82				
EIB-3	0.72	0.82				
EIB-4	0.75	0.74				
EIB-5	0.68	0.66				
EIB-6	0.79	0.74	4.22	0.70	0.86	0.84

Notes: Loadings = factor loadings, α = Cronbach alpha, C.R = composite reliability, square = square of item loading, S.S = sum of square.

In the next stage of data analysis, the authors validated whether the data-based model fits the theoretical model or not. To assess this, the authors performed CFA in AMOS and checked the results of different model-fit-indices (χ^2/df = 3.521, RMSEA = 0.059, NFI = 0.961, CFI = 0.928, IFI = 0.922, TLI = 0.957, and GFI = 0.927). The results of model-fit-indices are reported in Table 3 for the readers against their acceptability range. The results validated that there is a good fit between theory and the data. Thus, there is no issue of model-fit in the dataset of the current survey. Table 3 also presents the results of correlation analysis. According to these outcomes, all constructs are showing positive correlations. As a case, one can see that the correlation between CSR-E and SL is 0.27 **, which is positive and significant, confirming that these variables are positively related to each other. Next, the authors verified whether the criterion of discriminant validity (DSV) is established in the case of the dataset of the current study. To do this, the authors calculated the square-root of AVE (SQAVE) for each construct and compared it with the values of correlation in comparison. To explain further, the SQAVE value for CSR-E is 0.78, which is above the correlation values (0.27 **, 0.32 **). These results provide enough support to accept that the items of a construct discriminate with the items of other construct and, thus, the criterion of discriminant validity is established.

Table 3. Correlation, discriminant validity, and model fit indices.

Construct	Mean	S.D	CSR-E	SL	EIB
CSR-E	4.21	0.72	**0.78**	0.27 **	0.32 **
SL	4.07	0.68		**0.75**	0.35 **
EIB	4.29	0.53			**0.84**
Model fit indices	Range	Obtained	Model fit indices	Range	Obtained
χ^2/df	5.00	3.521	IFI	0.90	0.922
RMSEA	0.08	0.059	TLI	0.95	0.957
NFI	0.95	0.961	GFI	0.90	0.927
CFI	0.90	0.928			

Notes: S.D = standard deviation, ** = significant values of correlation, bold diagonal = discriminant validity results.

4.3. Hypotheses Testing

The authors continued with the data analysis to validate the hypotheses of the current survey. To do this, the authors used the structural equation modeling (SEM) technique in AMOS. SEM is an advanced level technique for data analysis to evaluate complex models, as is the case with the current research study. Further, SEM analysis is a co-variance-based analysis approach that is very popular among contemporary researchers [97–99], due to its advanced level features when compared to the conventional regression-based technique of data analysis. The authors in this connection performed SEM analysis in two stages. The first stage of SEM started with checking the direct effect analysis in which there was no intervention of any mediator in the model. Table 4 shows the results of the direct effect model. As per these results, the direct effect model produced significant results. These results confirmed that the first two Hypotheses (H1) and (H2) of the current survey are supported. These outcomes were declared on the basis of beta estimates and *p*-values ($\beta1 = 0.31$, $\beta2 = 0.38$, $p < 0.05$). The results further validated that the effect of SL on EIB is stronger as compared to the effect of CSR-E on EIB. Moreover, the model-fit-indices were also significant in this regard ($\chi^2/df = 3.192$, RMSEA = 0.051, NFI = 0.968, CFI = 0.936, IFI = 0.931, TLI = 0.960, and GFI = 0.931).

Table 4. The results for Hypotheses (H1) and (H2).

Path	Estimates	S.E	CR	*p*-Value	ULCI	LLCI	Decision
CSR-E → EIB	(β1) 0.31 **	0.046	6.74	***	0.210	0.639	Approved
SL → EIB	(β2) 0.38 **	0.051	7.45	***	0.315	0.521	Approved
Model fit indices	Criteria	Obtained	Model fit indices	Range	Obtained		
χ^2/df	5.00	3.192	IFI	0.90	0.931	R^2	0.24 * (H1) 0.28 * (H2)
RMSEA	0.08	0.051	TLI	0.95	0.960		
NFI	0.95	0.968	GFI	0.90	0.931		
CFI	0.90	0.936					

Notes: ULCI = upper-limit confidence interval, LLCI = lower-limit confidence interval, **, ***, * = significant values.

The second stage of SEM analysis was carried out with the inclusion of SL as the mediating variable. To test the effect of mediation, the authors use the bootstrapping method in AMOS by using a large bootstrapping sample of 2000. The bootstrapping method is more sophisticated as compared to the previous mediation analysis that was suggested by Baron and Kenny [100], which is criticized by different scholars, including Hayes [101] and Zhao, et al. [102]. The output of bootstrapping approach confirmed the mediation effect of SL between CSR-E and EIB. It is to be noted that the beta estimate, which was earlier 0.31 during the direct effect model (CSR-E → EIB), is reduced ($\beta3 = 0.037$ **), which is an indication that SL partially mediates between CSR-E and EIB. The further detail of bootstrapping is presented in Table 5 for the readers

Table 5. Mediation and moderation results for Hypotheses (H3) and (H4.)

Path	Estimates	S.E	Z-Score	*p*-Value	ULCI	LLCI	Decision
CSR-E → ELS → EPB	(β3) 0.037 **	0.017	2.18	***	0.119	0.216	Approved
Model fit indices	Criteria	Obtained	Model fit indices	Range	Obtained		
χ^2/df	5.00	1.86	IFI	0.90	0.940	R^2	0.32
RMSEA	0.08	0.033	TLI	0.95	0.968		
NFI	0.95	0.978	GFI	0.90	0.947		
CFI	0.90	0.952					

Notes: ULCI = upper-limit confidence interval, LLCI = lower-limit confidence interval, **, ***, = significant values, S.E = standard error.

5. Discussion and Implications

The current survey was carried out to serve two major objectives. The first objective of the current survey was to test the relationship between CSR-E and EIB in the healthcare sector of Pakistan in times of crisis. To this end, the empirical results of the current survey validated that CSR engagement of a hospital at the level of the employee helps to enhance the innovative behavior of employees at the workplace. The respondents of the current survey were of the opinion that, when they realize that their hospital is concerned to work for the betterment of society and the environment, they positively identify themselves with such a hospital. Thus, CSR-E positively relates to EIB in the context of the healthcare sector of Pakistan. Different researchers in the existing literature also support this argument that CSR-E and EIB are positively associated with each other [31,32,53,69]. This relationship can also be explained in the light of social identity theory. As per this theory, the employees working in a socially responsible hospital positively identify themselves as a member of the group (the hospital in this case). Thus, they put every effort into enhancing the effectiveness of their hospital via their engagement in different innovative activities. Further, the employees of a socially responsible organization develop a sense of security and fairness at the workplace and, hence, they do not hesitate to take risks for the betterment of their organization. Therefore, they think about new ideas without the fear of failure to better serve their organization and come up with new ideas especially in the time of crisis.

The second objective of the current study was to test the mediating effect of Servant leadership between CSR-E and EIB. The empirical results in this regard confirmed that servant leadership partially mediates the relationship between CSR-E and EIB. The respondents of the current survey established that the helping behavior of their leader (servant leader) encourages them to adopt such behavior on their part. Thus, a servant leader helps to transmit the sense of "servant employees" among the followers. A servant employee, like a servant leader, puts the organizational interest at the fore-front and wants to help his organization through extra-role behavior. One example of such extra-role behavior is the innovative work behavior of employees. The current study is not the first one to confirm this relationship, as different previous scholars have also confirmed that a servant leader inculcates innovative work behavior in employees [35,50,83,84]. The theory of social learning can also be related to further explain this finding. From the perspective of social learning theory, when employees see that their leader keeps the benefits and development of employees at the fore-front, they also learn this behavior on their part. Hence, after learning this behavior from their servant leader, they are motivated to perform extra-role for their organization and think of new ways to perform a task in a hospital. Likewise, the CSR orientation of a hospital also promotes a sense of caring for others among the employees. Therefore, both CSR-E and servant leadership encourage the workers to display innovative behavior in the workplace.

The current survey has some important theoretical implications to the existing literature on CSR and organizational management. In this regard, the first theoretical contribution of the current research study is that it enriches the existing literature to promote EIB through CSR-E. In this context, there have been some studies confirming that CSR activities at the employee level help an organization to positively influence the behavior of employees [26,27,86]. However, the relationship between CSR-E and EIB is sparse in the extant literature. Accordingly, this theoretical contribution adds significantly to the existing literature. The second theoretical contribution of the current research study is that it introduces the concept of servant leadership as a mediator between the relationship of CSR-E and

EIB. The majority of the previous studies have established the relationship of CSR-E and EIB [53,69] and servant leadership with EIB separately [35,50]. However, this study investigates their impact on EIB in a single model. Finally, the current study adds to the scant literature of CSR in the field of the healthcare sector, whereas the previous study in the majority, explored CSR in different sectors rather than focusing on the healthcare sector.

The practical implications of the current survey are also important for policymakers, especially from the healthcare sector. In this regard, the findings of the current research study are of utmost importance for the healthcare sector to consider their employees as a source of innovation. This implication has a special consideration for the healthcare sector which is under continuous pressure from patients to provide high-quality services. The authors' argument here is that, without innovation, this high-quality deliverance of service is challenging. The current state of innovation in the majority of healthcare organizations in Pakistan focuses on enhancing innovation through the adaptation of new technologies. Although it is important to consider the latest technology for a hospital to overrun the competitors, policymakers are suggested to note that employees are an even better and low-cost source of innovation. Moreover, as the employees in healthcare organizations interact with patients very closely, so it is likely to expect that, during this interaction, they can develop new ways (innovative) to better serve the patients. Another important practical implication of the current study is that it highlights the importance of servant leadership to encourage the employees at workplaces to be engaged in innovative work behavior. To this end, policymakers are suggested to arrange for special sessions and training with their managers to let them realize the importance of servant leadership for employee's innovative work behavior. Last but not least, the policymakers can benefit from the findings of the current study to upgrade their understanding of CSR to encourage the employees at workplaces to be engaged in innovative behaviors.

Limitations and Potential Research Directions

Although the existing study offers adequate grounds to accept the proposed research model and relationships among variables, some limitations will need to be addressed by future researchers. The first limitation of this analysis is that it attempts to explain employees' behavior through CSR-E and servant leadership. Although these variables are important to consider in explaining the behavior of employees, it is worth mentioning here that individual behavior is quite complex to understand. Hence, future researchers are suggested to consider other important variables in the proposed model of this study. For example, psychological contract and job autonomy may be important variables for future researchers to better explain employee innovative behavior. Likewise, this research study only considered hospitals that were located in Lahore city and, thus, the geographical concentration increases questions regarding the generalizability of this research. As a way to deal with this limitation, the prospective researchers are encouraged to consider a diverse sample of hospitals from different cities. Another limitation of this analysis is that it used cross-sectional data and, hence, forecasting causality based on cross-sectional data entails specific risks. Thus, future studies will need to consider the longitudinal data design.

6. Conclusions

The current study highlights the importance of CSR engagement of a hospital at the level of employees to foster workplace innovation. In this regard, the policymakers from the healthcare sector of Pakistan are encouraged to rethink CSR as a strategic enabler to foster the EIB of a hospital. Currently, in the majority of the healthcare institutions of Pakistan, CSR is kept limited to the extent of philanthropic orientation. This research argues that this is the time to shift from this thinking of philanthropic orientation of CSR to new areas, including workplace innovation. Moreover, the policymakers of the healthcare organizations are also encouraged to have a special focus on the style of leadership in their organizations, because, as per the empirical findings of the current survey, an appropriate leadership style, like servant leadership, is necessary to cultivate an environment in which employees are encouraged to display their innovative capability at the workplace.

Author Contributions: N.A., M.S., M.Z.A., S.K.A.J., R.I.S., W.A.K. and H.H. contributed to conceptualization, formal analysis, investigation, methodology, and writing and editing of the original draft. All authors have read and agreed to the published version of the manuscript.

Funding: This research received no external funding.

Institutional Review Board Statement: This study was conducted as per the ethical guidelines given in Helsinki Declaration. The authors also got approval from the ethical committee of Pakistan Kidney and Liver institute and research center, Pakistan.

Informed Consent Statement: Informed consent was obtained from the respondents of the survey.

Data Availability Statement: The data will be made available on request from the corresponding author.

Conflicts of Interest: The authors declare no conflict of interest.

References

1. Singh, A.; Anand, A.; Jaswal, N. Implementing University/Academicians' Social Responsibility Conceptual Framework in Medical Colleges. *Ann. Neurosci.* **2019**, *26*, 8–9. [CrossRef]
2. Silvius, A.G.; Kampinga, M.; Paniagua, S.; Mooi, H. Considering sustainability in project management decision making; An investigation using Q-methodology. *Int. J. Proj. Manag.* **2017**, *35*, 1133–1150. [CrossRef]
3. Manzoor, F.; Wei, L.; Nurunnabi, M.; Subhan, Q.A.; Shah, S.I.A.; Fallatah, S. The impact of transformational leadership on job performance and CSR as mediator in SMEs. *Sustainability* **2019**, *11*, 436. [CrossRef]
4. Khaskheli, A.; Jiang, Y.; Raza, S.A.; Qureshi, M.A.; Khan, K.A.; Salam, J. Do CSR activities increase organizational citizenship behavior among employees? Mediating role of affective commitment and job satisfaction. *Corp. Soc. Responsib. Environ. Manag.* **2020**, *27*, 2941–2955. [CrossRef]
5. Cho, S.J.; Chung, C.Y.; Young, J. Study on the Relationship between CSR and Financial Performance. *Sustainability* **2019**, *11*, 343. [CrossRef]
6. Hou, C.-E.; Lu, W.-M.; Hung, S.-W. Does CSR matter? Influence of corporate social responsibility on corporate performance in the creative industry. *Ann. Oper. Res.* **2019**, *278*, 255–279. [CrossRef]
7. Lin, Y.-E.; Li, Y.-W.; Cheng, T.Y.; Lam, K. Corporate social responsibility and investment efficiency: Does business strategy matter? *Int. Rev. Financ. Anal.* **2021**, *73*, 101585. [CrossRef]
8. Abbas, J. Impact of total quality management on corporate green performance through the mediating role of corporate social responsibility. *J. Clean. Prod.* **2020**, *242*, 118458. [CrossRef]
9. Kong, L.; Sial, M.S.; Ahmad, N.; Sehleanu, M.; Li, Z.; Zia-Ud-Din, M.; Badulescu, D. CSR as a potential motivator to shape employees' view towards nature for a sustainable workplace environment. *Sustainability* **2021**, *13*, 1499. [CrossRef]
10. Ahmad, N.; Ullah, Z.; Arshad, M.Z.; waqas Kamran, H.; Scholz, M.; Han, H. Relationship between Corporate Social Responsibility at the Micro-Level and Environmental Performance: The Mediating Role of Employee Pro-Environmental Behavior and the Moderating Role of Gender. *Sustain. Prod. Consum.* **2021**, *27*, 1138–1148. [CrossRef]
11. Ahmad, N.; Ullah, Z.; Mahmood, A.; Ariza-Montes, A.; Vega-Muñoz, A.; Han, H.; Scholz, M. Corporate social responsibility at the micro-level as a "new organizational value" for sustainability: Are females more aligned towards it? *Int. J. Environ. Res. Public Health* **2021**, *18*, 2165. [CrossRef]
12. Girschik, V.; Svystunova, L.; Lysova, E.I. Transforming corporate social responsibilities: Toward an intellectual activist research agenda for micro-CSR research. *Hum. Relat.* **2020**. [CrossRef]
13. Anwar, M.; Zaman Khan, S.; Ali Shah, S.Z. A study of the relationship between innovation and performance among NPOs in Pakistan. *J. Soc. Serv. Res.* **2020**, *46*, 26–40. [CrossRef]
14. Liu, M.; Cai, S.; Chadee, D.; Ren, S.; Wang, Z. Team reflexivity and employee innovative behavior: The mediating role of knowledge sharing and moderating role of leadership. *J. Knowl. Manag.* **2021**. ahead-of-print. [CrossRef]
15. Zhang, H.; Cao, F. Workplace friendship, psychological safety and innovative behavior in China. *Chin. Manag. Stud.* **2020**, *14*, 661–676. [CrossRef]
16. Teng, C.C.; Hu, C.M.; Chang, J.H. Triggering creative self-efficacy to increase employee innovation behavior in the hospitality workplace. *J. Creat. Behav.* **2020**, *54*, 912–925. [CrossRef]
17. Shanker, R.; Bhanugopan, R.; Van der Heijden, B.I.; Farrell, M. Organizational climate for innovation and organizational performance: The mediating effect of innovative work behavior. *J. Vocat. Behav.* **2017**, *100*, 67–77. [CrossRef]

18. Li, H.; Sajjad, N.; Wang, Q.; Muhammad Ali, A.; Khaqan, Z.; Amina, S. Influence of transformational leadership on employees' innovative work behavior in sustainable organizations: Test of mediation and moderation processes. *Sustainability* **2019**, *11*, 1594. [CrossRef]
19. De Jong, J.; Den Hartog, D. Measuring innovative work behaviour. *Creat. Innov. Manag.* **2010**, *19*, 23–36. [CrossRef]
20. Wisse, B.; van Eijbergen, R.; Rietzschel, E.F.; Scheibe, S. Catering to the needs of an aging workforce: The role of employee age in the relationship between corporate social responsibility and employee satisfaction. *J. Bus. Ethics* **2018**, *147*, 875–888. [CrossRef]
21. Wong, A.K.F.; Kim, S.S. Development and validation of standard hotel corporate social responsibility (CSR) scale from the employee perspective. *Int. J. Hosp. Manag.* **2020**, *87*, 102507. [CrossRef]
22. Kim, H.; Uysal, M.; Woo, E.; Kwon, N. The effects of corporate social responsibility (CSR) on employee well-being in the hospitality industry. *Int. J. Contemp. Hosp. Manag.* **2018**, *30*, 1584–1600. [CrossRef]
23. Ahmed, M.; Zehou, S.; Raza, S.A.; Qureshi, M.A.; Yousufi, S.Q. Impact of CSR and environmental triggers on employee green behavior: The mediating effect of employee well-being. *Corp. Soc. Responsib. Environ. Manag.* **2020**, *27*, 2225–2239. [CrossRef]
24. Kowalczyk, R.; Kucharska, W. Corporate social responsibility practices incomes and outcomes: Stakeholders' pressure, culture, employee commitment, corporate reputation, and brand performance. A Polish–German cross-country study. *Corp. Soc. Responsib. Environ. Manag.* **2020**, *27*, 595–615. [CrossRef]
25. Duthler, G.; Dhanesh, G.S. The role of corporate social responsibility (CSR) and internal CSR communication in predicting employee engagement: Perspectives from the United Arab Emirates (UAE). *Public Relat. Rev.* **2018**, *44*, 453–462. [CrossRef]
26. Zulfiqar, S.; Sadaf, R.; Popp, J.; Vveinhardt, J.; Máté, D. An examination of corporate social responsibility and employee behavior: The case of Pakistan. *Sustainability* **2019**, *11*, 3515. [CrossRef]
27. Lu, J.; Ren, L.; Zhang, C.; Wang, C.; Ahmed, R.R.; Streimikis, J. Corporate social responsibility and employee behavior: Evidence from mediation and moderation analysis. *Corp. Soc. Responsib. Environ. Manag.* **2020**, *27*, 1719–1728. [CrossRef]
28. Schaefer, S.D.; Terlutter, R.; Diehl, S. Talking about CSR matters: Employees' perception of and reaction to their company's CSR communication in four different CSR domains. *Int. J. Advert.* **2020**, *39*, 191–212. [CrossRef]
29. Akram, T.; Lei, S.; Haider, M.J.; Hussain, S.T. The impact of organizational justice on employee innovative work behavior: Mediating role of knowledge sharing. *J. Innov. Knowl.* **2020**, *5*, 117–129. [CrossRef]
30. Carlini, J.; Grace, D. The corporate social responsibility (CSR) internal branding model: Aligning employees' CSR awareness, knowledge, and experience to deliver positive employee performance outcomes. *J. Mark. Manag.* **2021**, 1–29. [CrossRef]
31. Afridi, S.A.; Afsar, B.; Shahjehan, A.; Rehman, Z.U.; Haider, M.; Ullah, M. Perceived corporate social responsibility and innovative work behavior: The role of employee volunteerism and authenticity. *Corp. Soc. Responsib. Environ. Manag.* **2020**, *27*, 1865–1877. [CrossRef]
32. Singh, S.K.; El-Kassar, A.-N.; Abdul Khalek, E. CSR, Entrepreneurial Orientation, Citizenship, and Innovative Work Behavior. In *Proceedings of Academy of Management Proceedings*; Academy of Management: Briarcliff Manor, NY, USA, 2020; p. 22108.
33. Mubarik, M.S.; Islam, T.; Khan, M.M. Leading the innovation: Role of trust and job crafting as sequential mediators relating servant leadership and innovative work behavior. *Eur. J. Innov. Manag.* **2020**. ahead-of-print. [CrossRef]
34. Dahleez, K.A.; Karatepe, O.M.; Aboramadan, M. Does climate for creativity mediate the impact of servant leadership on management innovation and innovative behavior in the hotel industry? *Int. J. Contemp. Hosp. Manag.* **2020**, *32*, 2497–2517. [CrossRef]
35. Zeng, J.; Xu, G. How Servant Leadership Motivates Innovative Behavior: A Moderated Mediation Model. *Int. J. Environ. Res. Public Health* **2020**, *17*, 4753. [CrossRef] [PubMed]
36. Carlucci, D.; Mura, M.; Schiuma, G. Fostering Employees' innovative Work Behaviour in Healthcare Organisations. *Int. J. Innov. Manag.* **2020**, *24*, 2050014. [CrossRef]
37. Majid, A.; Yasir, M. Boundary integration and innovative work behavior among nursing staff. *Eur. J. Innov. Manag.* **2019**, *22*, 2–22. [CrossRef]
38. Busch-Casler, J.; Haubner, S.; Pinkwart, A. Employee involvement in innovation activities in hospitals: How perception matters. *Health Serv. Manag. Res.* **2020**, 0951484820943600. [CrossRef]
39. Luengen, M.; Garrelfs, C.; Schulz, C. Employees' Acceptance of Health Care Service Innovations: A Study in the Field of Tele-audiology. In Proceedings of the 2020 IEEE International Conference on Healthcare Informatics (ICHI), Oldenburg, Germany, 30 November–3 December 2020; pp. 1–6.
40. Bammens, Y.; Notelaers, G.; Van Gils, A. Employees as a source of innovation: The role of perceived organizational support in family firms. In *Proceedings of Academy of Management Proceedings*; Academy of Management: Briarcliff Manor, NY, USA, 2013; p. 10400.
41. Harris, M.; Bhatti, Y.; Prime, M.; Del Castillo, J.; Parston, G. Low-cost innovation in healthcare: What you find depends on where you look. *J. R. Soc. Med.* **2018**, *111*, 47–50. [CrossRef]

42. Burns, L.R. *The Business of Healthcare Innovation*; Cambridge University Press: Cambridge, UK, 2012.
43. Porter, M.E. How competitive forces shape strategy. In *Readings in Strategic Management*; Springer: Berlin/Heidelberg, Germany, 1989; pp. 133–143.
44. Franco, S.; Caroli, M.G.; Cappa, F.; Del Chiappa, G. Are you good enough? CSR, quality management and corporate financial performance in the hospitality industry. *Int. J. Hosp. Manag.* **2020**, *88*, 102395. [CrossRef]
45. Halme, M.; Rintamäki, J.; Knudsen, J.S.; Lankoski, L.; Kuisma, M. When is there a sustainability case for CSR? Pathways to environmental and social performance improvements. *Bus. Soc.* **2020**, *59*, 1181–1227. [CrossRef]
46. Kraus, S.; Rehman, S.U.; García, F.J.S. Corporate social responsibility and environmental performance: The mediating role of environmental strategy and green innovation. *Technol. Forecast. Soc. Chang.* **2020**, *160*, 120262. [CrossRef]
47. Nakamura, E. The bidirectional CSR investment–economic performance relationship. *J. Glob. Responsib.* **2015**, *6*, 128–144. [CrossRef]
48. Ruggiero, P.; Cupertino, S. CSR strategic approach, financial resources and corporate social performance: The mediating effect of innovation. *Sustainability* **2018**, *10*, 3611. [CrossRef]
49. Cai, W.; Lysova, E.I.; Khapova, S.N.; Bossink, B.A. Servant leadership and innovative work behavior in Chinese high-tech firms: A moderated mediation model of meaningful work and job autonomy. *Front. Psychol.* **2018**, *9*, 1767. [CrossRef]
50. Opoku, M.A.; Choi, S.B.; Kang, S.-W. Servant leadership and innovative behaviour: An empirical analysis of Ghana's manufacturing sector. *Sustainability* **2019**, *11*, 6273. [CrossRef]
51. Jaiswal, N.K.; Dhar, R.L. The influence of servant leadership, trust in leader and thriving on employee creativity. *Leadersh. Organ. Dev. J.* **2017**, *38*, 2–21. [CrossRef]
52. Farrukh, M.; Ansari, N.Y.; Raza, A.; Meng, F.; Wang, H. High-performance work practices do much, but HERO does more: An empirical investigation of employees' innovative behavior from the hospitality industry. *Eur. J. Innov. Manag.* **2021**. [CrossRef]
53. Nazir, O.; Islam, J.U. Influence of CSR-specific activities on work engagement and employees' innovative work behaviour: An empirical investigation. *Curr. Issues Tour.* **2020**, *23*, 3054–3072. [CrossRef]
54. Mansoor, A.; Farrukh, M.; Wu, Y.; Abdul Wahab, S. Does inclusive leadership incite innovative work behavior? *Hum. Syst. Manag.* **2020**, *40*, 93–102. [CrossRef]
55. Gharleghi, B.; Afshar Jahanshahi, A.; Nawaser, K. The outcomes of corporate social responsibility to employees: Empirical evidence from a developing country. *Sustainability* **2018**, *10*, 698. [CrossRef]
56. Bandura, A.; McClelland, D.C. *Social Learning Theory*; Englewood Cliffs Prentice Hall: Hoboken, NJ, USA, 1977; Volume 1.
57. Tajfel, H. Social categorization, social identity and social comparison. *Differ. Between Soc. Group* **1978**, 61–76.
58. Čierna, H.; Sujová, E. Integrating principles of excellence and of socially responsible entrepreneurship. *Manag. Syst. Prod. Eng.* **2020**, *1*, 23–28. [CrossRef]
59. Carroll, A.B. The pyramid of corporate social responsibility: Toward the moral management of organizational stakeholders. *Bus. Horiz.* **1991**, *34*, 39–48. [CrossRef]
60. Curran, R.; O'Gorman, K.D.; Queenan, C.J.; Gori, K.; Farrington, T. Corporate social responsibility: Reviewed, rated, revised. *Int. J. Contemp. Hosp. Manag.* **2017**, *29*, 30–47. [CrossRef]
61. Donia, M.B.; Ronen, S.; Sirsly, C.-A.T.; Bonaccio, S. CSR by any other name? The differential impact of substantive and symbolic CSR attributions on employee outcomes. *J. Bus. Ethics* **2019**, *157*, 503–523. [CrossRef]
62. Farid, T.; Iqbal, S.; Ma, J.; Castro-González, S.; Khattak, A.; Khan, M.K. Employees' perceptions of CSR, work engagement, and organizational citizenship behavior: The mediating effects of organizational justice. *Int. J. Environ. Res. Public Health* **2019**, *16*, 1731. [CrossRef] [PubMed]
63. Stock, R.M. Is boreout a threat to frontline employees' innovative work behavior? *J. Prod. Innov. Manag.* **2015**, *32*, 574–592. [CrossRef]
64. Shen, J.; Benson, J. When CSR is a social norm: How socially responsible human resource management affects employee work behavior. *J. Manag.* **2016**, *42*, 1723–1746. [CrossRef]
65. Ghosh, K. How and when do employees identify with their organization? Perceived CSR, first-party (in)justice, and organizational (mis)trust at workplace. *Pers. Rev.* **2018**, *47*, 1152–1171. [CrossRef]
66. Ahmad, I.; Donia, M.B.; Shahzad, K. Impact of corporate social responsibility attributions on employees' creative performance: The mediating role of psychological safety. *Ethics Behav.* **2019**, *29*, 490–509. [CrossRef]
67. Javed, B.; Naqvi, S.; Khan, A.K.; Arjoon, S.; Tayyeb, H.H. Impact of inclusive leadership on innovative work behavior: The role of psychological safety. *J. Manag. Organ.* **2017**, *23*, 1–20. [CrossRef]
68. Zeffane, R.; Bani-Melhem, S.; Albaity, M. Determinants of employees' innovative behavior. *Int. J. Contemp. Hosp. Manag.* **2018**, *30*, 1601–1620. [CrossRef]
69. Li, G.; Li, L.; Chan, S.F. Corporate responsibility for employees and service innovation performance in manufacturing transformation. *Career Dev. Int.* **2019**, *24*, 580–595. [CrossRef]
70. Li, Y.-B.; Zhang, G.-Q.; Wu, T.-J.; Peng, C.-L. Employee's Corporate Social Responsibility Perception and Sustained Innovative Behavior: Based on the Psychological Identity of Employees. *Sustainability* **2020**, *12*, 8604. [CrossRef]
71. Mao, Y.; He, J.; Morrison, A.M.; Andres Coca-Stefaniak, J. Effects of tourism CSR on employee psychological capital in the COVID-19 crisis: From the perspective of conservation of resources theory. *Curr. Issues Tour.* **2020**, 1–19. [CrossRef]

72. Chaudhary, R.; Akhouri, A. CSR perceptions and employee creativity: Examining serial mediation effects of meaningfulness and work engagement. *Soc. Responsib. J.* **2019**, *15*, 61–74. [CrossRef]
73. Hur, W.-M.; Moon, T.-W.; Ko, S.-H. How employees' perceptions of CSR increase employee creativity: Mediating mechanisms of compassion at work and intrinsic motivation. *J. Bus. Ethics* **2018**, *153*, 629–644. [CrossRef]
74. Briones Peñalver, A.J.; Bernal Conesa, J.A.; de Nieves Nieto, C. Analysis of corporate social responsibility in Spanish agribusiness and its influence on innovation and performance. *Corp. Soc. Responsib. Environ. Manag.* **2018**, *25*, 182–193. [CrossRef]
75. Ratajczak, P.; Szutowski, D. Exploring the relationship between CSR and innovation. *Sustain. Account. Manag. Policy J.* **2016**, *7*, 295–318. [CrossRef]
76. Bibi, S.; Khan, A.; Hayat, H.; Panniello, U.; Alam, M.; Farid, T. Do hotel employees really care for corporate social responsibility (CSR): A happiness approach to employee innovativeness. *Curr. Issues Tour.* **2021**, 1–18. [CrossRef]
77. Szelągowska-Rudzka, K. CSR and Innovativeness of the Organisation. *Współczesne Probl. Ekon. Glob. Lib. Etyka* **2016**, 115–124. [CrossRef]
78. Mallén Broch, F.F.; Domínguez Escrig, E.; Chiva Gómez, R.; Lapiedra Alcamí, R. Promoting firm innovativeness through servant leadership and corporate social responsibility to employees. *Leadersh. Organ. Dev. J.* **2020**, *41*, 615–633. [CrossRef]
79. Korra, E.; Giotopoulos, I.; Tsakanikas, A. CSR Practices and SME Innovativeness in Greece. In *Entrepreneurship and the Sustainable Development Goals*; Emerald Publishing Limited: Bingley, UK, 2018; Volume 8, pp. 119–132.
80. Nart, S.; Yaprak, B.; Yildirim, Y.T.; Sarihan, A.Y. The relationship of diversity management and servant leadership with organizational identification and creativity in multinational enterprises. *Finans Polit. Ekon. Yorumlar* **2018**, *55*, 31–47.
81. Chen, H.; Lyu, B.; Zhang, Y.; Su, W. How does servant leadership influence employees' service innovative behavior? The roles of intrinsic motivation and identification with the leader. *Balt. J. Manag.* **2020**, *15*, 571–586. [CrossRef]
82. Brohi, N.A.; Jantan, A.H.; Qureshi, M.A.; Jaffar, A.R.B.; Ali, J.B.; Ab Hamid, K.B. The impact of servant leadership on employees attitudinal and behavioural outcomes. *Cogent Bus. Manag.* **2018**, *5*, 1542652. [CrossRef]
83. Karatepe, O.M.; Ozturk, A.; Kim, T.T. Servant leadership, organisational trust, and bank employee outcomes. *Serv. Ind. J.* **2019**, *39*, 86–108. [CrossRef]
84. Meng, L.; Cai, S.; Wang, Z. Servant leadership and innovative behavior: A moderated mediation. *J. Manag. Psychol.* **2019**, *34*, 505–518. [CrossRef]
85. Yu, M.-C.; Mai, Q.; Tsai, S.-B.; Dai, Y. An empirical study on the organizational trust, employee-organization relationship and innovative behavior from the integrated perspective of social exchange and organizational sustainability. *Sustainability* **2018**, *10*, 864. [CrossRef]
86. Fleischman, G.M.; Johnson, E.N.; Walker, K.B.; Valentine, S.R. Ethics versus outcomes: Managerial responses to incentive-driven and goal-induced employee behavior. *J. Bus. Ethics* **2019**, *158*, 951–967. [CrossRef]
87. Lau, P.Y.Y.; Tong, J.L.T.; Lien, B.Y.-H.; Hsu, Y.-C.; Chong, C.L. Ethical work climate, employee commitment and proactive customer service performance: Test of the mediating effects of organizational politics. *J. Retail. Consum. Serv.* **2017**, *35*, 20–26. [CrossRef]
88. Muenjohn, N.; McMurray, A. Design leadership, work values ethic and workplace innovation: An investigation of SMEs in Thailand and Vietnam. *Asia Pac. Bus. Rev.* **2017**, *23*, 192–204. [CrossRef]
89. Panuwatwanich, K.; Wipulanusat, W.; Stewart, R.A. Pathways to workplace innovation and career satisfaction in the public service. *Int. J. Organ. Anal.* **2018**, *26*, 890–914. [CrossRef]
90. Kucharska, W.; Kowalczyk, R. How to achieve sustainability?—Employee's point of view on company's culture and CSR practice. *Corp. Soc. Responsib. Environ. Manag.* **2019**, *26*, 453–467. [CrossRef]
91. Schaufeli, W.B.; Bakker, A.B. Utrecht work engagement scale: Preliminary manual. *Occup. Health Psychol. Unit Utrecht Univ. Utrecht* **2003**, *26*, 64–100.
92. Liden, R.C.; Wayne, S.J.; Meuser, J.D.; Hu, J.; Wu, J.; Liao, C. Servant leadership: Validation of a short form of the SL-28. *Leadersh. Q.* **2015**, *26*, 254–269. [CrossRef]
93. Hu, M.-L.M.; Horng, J.-S.; Sun, Y.-H.C. Hospitality teams: Knowledge sharing and service innovation performance. *Tour. Manag.* **2009**, *30*, 41–50.
94. Sun, H.; Rabbani, M.R.; Ahmad, N.; Sial, M.S.; Cheng, G.; Zia-Ud-Din, M.; Fu, Q. CSR, Co-Creation and Green Consumer Loyalty: Are Green Banking Initiatives Important? A Moderated Mediation Approach from an Emerging Economy. *Sustainability* **2020**, *12*, 10688. [CrossRef]
95. Raza, A.; Saeed, A.; Iqbal, M.K.; Saeed, U.; Sadiq, I.; Faraz, N.A. Linking corporate social responsibility to customer loyalty through co-creation and customer company identification: Exploring sequential mediation mechanism. *Sustainability* **2020**, *12*, 2525. [CrossRef]
96. Harman, H.H. *Modern Factor Analysis*; University of Chicago Press: Chicago, IL, USA, 1976.
97. Richter, N.F.; Schubring, S.; Hauff, S.; Ringle, C.M.; Sarstedt, M. When predictors of outcomes are necessary: Guidelines for the combined use of PLS-SEM and NCA. *Ind. Manag. Data Syst.* **2020**, *120*, 2243–2267. [CrossRef]
98. Matthews, L. Applying multigroup analysis in PLS-SEM: A step-by-step process. In *Partial Least Squares Path Modeling*; Springer: Berlin/Heidelberg, Germany, 2017; pp. 219–243.
99. Thakkar, J.J. Applications of structural equation modelling with AMOS 21, IBM SPSS. In *Structural Equation Modelling*; Springer: Berlin/Heidelberg, Germany, 2020; pp. 35–89.

100. Baron, R.M.; Kenny, D.A. The moderator–mediator variable distinction in social psychological research: Conceptual, strategic, and statistical considerations. *J. Personal. Soc. Psychol.* **1986**, *51*, 1173. [CrossRef]
101. Hayes, A.F. Beyond Baron and Kenny: Statistical mediation analysis in the new millennium. *Commun. Monogr.* **2009**, *76*, 408–420. [CrossRef]
102. Zhao, X.; Lynch, J.G., Jr.; Chen, Q. Reconsidering Baron and Kenny: Myths and truths about mediation analysis. *J. Consum. Res.* **2010**, *37*, 197–206. [CrossRef]

MDPI AG
Grosspeteranlage 5
4052 Basel
Switzerland
Tel.: +41 61 683 77 34

International Journal of Environmental Research and Public Health Editorial Office
E-mail: ijerph@mdpi.com
www.mdpi.com/journal/ijerph

www.ingramcontent.com/pod-product-compliance
Lightning Source LLC
Chambersburg PA
CBHW040749250926
51850CB00007BB/1451